'This unique collaboration between a dream resear[cher...] a comprehensive summary of decades of dream re[search...] a function of dreaming, while at the same time cel[ebrates the] uniqueness of our dreams, along with beautiful art[...]'
— **Katja Valli**, *Professor of Cognitive Neuroscience,
University of Skövde, Sweden*

'Why we dream is a major question in neuroscience and psychology. Blagrove and Lockheart provide novel and compelling insights into this debate and extend it to the realms of our social world, art and evolution.'
— **Antonio Zadra**, *PhD, University of Montreal,
co-author of* When Brains Dream

'Each chapter of this book presents major research findings while maintaining the personal touch of a dream relevant to each topic and Julia Lockheart's evocative paintings to remind us how predominantly visual dreams are.'
— **Deirdre Barrett**, *PhD, Harvard Medical School, author
of* The Committee of Sleep *and* Pandemic Dreams

'An innovative multidimensional work that dovetails highly creative artistic renderings of dreams with an authoritative account of current trends in dream research and theory.'
— **Tore Nielsen**, *PhD, Dream and Nightmare
Laboratory, University of Montreal*

'This book accomplishes the rare feat of being delightful, informative, and provocative all at the same time. As one small example of its many insights, it argues that dreams may not have a function during sleep, but nonetheless may have been important in human evolution because our ancestors increasingly shared and discussed their dreams when they gathered around their nightly fires.'
— **G. William Domhoff**, *PhD, University of California Santa Cruz,
author of* The Neurocognitive Theory of Dreaming:
The Where, How, When, What, and Why of Dreams

'*The Science and Art of Dreaming* constitutes an utterly unique project. For centuries, poets and philosophers have explored how art functions like dreams; psychologists have analyzed how dreams resemble art. But has anyone till now both methodically and creatively responded to the universal phenomenon of dreaming by marrying art to research and theory, and putting science to the service of creative expression? Blagrove and Lockheart's work literally illustrates our most common questions about dreams and dreaming with a selection of 22 dreams, accompanied by artworks that in their own way address the same issues as the explanatory text: Why are dreams so often bizarre? Why do they transport us to the past, and in such detail? Is Freud's view still relevant? This book vividly justifies the appreciation of art associated with dreaming – Surrealism and oneiric cinema, for example – as intellectually on a par with the theoretical contributions and empirical research of science, and convincingly demonstrates the benefits of recalling and sharing dreams, especially for people in creative endeavors.'

— **Bernard Welt**, *PhD. Professor Emeritus, The Corcoran School of the Arts and Design, George Washington University. Author of* Mythomania: Fantasies, Fables, and Sheer Lies in Contemporary American Popular Art; *Co-author of* Dreaming in the Classroom: Practices, Methods, and Resources in Dream Education

The Science and Art of Dreaming

The Science and Art of Dreaming is an innovative text that reviews the neuroscience and psychology of how dreams are produced, how they are recalled and their relationship to waking life events and concerns of the dreamer. Featuring beautiful original artwork based on dream representations, the book delves deeply into what happens when we dream, the works of art we produce when asleep and the relevance of dreaming to science, art and film.

The book examines the biological, psychological and social causes of dreaming, and includes recent advances in the study of nightmares and lucid dreaming. It shows how sleep can process memories and that dreams may reflect these processes, but also that dreams can elicit self-disclosure and empathy when they are shared after waking. The playfulness, originality and metaphorical content of dreams also link them to art, and especially to the cultural movement that has most valued dreams – Surrealism. The book details the history of scientific research into dreams, including a re-reading of the two dreams of Freud's patient, the feminist hero Dora, and also the history of Surrealism and of films that draw on dreams and dream-like processes. Each chapter starts with a dream narrative and accompanying painting of the dream to highlight aspects of each of the chapter themes.

This highly engaging book will be relevant to researchers, students and lecturers in the fields of psychology, neuroscience, psychoanalysis, consciousness and social evolution. It will also be of value within the study and practice of visual art, design and film, and will be of interest to the general reader and anyone who holds a personal interest in their own dreams.

Mark Blagrove is a Professor of Psychology and the Director of the Sleep Laboratory at Swansea University, UK.

Julia Lockheart is an Associate Professor at Swansea College of Art, University of Wales Trinity Saint David, and an Associate Lecturer in the Department of Design, Goldsmiths, University of London, UK.

The Science and Art of Dreaming

Mark Blagrove and Julia Lockheart

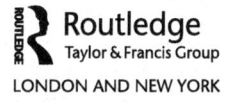

Routledge
Taylor & Francis Group
LONDON AND NEW YORK

Designed cover image: Julia Lockheart

First published 2023
by Routledge
4 Park Square, Milton Park, Abingdon, Oxon OX14 4RN

and by Routledge
605 Third Avenue, New York, NY 10158

Routledge is an imprint of the Taylor & Francis Group, an informa business

© 2023 Mark Blagrove and Julia Lockheart

The right of Mark Blagrove and Julia Lockheart to be identified as authors of this work has been asserted in accordance with sections 77 and 78 of the Copyright, Designs and Patents Act 1988.

All rights reserved. No part of this book may be reprinted or reproduced or utilised in any form or by any electronic, mechanical, or other means, now known or hereafter invented, including photocopying and recording, or in any information storage or retrieval system, without permission in writing from the publishers.

Trademark notice: Product or corporate names may be trademarks or registered trademarks, and are used only for identification and explanation without intent to infringe.

British Library Cataloguing-in-Publication Data
A catalogue record for this book is available from the British Library

Library of Congress Cataloging-in-Publication Data
Names: Blagrove, Mark, author. | Lockheart, Julia, author.
Title: The science and art of dreaming / Mark Blagrove, Julia Lockheart.
Description: Abingdon, Oxon; New York, NY: Routledge, 2023. | Includes bibliographical references and index.
Identifiers: LCCN 2022030900 (print) | LCCN 2022030901 (ebook) | ISBN 9780367479961 (hardback) | ISBN 9780367479947 (paperback) | ISBN 9781003037552 (ebook)
Subjects: LCSH: Dreams.
Classification: LCC BF1078 .B555 2023 (print) | LCC BF1078 (ebook) | DDC 154.6/3—dc23/eng/20220824
LC record available at https://lccn.loc.gov/2022030900
LC ebook record available at https://lccn.loc.gov/2022030901

ISBN: 9780367479961 (hbk)
ISBN: 9780367479947 (pbk)
ISBN: 9781003037552 (ebk)

DOI: 10.4324/9781003037552

Typeset in Bembo
by codeMantra

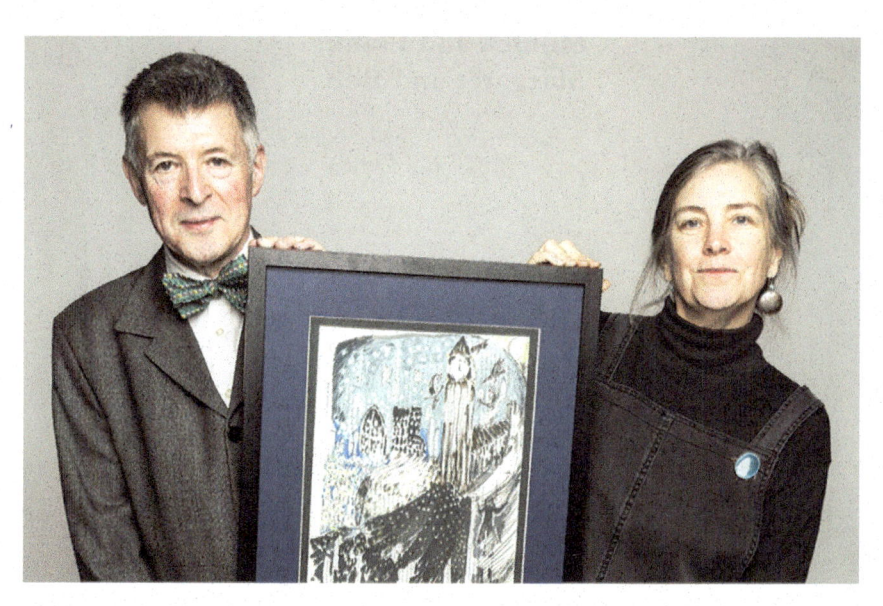

Mark Blagrove and Julia Lockheart, with painting of flying dream with lucidity (see Chapter 7). Photo: Paul Duerinckx

For our parents,
Monica and Frank,
Margaret and Bob.

Contents

List of diagrams   xi
List of figures   xii
Preface   xiii
Acknowledgements   xv

1 What are dreams and what affects dream content?   2

2 Why do some people recall dreams more than others?   18

3 Nightmares   28

4 Sleep   36

5 Sleep and memory   46

6 Dreaming and the brain   58

7 Lucid dreams   68

8 Freud, psychoanalysis and dreams   80

9 Freud and Dora   90

10 How to find meaning in dreams: The Montague Ullman dream appreciation method   104

11 Dreaming and insight   116

12 Functions and theories of dreams   128

13 Dream-sharing and empathy, a new theory of dream function 142

14 The DreamsID science and art collaboration: Surrealism
   and the socialising of dreams 154

15 Sleep and dreaming during the Covid-19 pandemic:
   Exploring and painting Covid-19 and Lockdown dreams 172

16 Dreaming, films and Surrealism 186

17 Dream-sharing, evolution and human self-domestication 204

18 Conclusions and summary 218

References 223
Index 247

Diagrams

4.1 Placement of electrodes on the head to measure sleep   39
4.2 Brain waves and eye movement traces found in wake and
     sleep stages   40
4.3 Hypnogram showing the stages of sleep across the night   43

Figures

1.1	Dream of briefly seeing mother again, 2018	2
2.1	Dream of my brother's operation, 2019	18
3.1	Nightmare of suffocating after a party during Covid-19, 2020	28
4.1	Dream of cradling my dying brother by the side of a road, 2019	36
5.1	Dream of new life by a beach, 2020	46
6.1	Dream of three stages of woman, 2018	58
7.1	A flying dream with lucidity, 2018	68
8.1	Dream of walking alone and then dancing with friends, 2020	80
9.1	Dora's first dream, of escape from a burning house, 2020	90
9.2	Ida Bauer, aged 6, and Otto Bauer, aged 7; photograph taken 1 January 1889, unknown photographer	93
9.3	Dora's second dream, of travelling to her father's funeral, 2021	102
10.1	Dream of choosing between known and unknown keys, 2022	104
11.1	Dream of pulling through from Covid-19, 2021	116
12.1	Dream of mother and daughter attacked on freeway, 2019	128
13.1	Dream of 'where is my home?', 2017	142
14.1	Dream of cop and apocalypse spores, 2021	154
14.2	Julia Lockheart and Mark Blagrove at the Freud Museum London in 2018 (Courtesy of the Freud Museum London)	158
14.3	Julia Lockheart at the Freud Museum London in 2018 (Courtesy of the Freud Museum London)	158
14.4	Julia Lockheart at the Paris Institute of Advanced Study in 2019	159
15.1	Dream of peeling quails' eggs for cure for Covid-19, 2020	172
15.2	Dream of gift including death preparation kit, 2020	178
15.3	Dream of failing to drive up incline, 2020	179
15.4	Dream of robin pecking Covid-19 from lungs, 2020	181
15.5	Dream of emerging from shell and seeing seal pup in the ocean, 2020	182
16.1	Dream of snowy beach, underclothes and ferry, 2022	186
17.1	Dream of unfair blame, 2017	204
18.1	Dream of boss on stage at festival, 2019	218

Preface

Dreams are related to our brain, mind and waking life circumstances, and so are a major topic for science. They are also a creative series of images that can fascinate us all, and intrigue and inspire creative practitioners. Indeed, dreams are works of art that we all produce when asleep. This book addresses the science and art of dreaming, with texts of dreams that are relevant to the theme of each chapter, and with a painting of each dream that returns it to a visual form. This book has resulted from the collaboration, since 2016, between sleep scientist Mark Blagrove and artist Julia Lockheart, which has explored the science, art and personal relevance of dreams and dreaming.

Mark Blagrove's interest in dreaming started with being given Charles Rycroft's book *The Innocence of Dreams* in 1982. The book proposed that dreams innocently and metaphorically depict the waking life concerns of the dreamer. This led to a PhD in dreaming and then many years doing experiments on sleep, memory and dreaming, which continue, in the Swansea University Sleep Laboratory. But this work led to a question. What if, after the dream is studied as part of an experiment, it is returned to the dreamer and discussed in an open-ended way, asking where its components might have come from, and what sense the dreamer could make of the dream? And so, highly controlled, often physiologically related studies of sleep and dreaming were complemented by research on how the dreamer, with the help of others, can make sense of the dream. This research was encouraged by discussions with the eclectic mixture of disciplines and people at the conferences of the International Association for the Study of Dreams, which also publishes the academic journal *Dreaming*.

Julia Lockheart has an eclectic background in art, design and performance. She studied fine art to M-level and, after an art fellowship in Japan, became interested in the impact of art on language. Growing up, her brother, Robert, who was an illustrator, introduced Julia to *A Humument*, a found book *Gesamtkunstwerk* by Tom Phillips (1980), in which each page is drawn on, painted and collaged so that a found epic poem unfolds across the pages. From childhood she dreamt vividly in colour, waking regularly with images and surreal narratives that became embedded in her large canvasses. Dreaming made sense in relation to the symbols and imagery when it flowed directly into her painting practice. Julia's PhD research and academic career led her to offer performative workshops in which collaborative writing practices were aired and explored in communities of practice. She is co-editor of the *Journal of Writing in Creative Practice* and Director of the Metadesign Research Centre at the University of Wales Trinity Saint David. She writes and performs songs with her band and is a published poet.

As Mark was researching the outcomes of group discussions with people about their dreams, Julia suggested that she could paint each dream quickly during each discussion. The dreamer could then be given an artwork so as to elicit further consideration of the dream with family and friends. Their first event was at the 2016 British Science Festival. To make a further connection with the science of dreaming, Julia decided to paint each dream onto pages torn by her from Freud's book *The Interpretation of Dreams*. Each painting is thus a palimpsest. We are grateful for the kind permission of the publishers (Wordsworth Editions, Hertfordshire, UK) to use the first English translation of the book in the production of these artworks. By chance, words that Freud wrote in his book are incorporated, as objets trouvés, found objects, into each of these paintings. In some instances, the site-specific performance of painting the dream results in found poems combining words of Freud that resonate with the dream, and with the live discussion of the dream.

We named our science art collaboration DreamsID, this being a contraction of Dreams Illustrated and Discussed, and Dreams Interpreted and Drawn, but also with reference to Freud's notion of the *id,* and with ID also referring to the identity of the dreamer, which is explored in each discussion. We started to have performances worldwide, and later online. This has been a true and synergistic collaboration, in that holding the public performances, comprising dream discussions and art, was inspired by the previous research on dreams and dream-sharing, and our subsequent research on dream-sharing and empathy arose as a result of the experience of undertaking those public dream and art performances.

We hope that you enjoy learning more about the science *and* art of dreaming, which to us come together in the creative, collaborative and co-operative act of the sharing of dreams between people, whether publicly or privately.

Acknowledgements

We thank Swansea University, University of Wales Trinity Saint David and Goldsmiths, University of London, for their support for our science art collaboration and research. We also thank the British Science Association, which hosted our first public event at the British Science Festival in 2016, and the International Association for the Study of Dreams, and the International Society for the Study of Surrealism for their continuing support. We are grateful to the many venues for hosting our performative events and/or showing the artworks in exhibitions: these include all the venues and institutions worldwide mentioned in this book, and in particular those that have supported us from the start of our collaboration: the Freud Museum London, Glynn Vivian Art Gallery, Oriel Science, the many annual Swansea Science Festivals, and the Royal Society of Arts, Manufacturing and Commerce (the RSA). Above all, we give heartfelt thanks to those individuals worldwide who have shared their dreams with us in our public events, whether in venues or online, and to the many people, friends and colleagues, who have taken part and contributed as empathic and insightful audience members. We also thank everyone at Routledge, and at Taylor & Francis, involved in the commissioning, editing and production of this book, for their diligence, advice and support throughout.

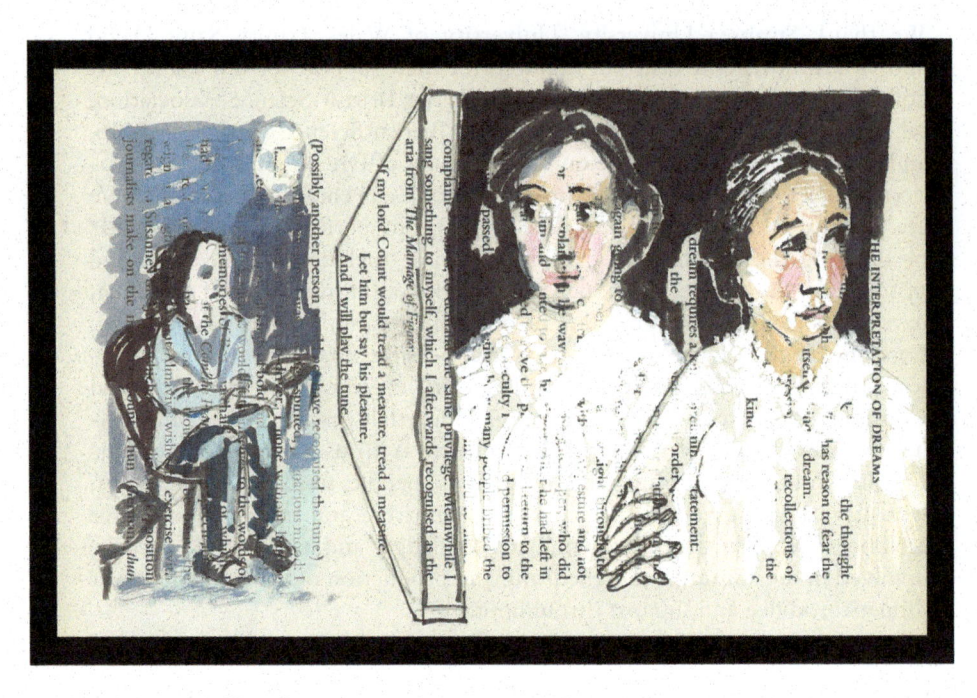

Figure 1.1 Dream of briefly seeing mother again, 2018.

1 What are dreams and what affects dream content?

This chapter addresses how highly emotional experiences and concerns are often incorporated into dreams. We illustrate this with a dream of bereavement that was told to us at a science festival.

DREAM NARRATIVE: *The dream is about me sitting in a waiting room, while some member of my family has asked me (a voice that I know, but I didn't see the face) why I look so happy, and also why I am so excited. I reply that I have an appointment with my mum who died when I was 2 years old. My mum and my maternal grandmother appear a few minutes later standing by the door, looking young and very healthy, white faces, red cheeks and black hair, tied up at the back. But it was only for a few minutes if not a few seconds when my grandmother keeps telling my mum, 'Time is up, let's go,' and pulling her by her hand. I am so disappointed, and the same voice asks why I don't look happy and I say I was so excited to see my mum and have a chat with her but my grandmother took her away from me and didn't let her stay longer with me.*

DISCUSSION: The dreamer, Zoubida, as an adult, had this dream of her mother, who died when she was very young. Zoubida had only one fleeting memory of her mother, seeing her body in a darkened room, surrounded by candles. Shortly before the dream she had thought of her mother on hearing of the death of a relative.

JULIA: (Painting shown as Figure 1.1.) As the narrative of the dream has quite a simple spatial structure and plot, I chose one page with two paragraphs and a centrally dividing poem. I turned the page on its side and created two interior spaces on the page. I used the poem to create the perspective for the open door separating the dreamer from her mother. The door and opening took up quite a large proportion of the composition because they formed an important threshold for the action in the dream.

This chapter explores the characteristics of our dreams, the factors that affect the content of our dreams and what methods are used to investigate them.

DOI: 10.4324/9781003037552-1

Characteristics of dreams

Dreams are fascinating to many people. Much of this is because they seem to happen to us and we create whole scenarios apparently without any intention or knowledge of how they are created. And we also live and act in the dream. It is usually presented to us not as a film, but, even when we are an observer, as a world in which we are one of the characters. These characteristics are some of the reasons why dreams are intriguing.

We have many types of experiences when we are asleep, and sometimes no experience at all, what is called dreamless sleep. But it is the longer, plot-type experiences, often with ourselves taking part or at least being present, which have fascinated humans for centuries. For Fox and colleagues (2013), these are intensified versions of the daydreams we have when awake. For Windt (2015), a dream is an 'immersive spatiotemporal hallucination'. And this is what intrigues people so much, we believe the dream is real while it occurs, and we are part of it. We are also intrigued because dreams are so novel. Fosse and colleagues (2003) collected dream reports and asked participants to describe whether similar or exact same events had occurred in waking life. In only 2–3% of reports was there an exact copy of a waking life episode, with characters, environment and actions the same in the dream as in waking life.

And so almost all of us are creating our own novel worlds when asleep, worlds in which we take part. And these are emotional worlds. Although individuals may differ in the emotions in their dreams, and the relative proportion of positive and negative emotions, across a large sample of people there tends to be equal proportions of positive and negative emotions (Schredl & Doll, 1998). And we tend not to dream of mundane activities. In his paper, 'We do not dream of the 3 Rs,' Hartmann (2000) found that people in general do not dream of reading, writing or arithmetic, as these are usually not important or emotional activities to us, even though people can spend many hours doing these each day. By contrast, walking, talking with friends and sexual activity occurred much more often in dreams.

We also usually dream of other people, some of whom we know. Social Simulation Theory (SST; Revonsuo, Tuominen, & Valli, 2016) considers dreaming to be the simulation of social events, with people interacting with each other in realistic and sometimes unrealistic ways. Using a Social Content Scale (SCS), developed to quantify social events in wake and dream reports, Tuominen and colleagues (2019) found that dreams overrepresent social events compared to reports of our waking life, which they term a Sociality Bias for dreams.

The above characteristics might be well known to the reader and the general public. We will now address other characteristics, and consider how these are investigated.

Bizarreness

There have been many investigations of bizarreness in dreams. Some of these have involved asking the dreamer, or an independent judge reading the dream report, to rate the dream on a scale ranging from the dream being realistic, in that events in it could have happened in waking life, to the dream events being unlikely to occur in waking life, to the events of the dream being impossible in waking life.

Domhoff (2007) acknowledged that aspects of dream content can be unusual and perhaps nonsensical, but emphasised the rareness of dream bizarreness, in comparison to how people often think dreams are. He cites Dorus et al. (1971), who found that 8.9% of sleep lab dreams were highly improbable by waking standards, and Strauch and Meier (1996), who found for home dreams that there were no bizarre elements in 23.9% of the reports, and only one bizarre element in another 39.3%. Others, however, find a greater prevalence of bizarreness. In Williams et al. (1992), 55% of home-reported dreams had an incongruity of place, action, characters, objects or time, and 25% of dreams had cognitive uncertainty of the dreamer or uncertain qualities of dream content, including objects, characters or place. Bizarreness was twice as prevalent in dream reports as in wake-state fantasy reports of the same subjects: 22% of dream report sentences contained an instance of bizarreness, compared to 9% of waking fantasy report sentences.

The most extensive quantitative review (Colace, 2003) calculates average scores across many studies as showing 38% of sleep onset dreams as bizarre, 61% of N2 dreams, 51% of N3 dreams and 74% of REM dreams, but this measure does combine impossibility and improbability. (These N2 and N3 stages of Non-Rapid Eye Movement sleep, and Rapid Eye Movement sleep, are described in Chapter 4.)

Relationship of dreams to our memories

As stated above, we very rarely replicate waking life experiences in our dreams. But there is also only rare use of memory within dreams. Baird and colleagues (2022a) addressed whether episodic thoughts of the past and future differ between waking, NREM sleep and REM sleep. They designed an experiment in which 138 individuals underwent experience-sampling during wakefulness as well as serial awakenings in sleep. Experience sampling is when participants are alerted periodically to record what had just been going through their minds. Baird and colleagues found that episodic thoughts were more common during waking spontaneous thought than in either N2 or REM sleep, and had a strong bias towards future planning. This suggests that waking life experiences and dreams differ in the occurrence of spontaneous episodic thoughts. Somehow the person when dreaming is not thinking as much about their past or future within the dream than they do when awake. Arguably this is the basis for the feeling that our dreams happen to us, that we are there, reactive and in the moment, rather than the dream being a product of deliberate thought and action.

Factors affecting dream content

Soon after experimental work on dreaming began in the 1950s, attempts were made to influence dream content. There was some success. For example, in 1958, Dement and Wolpert found that, if water was sprayed on sleeping participants, 40% of the time the water spray was incorporated into the dream, either directly, such as dreaming of being caught in a rainstorm, say, or indirectly, such as dreaming of watching a TV programme or film about rainstorms. The sound of a bell was only incorporated 10% of the time, and a tone not at all. The conclusion was that natural or important stimuli are incorporated, but unnatural or irrelevant sounds are not.

The influence during sleep of the outside environment, and the bodily environment, can be seen in dreams of pain. Pain sensations are known to occur in about 1% of dreams in healthy persons and about 30% of patients with acute, severe pain. Schredl and colleagues (2017) undertook the first study of pain dreams in patients with chronic pain. Chronic pain patients reported more pain dreams and more negatively toned dreams compared to healthy controls. Such pain dreams might be instigated by actual pain whereas, for healthy persons, pain dreams might be pain memories (self-experienced pain and/or seeing persons in pain).

There has been extensive research on how our waking life affects or is reflected in the content of our dreams. One method to address the influence of waking life events and concerns on dreams is to collect dreams, either in the sleep laboratory or at home, and to then interview participants about where the different components of the dream came from in their waking life. This is similar to the free association method devised by Freud, which we detail in Chapter 8. For seven days, Vallat and colleagues (2017a) asked participants upon awakening at home to report their dreams, and then to identify the waking life elements that they could think of that were related to their dream content. The participants then rated these waking life elements and their dream content on several scales.

The participants were allowed to report waking life elements from the whole lifespan, and on average 83% of the dream reports were related to one or more waking life elements. Among all the waking life elements incorporated into dreams by participants, 20% of them happened the day before the dream, so there seems to be a preferential incorporation into dreams of experiences that happened the day before the dream, compared to experiences that occurred before that. Interestingly, the environment of each dream was more likely to be imaginary than copied from waking life. In addition, 23% of the dream reports incorporated a current concern of the participant.

A second method has participants keep daily diaries of their waking life experiences, and the contents of the diaries are then compared to dream content. With participants matching diary reports from the day before a dream with dream reports, Eichenlaub et al. (2019) found that home dreams refer to an average of 0.35 current concerns from the previous day, and approximately 0.5 events from the previous day. And so, on average, one in every three dreams refers to a waking life current concern, and one in every two dreams refers to an event from the previous day.

However, although some dream content can be related to waking life experiences and concerns, there is the question of how much of the dream can be related to waking life experiences. With Chris Edwards, Mark Blagrove held dream group discussion sessions in which a dream is discussed in detail for about an hour, with the dreamer giving information about how their recent waking life relates to the dream. The method is described in detail in Chapters 10 and 11. They found that waking life sources could be identified for an average of only 14.4% of dream report text (Edwards et al., 2013). So, a very large amount of dream report text does not seem to be relatable to anything in the participants' waking life.

One way to address the influences of waking life on dreams is to investigate the effects of specific events. This was achieved by Propper and colleagues (2007) who had been collecting dream diaries from people in the weeks before 9/11, and so fortuitously had collected control data of dreams that occurred shortly before 9/11. They found that dreams in the weeks after 9/11 had more references (which could be literal or metaphorical/non-literal) to the events of 9/11 than did dreams from before 9/11. For example, there were more threats in the dreams after 9/11 than there were before. Interestingly, the amount of reference to 9/11 in dreams each individual had was correlated with the amount of TV coverage of 9/11 that the person watched that day, but it was not correlated with the amount of time they had spent talking about the 9/11 events that day. Propper and colleagues proposed that the dream content was related to unresolved emotion from TV watching, as TV watching is more passive than talking to other people.

Dreams and emotional experiences

The studies reported so far in this section support the view that we dream of what is emotionally important to us. However, in order to take into account how much we dream of experiences that are not emotional, data need to be collected on a variety of emotional and non-emotional experiences. This was done by Schredl in 2006 in a study of 46 psychology students who kept a structured diary over a two-week period. The diary consisted of 14 sheets for recording daytime events and 14 sheets for recording dreams. The participants were asked to list the five most important events of each day and to rate them on a five-point scale about their emotional tone, from very negative to very positive, and on another scale to measure their emotional intensity, from not at all intense to very strong. Over the two-week period, 254 dreams were recorded; 64 of those dreams included daytime events that were recorded previously on the structured list in the diaries. Importantly, of the events from each day that were recorded in the diaries, some of them then become incorporated into the following dreams, and other ones were not incorporated. Schredl took all the events that were incorporated into a dream, and worked out their average emotional score, and then took all the events that were not incorporated into a dream and worked out their average emotional score. It was found that the events in the diaries that were incorporated into dreams were significantly more emotional than events that were not incorporated into dreams, and that this held for positive and negative emotional events.

We (Eichenlaub et al., 2018) followed up Schredl's home dream study by collecting REM and Slow Wave Sleep (also known as N3) dreams in the sleep lab, with participants having kept a diary of waking life experiences for the week before sleeping in the sleep lab. For an individual to be included in the analysis they had to have at least one experience recorded in their diary that was incorporated into a dream and at least one that was not incorporated into a dream, and we calculated the average level of emotion for these two types of diary items. We found that experiences from waking life that were incorporated into a dream were significantly more intense emotionally than were experiences that were not incorporated, and that this occurred for positive emotional items and negative emotional items, and occurred for REM dreams as well as Slow Wave Sleep (SWS, or N3) dreams. So, these studies show that we do tend to dream of what is emotional to us in waking life. Somehow our dreams sift through our waking life experiences and prioritise the emotional ones to include in dreams, whether they are emotionally positive or emotionally negative.

We can give an example of dreaming of a highly emotional real-life situation, taken from Kelly Bulkeley and Patricia Bulkley's (2005) work on the often metaphorical content of dreams of people who are close to death. In these instances, there are dreams of deceased relatives, or guides, who are often deceased relatives, and dreams of journeys, such as preparing for a train journey or a flight, often without friends or relatives with them. Bulkeley and Bulkley give an example of Scott (pp.59–61), a terminally ill young man, who knew he would never reach the age of having a driving licence, and they relate how he dreamt of seeing a deceased but admired schoolmate alive again, sitting in a red convertible car, and offering Scott a ride. Happy, Scott said yes, got in the car and drove away. This is a highly poignant dream, metaphorically depicting Scott's tragic waking life circumstances.

A prospective study on end-of-life dreams was published by Kerr and colleagues (2014) in the *Journal of Palliative Medicine*, which is the major medical journal about end-of-life care. They asked 59 patients in a hospice about the content and frequency of their dreams and visions, and the level of comfort and distress that occurred due to the dreams and visions. Eighty-eight per cent of the patients reported having had at least one dream or vision in the hospice, mostly during sleep. This was a higher prevalence than previously thought, possibly due to these interviews being first-hand rather than of health care staff or relatives. Forty-six per cent of the dreams or visions were of deceased loved ones, 17% of living friends and relatives, and 39% of going or preparing to go somewhere. Dreaming of a deceased friend or relative was the most comforting kind of dream, and these became more prevalent as the end of life drew nearer. The authors caution that although such dreams and visions can be a profound source of meaning and comfort to the dying, the dreams may be ridiculed or dismissed by family or health workers as delirium, and Kerr and colleagues thus called for more attention to these types of dreams.

Related to these end-of-life dreams are grief dreams, in which we dream of the deceased. Bereaved persons often experience vivid and deeply meaningful dreams of the deceased, which may reflect the process of mourning. In a study by Wright and colleagues (2014), that surveyed 278 bereaved persons regarding their dreams, 58% of respondents reported dreaming of their deceased loved ones, with varying levels of frequency. Most reported that the dreams were either pleasant or both pleasant and disturbing, with few reporting purely disturbing dreams. Prevalent dream themes included pleasant past memories with the deceased, dreaming of the deceased free of illness, memories of the deceased's illness or time of death, the deceased in the afterlife, often appearing comfortable and at peace, and the deceased communicating with the dreamer, including giving messages. Sixty per cent of respondents felt that their dreams affected their bereavement process, including increased acceptance of the loved one's death, and also having comfort and sadness. The authors conclude by emphasising the importance of grief counsellors having an awareness of such dreams. Grief dreams also occur after the death of a pet. For people whose cat or dog had died, Black and colleagues (2019) found that 78% dream of the pet, with the majority dreaming of the cat or dog being healthy or happy, and a majority being comforted by these dreams. Dreaming of the pet was related to the level of grief.

Another highly emotional experience for people can be sleeping in the sleep lab. Participants might dream that they have already been woken up, or that they are talking to the people in the lab. They may even dream of having their hair washed because in the sleep lab the participant will spend about half an hour having electrodes put onto their scalp. So there are direct and indirect references in dreams to being in the sleep lab. This effect was noticed early on in sleep lab studies of dreaming, with Dement and colleagues (1965) finding that lab references decrease in dreams across the night, and decrease as the person spends more nights in the lab. Picard-Deland and colleagues (2021) found that these lab incorporations occur in over a third (35.8%) of all sleep lab dreams. They found that common themes associated with lab incorporation were: meta-dreaming, including lucid dreams and false awakenings (40.7%); sensory incorporations (27%); wayfinding to, from or within the lab (24.3%); sleep as performance (19.6%); friends/family in the lab (15.9%); and being an object of observation (12.2%). Finally, 31.7% of the lab incorporation dreams included projections into a near future (e.g., the experiment having been completed), but very few projections into the past (2.6%).

Obtaining an unbiased sample of dreams: the most recent dream method

The Most Recent Dream (MRD) method for studying dream content is detailed by Bill Domhoff in his (2003) book *The scientific study of dreams: Neural networks, cognitive development, and content analysis* and on his website dreamresearch.net. The method asks individuals to write down the most recent dream they can remember. The method has the aim of not allowing the person to choose which dream to report, either to fit what the person thinks might be a hypothesis for the study, or to choose a dream that looks more interesting or important. The sample of dreams that results should thus be unbiased by participant selection of the dream. The dreams are then scored by the experimenters very much on the surface level, simply coding the content. So, for example, whether there is an instance of good fortune in the dream, or an aggression, or the number of characters.

The MRD method aims also to reduce the influence of individual's beliefs about their dreams, which can affect individuals reporting on questionnaires about their dreams in general. In a study in which participants completed dream diaries for up to five consecutive weeks, and a questionnaire about their dream content in general, it was found that people with high dream recall frequency have accurate beliefs about their general dream content; such people know what their dreams are like because their memories of them are easily available (Beaulieu-Prévost & Zadra, 2005). However, the researchers found that if dream recall frequency is low, people's beliefs about their general dream content are influenced by their current emotional state, and do not accord with what was reported in the few dream diaries. Thus, anxious people overestimate how many anxious dreams they have, if they only rarely recall dreams.

In studies that use the MRD method, Domhoff and Schneider (1998) specify that for a study of groups, 100–125 individuals should each provide a dream so as to ensure reliable coding, and that if the dreams of one person are being studied, a minimum of 75–100 dreams should be provided. For the dreams of one individual, a diary will produce an unselected sample of dreams if the person has documented all their dreams across a period. Many people have left volumes of dream diaries to Domhoff and his team, some diaries spanning decades, and these have been coded by Domhoff's team. In the case of one dream series, that of a young adult male who kept a diary of his dreams from the age of 18 to 32, his dreams have a constant level of sexuality in them, about 10% of his dreams have at least one instance of sexuality across that period, and about 35% of his dreams have at least one instance of aggression across that period. An advantage of such diaries is that they will often have been completed for many years without the expectation that somebody later on was going to scientifically study them.

The scoring system used by Domhoff and many other researchers is called the Hall and Van de Castle system, named after Calvin Hall and Bob Van de Castle, who were early dream content researchers. The system is very comprehensive and each study will often only use some of the possible variables, such as whether:

- an animal is present in the dream,
- there are family members present in the dream,
- the dream has a familiar or unfamiliar setting.

Also,

- is there a success?
- is there a failure?
- how many characters are present?
- what proportion of characters are friendly?

There are then personal interactions, such as victimisation, or befriending, and many other variables. Statistical analyses can be conducted on these variables, so as to compare one sample of dreams with another. For example, there are fewer familiar characters and more physical aggression in male dreams than in female dreams. Male dreams also tend to have two-thirds of characters being male, whereas female dreams tend to have an equal number of male and female characters (Domhoff, 1996).

The method can also be extended to comparing samples of dreams taken from one person's series of dreams. Domhoff (2003, Chapters 3 and 5) reports analyses of one series of dreams, the 3,116 dreams donated to Domhoff by a woman given the pseudonym Barb Sanders, the dreams were from a period of over 20 years of her life. In waking life Barb Sanders had had a husband called Howard and later a close friend called Derek, to whom she was attracted but did not have a sexual relationship. For one analysis Domhoff took a sample of 250 of Barb Sanders' dreams. He compared Hall Van de Castle (HVdC) variable scores on dreams that included Derek with those that included Howard, and these were also compared to a baseline sample of her dreams which had neither man in them. In the dreams that Derek was in, there were more instances of friendliness and also of sexuality, than in dreams that included her husband. In both Derek's and Howard's dreams, there was a much lower amount of physical aggression compared to her dreams in general. In some respects, these analyses are laying the dream open to a type of interpretation, in that these results can be compared to facts known about Bard Sander's waking life and the autobiography that she told Bill Domhoff. But these scores are very different from traditional clinical or psychoanalytic interpretation because, for example, if there is friendliness in the dream, it does not matter which character displays it, it would simply be scored as one instance of friendliness. So, for the Barb Sanders series, the presence of friendliness would be scored if it was Derek being friendly, Howard being friendly, or another person, or even Barb being friendly. Nevertheless, despite there being no consideration of who is exhibiting the instance of friendliness, the dream data are relatable to the dreamer's waking life circumstances.

The theoretical conclusion of this work on coding dreams is detailed by Domhoff (2011, 2017). Domhoff holds that the content of dreams is continuous with the dreamer's conceptualisations in their waking life. Dreams are thus simulations of waking life, embodied in that the whole environment is like virtual reality (VR), in which the dream character interacts, and with this simulation dramatising waking life concerns and conceptualisations of the dreamer. For the Barb Sanders series, this means her general conceptions of how she saw and thought of Derek and how she saw and thought of Howard. Importantly, this view emphasises the incorporation of current concerns and waking life conceptualisations into dreams, rather than recent specific events.

The above findings, and findings in previous sections of this chapter, can be summarised as dreaming being continuous, in many respects, with waking life cognition, rather than being separate and unrelated to waking life. This was termed the *continuity hypothesis* by Hall and Nordby (1972, p.104). The development of that term and research programmes derived from it are described in detail by Domhoff (2017), and the relationship of the continuity hypothesis with the incorporation of waking life experiences into dreams is reviewed by Schredl (2003, 2006). We now proceed to describe research that addresses the timescale of the incorporation of waking life experiences into dreams.

The dream-lag effect

Freud (1900/1997) used the term 'day-residue' to refer to the greater incorporation into dreams of experiences from the day before a dream, in comparison to incorporation of experiences from days before that. This is a well-known phenomenon, shown by Vallat et al. (2017a) as mentioned above, and which has led to the assumption that incorporations become less frequent with increasing time between the occurrence of the experiences and the occurrence of the dream. However, having heard of tragic events such as suicides and shootings being copied after a delay of several days, Tore Nielsen wondered whether waking life events might also be incorporated into dreams after a delay, as well as in dreams on the night following the event. He thus investigated what became termed the 'dream-lag effect', finding in several papers that we tend to dream of events that occur five to seven days previously (delayed incorporations), as well as one day previously (immediate incorporations) (Nielsen & Powell, 1989; Nielsen, et al., 2004; Powell et al., 1995).

There was, however, doubt from some of the scientific community about the reality of this effect, because of the possibility that as the schedules in people's lives are regular, it may be that individuals are dreaming of an event because it happened the day before, but, because these events might occur every week for the person, it would appear that they are dreaming of an event that occurred a week previously. This was a famous one-week, or seven-day, confound. And so, Mark Blagrove, Josie Henley-Einion and colleagues (2011b) conducted a large-scale data collection study to test for this confound. Participants kept a daily diary and a dream diary for 14 days. At the end of the two weeks, each participant was given a large batch of sheets, each with a dream report on the left side and a daily diary on the right, so that every dream report could be compared to every daily diary. Dream reports were even compared to daily diaries for each of the days after the dream had occurred. Participants then rated how similar each dream report was to each diary record. On the dream diary/daily diary sheets, the days of the diary and of all the dreams were randomised, so that participants could not spot or create any scoring patterns on the basis of how close in time the dream and diary day had been.

An advantage of this method was that there were many instances of particular time periods between a dream and a diary day. For example, a diary on day 3 compared to a dream on day 6 has the same time period between them as for, say, a diary on day 8 and a dream on day 11. We were thus getting an advantage of a large sample of data for each time period between diary day and dream. We also had a vast number of comparisons of dreams with diary records in the future, so as to assess the baseline level of similarity for any particular person between dreams and daily life. As expected, those similarities were small, and indeed we did not expect dreams to be significantly predictive of people's future. The main results were that we found a day residue effect, with a high level of immediate incorporation of daily experiences into dreams, then a lower level of similarity between dreams and waking life experiences where the experiences occurred two, three or four days before the dream, and then a high level of delayed incorporation of experiences from five, six or seven days before the dream. The study thus found the same U-shaped time course of incorporation of waking life experiences into dreams as was obtained in the papers by Nielsen and his colleagues.

Nielsen and Stenstrom (2005) had published a review article in the science journal *Nature* on the dream-lag effect, proposing that the effect showed that memories were being processed and consolidated over the course of a week, and that dream-content reflected this processing. There is sense in this speculation because it is difficult otherwise to explain the delayed incorporation. Immediate incorporation is relatively easy to explain, because unfinished business from the day may still be on one's mind during sleep. Researchers who hold that dreaming has a function and those who think it has no function would equally accept that our dreams would be composed of emotional material from the previous day. But it was difficult to think of why there would be this delayed incorporation unless it was due to some memory processing effect. Nielsen and Stenstrom suggested that it takes time for the hippocampus, which stores new memories, to pass those memories to the cortex for permanent storage. They proposed that there is some feature of the consolidation that can take up to a week to occur.

To test this speculation, Blagrove, Fouquet and colleagues (2011a) investigated whether the dream-lag effect might be specific to Rapid Eye Movement (REM) sleep dreams, because, as we will see in Chapter 5, REM sleep appears to be more involved with emotional memory consolidation than is non-REM (NREM) sleep. This had not been studied before because all dream-lag studies until then had involved dreams that people had recorded on awakening at home. We had participants keep a daily diary for ten days before coming to sleep in the sleep lab. We woke them from REM sleep and from the N2 stage of NREM sleep, to obtain REM and N2 dreams. We then had participants compare their dream reports with each of the diary records from the ten days before the dream, and to rate the similarity between each diary record and each dream report. Of course, participants did not know if a dream was from REM or N2 sleep, and we were able to plot the time course of waking life incorporations into dreams for REM and N2 dreams separately. Our results were that, again, delayed incorporation of daily life experiences into dreams was found, but only for the REM dreams and not for N2 dreams.

It did therefore appear that the dream-lag effect is part of memory consolidation during sleep. But we had not yet tested what it is about each dream report and waking life diary that results in them being matched. So, rather than asking participants to write a narrative diary each day, we gave them a structured diary, so that for each day they recorded their major daily activities, such as travelling to work, their personally significant events, such as watching an emotional film or meeting with someone, and their major concerns. Then, when dream reports were compared to each diary, rather than a global score of similarity between the dream and diary record, participants had to identify what parts of the dream had a similarity to what structured diary item. This resulted in separate scores for the incorporation into dreams of daily activities, personally significant events and major concerns. We collected REM dreams using a sleep monitor that could be used in participants' homes, and we found that the day-residue and dream-lag effects occurred, but only for personally significant events, and not for major daily activities, nor major concerns (van Rijn et al., 2015, study 1 on home collected REM dreams). This may be because personally significant events can be emotional or important and specific to a day, whereas major daily activities are relatively unemotional, and major concerns tend to be spread out over several days, so their effects are more difficult to identify.

We thus showed that it is personally significant events that account for immediate incorporations and delayed dream-lag incorporations in dreams. But there were two problems here. The first was that, whereas this was found for participants' ratings of the similarity between dream reports and diary records, we wanted to check if independent judges could also identify dream-lag relationships between dream reports and diary records. The second was that using naturalistic events from daily life does introduce randomness and variability into the data because some days might have a more captivating or significant event than another day. We therefore wanted to give participants a single standardised stimulus, and to see how it was incorporated into their dreams. Our stimulus for this aim was a night of sleeping and being experimented on in the sleep lab. This standardised stimulus had the additional advantage that independent judges could assess dreams for the presence of references to this experience, without the need for biographical information about each participant.

And so after being in the sleep lab for a night, participants kept a daily dream log for the following ten consecutive days at home. After these ten days, participants and independent judges were given the reports of the dreams and a general but detailed account of what happened to all the participants for the night in the sleep lab. They were instructed to rate the extent to which each dream referred to the account of what occurred on the night in the sleep lab. The ratings by participants and by independent judges, who were given the dream accounts in random order, did show the 5–7 day dream-lag effect (van Rijn et al., 2015, study 2), although only for the participants who had expressed concern about being in the sleep lab.

Then, in 2019, with lead author Jean-Baptiste Eichenlaub, we published a study that took account of how people differ in their general number of correspondences they find between each dream and each diary record, and with the largest number of participants in a dream-lag study where participants were trained to match diary records and dream content; we again confirmed the day-residue and dream-lag effects. Perplexing though the dream-lag effect is, it does seem to be a robust finding, and an important determinant of dream content.

More recent work has attempted to experimentally alter the dream-lag effect. Picard-Deland and Nielsen (2022) gave participants a Virtual Reality (VR) task in the sleep laboratory, after which they either had a two-hour nap or a two-hour period reading. Auditory cues associated with the VR task were replayed in either wake, or REM sleep, or SWS (N3), or were not replayed. Participants then recorded their dream reports at home for ten days after being in the sleep lab. It was found that participants dreamed more about the task 1–2 days later when auditory cues had been applied in REM sleep and 5–6 days later when they were applied in SWS sleep, compared to participants with no cueing. These findings may help explain the mechanism behind the intriguing dream-lag phenomenon, in that SWS and REM sleep may be involved in causing the effect, even if the effect is only seen in REM sleep dreams.

Summary

Dreams tend to refer to emotional experiences from waking life more than to our non-emotional experiences. Scenarios in dreams are highly novel and very rarely copy exactly waking life events. Such scenarios can be realistic, or unlikely, or impossible and bizarre. There has been so far a conclusion that the dream-lag effect has a role in or is a consequence of memory processing during sleep, but a very different explanation will be suggested in Chapter 13.

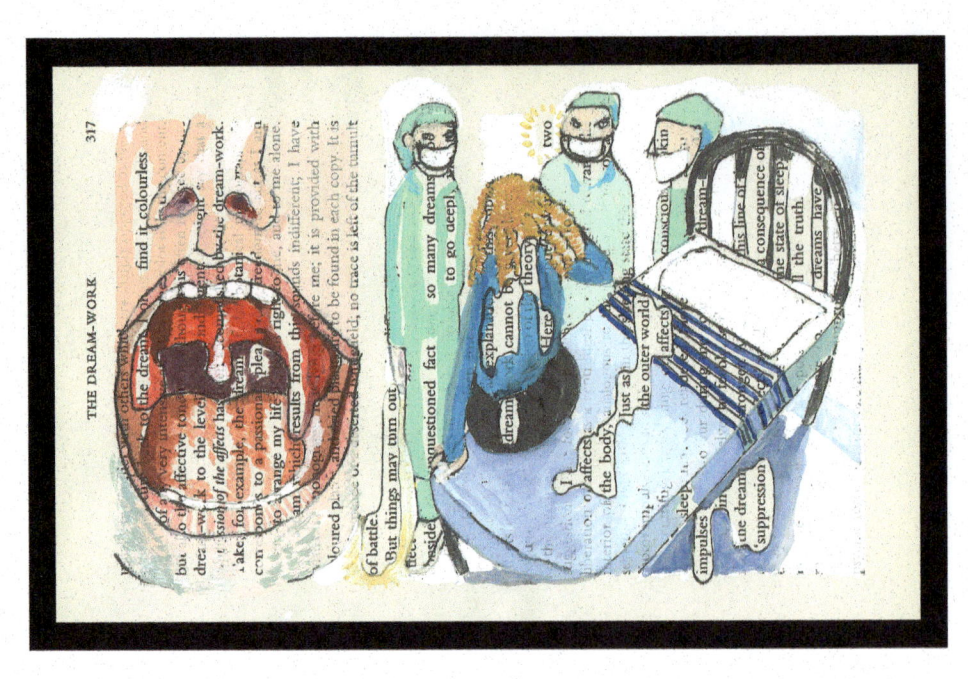

Figure 2.1 Dream of my brother's operation, 2019.

2 Why do some people recall dreams more than others?

This is a dream of a neuroscientist who studies what happens in the brain when dreams are produced. The dream was told to us as part of a sleep conference at the Paris Institute for Advanced Study.

DREAM NARRATIVE: *I am in a hospital in a city in Switzerland. I have arranged for my brother to have two operations, at separate hospitals. He has travelled to the city so as to have both operations in one day. The first is on his mouth and throat. I am then waiting at the second hospital. I am in a room with the doctors. My brother phones me and says that he cannot make the second operation. I realise that a person can't be intubated twice in one day. I am annoyed with myself for organising so much for him to do.*

DISCUSSION: The dreamer had been on vacation when she had the dream. Despite being on vacation she had brought along two grant applications to complete. We related this to being unable to complete two operations in the dream.

JULIA: (Painting shown as Figure 2.1) As the narrative of the dream required two main plot components, I chose one page with three paragraphs. I used a central four-line paragraph to contain one of the masked doctors. This means the doctor stands alone. His body contains the found poem:

unquestioned fact
so many dreams
to go deep

I used the paragraph at the top of the page to contain the dreamer's brother's open mouth and tonsils. The red colour range and visceral imagery dominate the composition, even though it is not the largest compositional component. The tonsils and tongue contain the found poem:

affective
to the level
of the affects
to arrange my life

DOI: 10.4324/9781003037552-2

This is contrasted with the green of the doctor's scrubs and the blue of the bed. The dreamer's body contains the found poem:

explained
dream
cannot be theory
Here

This chapter looks at why people differ in how often they remember or recall their dreams. We will first examine psychological and personality reasons for these differences, and then consider whether there are differences in the brains of people with high and low dream recall, and how dream recall and dream content change from childhood to adulthood.

Personality differences between high and low dream recallers

Surveys have found that on average about one-third of people recall dreams a few times per week, about one-third a few times per month, and one-third recall dreams less than once per month, and with dream recall decreasing with age (e.g., Stepansky et al., 1998). Although many people claim never to dream, Jim Pagel (2003) found that whereas 6.5% of patients at his sleep clinic on a questionnaire reported never dreaming, only 0.4% of patients reported no dreams when awakened from sleep (including REM sleep) in the sleep lab and immediately queried about dream recall. This shows it is very rare for people to report having no dreams at all.

After several decades of research into the relationship between dream recall and memory ability, the conclusion is that high dream recallers do not have better short-term or long-term verbal memory than low recallers, but might have better visual memory (Blagrove & Pace-Schott, 2010). Another hypothesis has been that low dream recallers might be more distractible, so that failing to recall a dream in the morning may be due to thinking about or ruminating on other things when one wakes up. To test this, Cohen and Wolfe (1973) asked participants, who were sleeping at home, to phone the weather report phone number immediately upon waking and to write down the weather forecast. Cohen and Wolfe found that this decreased recall of dreams, compared to participants who were told to remain in bed without this distraction. Dream recall can also decrease for people distracted by stresses they are under, because, in general, recalling and thinking about a dream is needed immediately on waking so as to transfer the dream to long-term memory (although sometimes spontaneous recall can occur later in the day if someone experiences a reminder of the dream). Another possibility for poor recall is that because dreams are often disorganised, rather than a linear plot, it can be difficult to recall the full dream, much as a stand-up comedian's performance containing digressive interactions or jokes can be difficult to reconstruct afterwards.

Differences in dream recall, either trait differences between people or night-by-night differences for a person, might also be due to the content of dreams. For Freud (1900/1997, chapter VII (A)), dream content is repressed and forgotten because of its taboo nature. In contrast, the salience hypothesis (reviewed in Parke & Horton, 2009) holds that frequent dream recallers have more memorable, interesting or striking dreams, and so content is not being repressed, but rather for some people is not interesting or captivating enough to recall or lay down as a long-term memory. There have been attempts to test this, with findings such as a relationship between irregular breathing during sleep and increased dream recall, with the respiratory irregularity being taken as showing that a dream is vivid or emotional (Shapiro et al., 1964). Further evidence is seen in Cohen (1974), who had participants complete mood rating sheets each evening and dream diaries each morning at home for five days. Cohen found that dream recall was more likely to occur when the person had a negative mood before going to sleep, and concluded that this supports the hypothesis that pre-sleep mood affects the salience of dreams, and thus their likelihood of being recalled.

Another area of explanation for differences in dream recall is personality. Rosalind Schonbar's (1965) 'lifestyle hypothesis' for dream recall proposed the existence of two lifestyles, the inner-acceptance type of person, and the inner-rejectant type, who instead represses emotions. She held that the former are more likely to be high dream recallers, as they have more access to their own psychic world, with cognitive flexibility and creative responsiveness, whereas low dream recallers are more likely to repress their emotions, and have a blander fantasy life, dealing with the world on concrete terms. The lifestyle hypothesis can be linked to the personality characteristic of absorption, which is the ability to be absorbed in imaginings, including films and books. This greater acceptance of and interest and engagement in fictions might lead to better recall of dreams, or even a greater production of dreams, and the relationship is supported by Schredl et al. (1997). Fitch and Armitage (1989) addressed another personality measure, finding that high dream recallers score higher on a test of creativity in which people are asked to devise multiple uses for an object, such as a brick. High recallers were found to generate more elaborate and original uses for objects than were low recallers.

A prominent personality correlate of dream recall frequency is Ernest Hartmann's (1991) construct of 'thin boundariness', which combines creativity, acceptance of ambiguity, and openness to experience. This has such items as 'I am easily hurt', 'I spend a lot of time daydreaming, fantasising or in reverie', 'I think I would enjoy being some kind of creative artist', where high scores indicate thin boundaries, and items such as 'I like stories that have a definite beginning, middle and end', for which a high score indicates thick boundariness, in other words, that the person is more down-to-earth or 'no nonsense'. In many studies, frequent dream recall has been found to correlate with thin boundariness (e.g., Schredl, Schäfer, Hofmann, & Jacob, 1999). The latter authors also found that thin boundaried people regard their dreams as more meaningful and creative than do thick boundaried people, and might thus have more interest in their dreams when they wake up, and a greater incentive for recalling and remembering them. Thin boundaried people also tend to have longer, and more vivid, emotional and bizarre dreams, with more interaction between characters (Hartmann et al., 1991), and so they might have dreams that are more memorable because of these content differences.

Much of the work above involves what are called retrospective assessments of dream recall, where individuals answer one questionnaire that asks how often they dream, with options such as, for example, several times per week, or once per month or once per year. Beaulieu-Prévost and Zadra (2007) extended this by asking participants to complete a retrospective questionnaire on their dream recall but to also keep a log each morning of whether they had had a dream. Beaulieu-Prévost and Zadra found that whereas thin boundaries and absorption correlated with the retrospective assessment of dream recall, it did not correlate with the log method. The implication of this is that people who score high on absorption and thin boundariness don't actually have more dreams; instead, they see themselves as being a frequent dream recaller, even if objectively this is not true. This might also be an example of the availability heuristic, which describes the tendency for people, when asked to estimate the frequency of events, such as car crashes or plane crashes, to base their estimate on how many such instances they can remember. How easily available examples are to memory, affects the estimate of the frequency of their occurrence. Thin boundaried or high absorption people might thus have a higher number of dreams that they can think of, and thus give a higher estimate to their frequency of occurrence of dreams than do people scoring low on these personality measures.

Beaulieu-Prévost and Zadra did however find one personality correlate of retrospective and log dream recall, this was Attitude towards Dreams. Attitude towards Dreams measures whether or not a person appreciates dreams, is interested in them, or in contrast, does not value them and indeed might have a low opinion of people who are interested in dreams. It is not clear whether this correlation means that people with many dreams develop a positive attitude towards dreams, or whether people with a very positive attitude towards dreams are then motivated to recall more of their dreams.

To conclude so far, there has been very little success in finding personality correlates of dream recall, apart from individuals' Attitude towards Dreams. Recently, however, there is evidence that Sensory Processing Sensitivity (SPS) is related to dream recall. SPS is a personality trait that is the basis for the Highly Sensitive Persons Scale (Aron & Aron, 1997), high scorers on which have a deep processing of stimuli, like to think about intellectual and philosophical issues, get upset if overstimulated, such as when too much is happening around them, and jump at sudden noises like somebody dropping a milk bottle or sneezing loudly! Highly Sensitive Persons (HSPs) also do not like violent videos and scenes of cruelty, appreciate the arts, and think deeply and slowly. HSPs are more distressed in adverse circumstances than are non-HSPs, but can flourish in positive environments. HSPs also have higher brain reactivity and can more accurately detect degraded auditory words than non-HSPs (Williams et al., 2021). With Jess Williams and Michelle Carr, we have found higher dream recall frequency, and, as we will see in the next chapter, higher frequency of nightmares, for HSPs than for non-HSPs (Carr et al., 2021). Furthermore, findings from Schredl, Blamo, Ehrenfeld, and Olivier (2022) suggest that this relationship may be predominantly due to the Aesthetic Sensitivity component of SPS, rather than components more related to being overwhelmed or annoyed by stimuli. This biopsychological trait and the brain excitation associated with it thus do seem to cause some people to be higher dream recallers. However, these findings do need to be confirmed with dream recall assessed by logs rather than retrospective questionnaire, so as to remove the issue of someone's self-concept of being a thoughtful sensitive person affecting their estimate of how often they recall dreams. We also do not know if HSPs spend more of the night dreaming, or whether they just recall dreams better than do non-HSPs, or whether they do both, that is, have higher dream formation and better memory for dreams. As SPS is partly a brain activity trait, this brings us to whether there are differences in the brains of people who frequently recall dreams.

Differences in the brain and sleep of high and low dream recallers

Eichenlaub, Bertrand and colleagues (2014a) played to participants their first name or a different first name when they were awake and when asleep. These names were presented randomly and rarely among repeated pure tones. This is called the novelty oddball paradigm. Eichenlaub and colleagues measured the brain activity responses to the names. The response is termed an evoked response potential, which is a brain wave pattern lasting approximately one-fifth of a second. They recruited people so as to have high dream recallers (more than three dreams recalled per week) and low dream recallers (less than two dreams recalled per month). They found that there was greater brain reactivity of high dream recallers to the names played during wake and sleep compared to low dream recallers. They concluded that the different brain reactivity might facilitate either the production or encoding of dreams.

There was a replication of these findings by Vallat et al. (2017b), who presented 18 high dream recallers and 18 low dream recallers with sound stimuli during a night of sleep in the lab. Response to stimuli was again measured by evoked response potential, showing the brain's immediate response to a stimulus. The high recall participants showed higher evoked response potentials to arousing stimuli and more long awakenings during the night compared to low recallers. Vallat and colleagues (2022) then assessed the connectivity between areas of the brain involved in the Default Mode Network (DMN), which is the network of connections found between brain areas when the brain is not attending to any task, and is the basis to mind wandering. High recallers demonstrated a greater connectivity between areas of the brain involved in the DMN than did low recallers. These results demonstrate that there are neurophysiological trait differences between individuals who frequently recall their dreams and those who do not.

Further information about areas of the brain involved in differences between people in dream recall frequency was found by Eichenlaub, Nicolas and colleagues (2014b). This study used a positron emission tomography (PET) scan to detect active areas of the brain by their increased blood flow. In PET scans, a mildly radioactive type of sugar is ingested and builds up in areas of the brain when they are active. The radioactivity is detected and a 3D map of the brain is produced, showing where the activity is taking place. Participants with high and low dream recall frequency were studied during wakefulness and during Rapid Eye Movement sleep, and in stages N2 and N3 of non-REM sleep. Participants were deprived of sleep for one night so that they would be able to sleep in the PET scanner. They were also asked to provide a dream report at the end of the night, so as to validate the division into high and low recallers. The high recallers were found to have higher blood flow compared to low recallers in the temporal parietal junction during REM sleep, N3 and wakefulness, and in the medial prefrontal cortex during REM sleep and wakefulness. These two areas are similar to the ones found by Mark Solms (1997, 2000) to be supporting dreaming; Solms' work is covered in Chapter 6. For this chapter, the implication is that activity in these two areas differs between people, and causes differences in either dream production, dream recall or both of these.

Child development and dreaming

There are also effects of age on dream recall and dream content. The most extensive work on children's dreams was done in the 1970s and 1980s by David Foulkes in a very large series of studies in which he studied children and teenagers in the sleep laboratory (Foulkes, 1999). These were longitudinal studies, following each child for many years. For children aged 3–5 years, he found that 27% of REM awakenings yielded a dream report, which is much less frequent than for adults, and with an average length of dream reports of just 14 words. He also looked at the content of the reports. He found there were no strangers in these dreams. Though there were animals, there were no interactions with people, and there were often body state descriptions, with concerns such as being cold or hungry. However, at ages 5–7, Foulkes found that dreams become more of a novel, mentally skilled experience. He found that 31% of REM awakenings were followed by a dream report, that the length of reports tripled to about 41 words, and that at this age there were now social interactions in the dreams. Humans were now more frequent in these dreams than animals, but the self-character in the dream was watching what was happening, rather than participating. At this point, dreams took on a linear story, with a plot and some characters not known from waking life.

At ages 7–9 years, the recall rate from REM sleep was now 48%, and 21% from NREM sleep, and there was self-participation of the dreaming child in the dream. The main emotion felt was happiness, but there were some nightmares. At this age, he found the frequency of known persons in their dreams increased. Foulkes concluded that children differ in their ability to represent people that they know in the dream.

At ages 9–13 years, dreams begin to show diverse emotions and an increase in novel characters being produced; these are now true strangers, people who are not real or based on anyone known in waking life. Additionally, he found that the number of strangers in dreams is higher for children who are scoring high on a cognitive task of block design. This visuospatial task involves putting blocks together, each block having a design on, so as to copy a single large design. He found that only at ages 11–13 are there sex differences other than the most prominent sex difference which happens in dreams, which is that females tend to dream equally of male and female characters, whereas males dream more of male characters. At ages 11–13 there are sex differences such as of the level of aggression in dreams, and at ages 13–15 years, there are frequent novel characters and novel settings, with dreams becoming very much like adult dreams, with great originality.

For Foulkes, the relationship of dream content to cognitive ability showed that children at each age differ in their abilities to create complex dreams, and that it is only in the youngest age group of 3–5 years that dream recall was related to verbal and social abilities. From the longitudinal studies, he concluded that children slowly learn the cognitive skill of dreaming, and that it develops in stages. He drew a comparison with the work of Piaget on the stages by which children develop their cognitive skills. Piaget (1936, 1945) showed that at any one age there are certain skills that are beyond the child, that they cannot do, and that they have to slowly develop concepts and skills, such as conservation, where with age and experience the child appreciates that there may be the same amount of liquid in a tall thin jar as in a short fat jar. Similarly, for Foulkes, there is a neurocognitive ability to produce and recall dreams that develops over time. As we will see in Chapter 6, this view de-emphasises the differences between sleep stages, and even the difference between dreams and daydreams.

However, Resnick, Hobson and colleagues published a study in 1994 on self-representation and bizarreness in children's dream reports collected in the home setting. They found active self-representation in 85% of the dreams of 4–5-year-olds and in 89% of the dreams of 8–10-year-olds. There were also bizarre elements in about half the dreams of 4–5-year-olds, and in 71% of the dreams of 8–10-year-olds. This is very different from Foulkes' findings of quite simple dreams in young children. In contrast, Resnick and colleagues (1994), with a more physiological rather than a psychological view of dream formation, were finding that these young children have dreams that are like adult dreams. Foulkes' (1996) response to this was that his collecting of dreams was done in the sleep laboratory so as to diminish possibilities for confabulation, that is, the imagining or inventing of content once awake, and the waking elaboration of reports, and that he had also collected dreams in children's homes, and found no differences between dreams collected in the two settings.

There has been recent work that has conducted interviews of children at home to a rigorous standard. Sándor and colleagues (2015) found dream recall frequencies of 19%, 26% and 18% per night for children aged 3.8–5.5 years, 5.51–7 years, and 7.01–8.5 years, respectively, waking naturally at home. On average there were 3.13 characters per dream (not including the self), and 7.9% of the characters were animals. The dreamer's own self appeared in an active role in 77.6% of the dreams, which did not differ significantly between the age groups. Eighty-six per cent of all dreams were cinematic, out of those dreams where cinematic or static nature was explicitly reported by the dreamer, and this did not change with age. These findings are thus of high levels of complexity in children's dreams in terms of self-representation and interactions of characters, and self-initiated actions, and almost one emotion per dream: all of these are higher than in the work of Foulkes. Sándor and colleagues (2016) found in children aged four to eight years that dreamer's self-effectiveness, wilful effort and cognitive reflections in dreams were correlated with executive control in waking life (measured by the ability to ignore distractions on the Stroop task, in which font colour of words is responded to while ignoring the meaning of the word), thus showing that cognition in dreams is related to cognitive abilities when awake. However, they failed to replicate Foulkes' finding of a relationship between dream recall and visuospatial ability.

Summary

The main reason for differences between people in dream recall seems to be due to different levels of activity of the brain during sleep, but there is also a relationship with whether people have a positive or negative attitude towards dreams, although the direction of causality for the latter relationship is not clear. If the attitude towards dreams could affect dream recall then it is plausible that becoming interested in dreams could lead to an increase in how often one recalls dreams. The findings on children's dreams reviewed here do show the considerable cognitive skill involved in dream formation, despite differences in the literature about how early the more adult type of dreaming occurs.

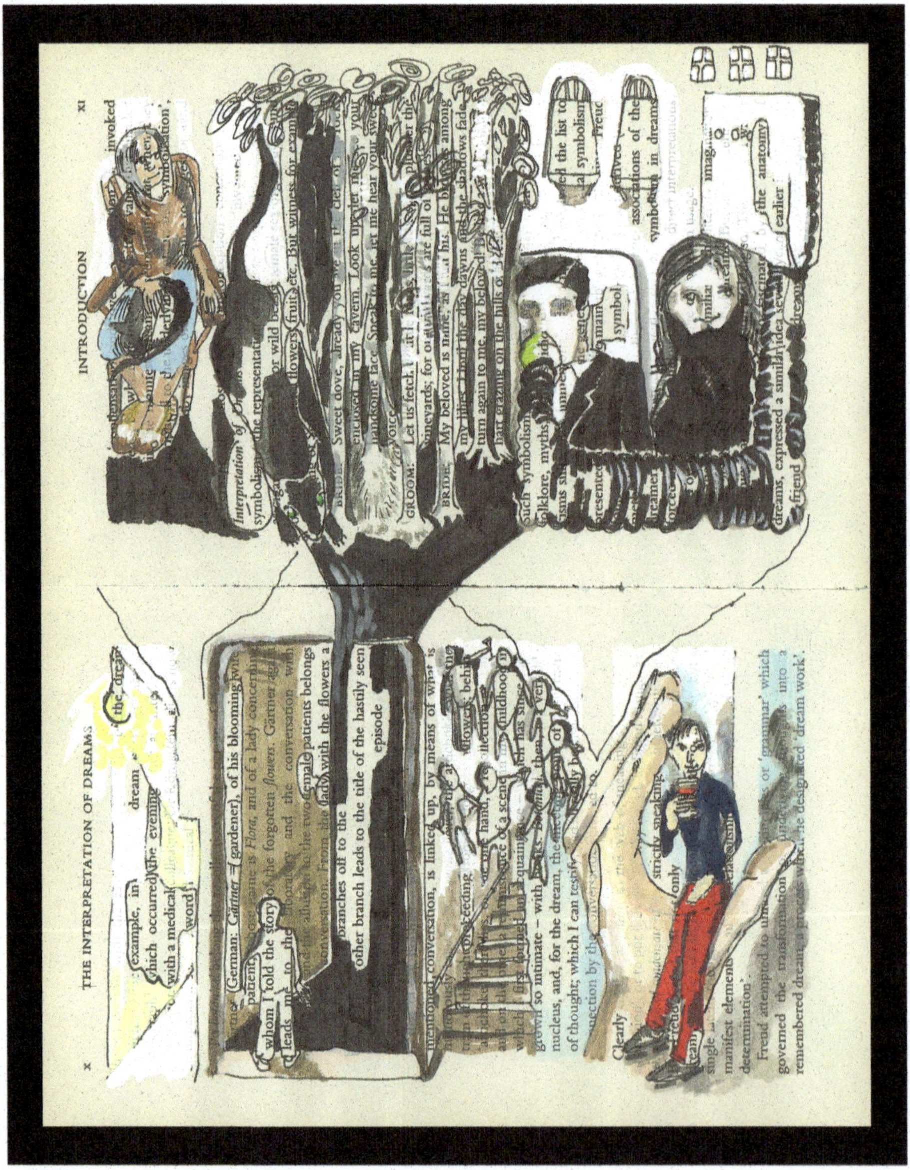

Figure 3.1 Nightmare of suffocating after a party during Covid-19, 2020.

3 Nightmares

A nightmare of Libby, a nurse who was isolating from Covid-19 in the first Lockdown in 2020, and who told the nightmare to us and the audience online.

DREAM NARRATIVE: *I stand at the open door of a house and can see strange trees outside with strange leaves. I know it is very dangerous outside and the danger will soon come into the house. I can't close the door as it is so large. I go inside to warn people. I go into a large hall with stairs. A party is happening and everyone ignores my warnings, they don't look at me and seem not to have faces. I then see a man with red trousers who is a composite of all my past loves, he looks at me and knows what I am warning about, but with a smile, he says without words that all is actually fine and that I should not worry. I go into a side room, which is a hospital room with a dead man on the bed and an old noisy ventilator. My deceased mother is there with a cat on her lap. The cat jumps onto me and onto my mouth and stops me from breathing.*

DISCUSSION: Libby had Covid-19 when she had this nightmare and was quarantined separately from her family. She described her difficulties breathing due to Covid-19. She said how during the Lockdown people are being divided between those who are at home drinking wine and those who need to go out to work.

JULIA: (Painting shown as Figure 3.1) For this highly complex dream narrative, I painted on two pages. I chose them for the seven paragraphs, which I wove together with the branches of trees, and included Freud's words *branches off to the other branch* in the trunk of the tree. There is a dark, broodingly eerie feel to the image. I incorporated many of Freud's words which take on a living meaning beyond his original text: in reference to the red-trousered man, *My beloved is mine, turn again to me my beloved* is in the branches of the tree, and in reference to her quarantine, *Sweet dove, already you are enclosed in my cavern*, is also in the tree.

This chapter explores what nightmares are, who gets them, theories of how they are formed, and methods to reduce their occurrence.

DOI: 10.4324/9781003037552-3

What are nightmares?

In the Diagnostic and Statistical Manual of Mental Disorders (DSM-5) and the International Classification of Sleep Disorders (ICSD-3), the medical definition of a nightmare is an 'extended, extremely dysphoric' dream that 'usually involves efforts to avoid threats to survival, security, or physical integrity' (Gieselmann et al., 2019). Nightmare disorder is further defined as 'the repeated occurrence of nightmares that cause clinically significant distress or impairment in social, occupational or other important areas of functioning', that is not due to other conditions or substance use. Nightmares are distinguished from night terrors which are a disorder of arousal from non-REM sleep, and from which dreams are not recalled, but where there can be visions on waking, such as of seeing an ominous or threatening figure in the room. The average incidence of nightmares is 1–2 per year, and about 4–8% of people have a 'current problem' with nightmares, with this being greater in females than males (Spoormaker et al., 2006).

The definition of nightmares presented above does not include a criterion that had been used previously, that the nightmare wakes the sleeper. That criterion is now a matter of debate. The criterion had been used because nightmares that wake the dreamer seem to be a rarer and more severe type of dysphoric dream than those where waking is caused for another reason. For example, in Robert and Zadra's (2014) thematic and content analysis of nightmares, very disturbing dreams that wake the sleeper were found to be more likely to include physical aggression, bizarreness and unfortunate endings, than did very disturbing dreams where waking was not caused by the dream.

Nightmares can be divided into two categories: idiopathic and post-traumatic. Idiopathic nightmares are those which are spontaneous or of unknown cause; post-traumatic nightmares are a feature of post-traumatic stress disorder (PTSD). Ernest Hartmann (1996) compared these types of nightmare and showed that PTSD nightmares can replay what occurred during the trauma, which is different from the more ordinary idiopathic nightmares where the plot may change each time. PTSD nightmares are more likely to be repetitive, to occur on many nights, involve physical bodily movements, and to occur earlier in the night, than idiopathic nightmares.

There is an issue about how to measure people's frequency of nightmares. One method is to ask for a retrospective estimate, by giving people a single questionnaire that asks how many nightmares they have per month or per year. The second method is a nightly log, where each morning people report whether they have had a nightmare or not. Robert and Zadra (2008) found that the daily log method results in a higher number of nightmares being reported than do retrospective measures. So, people may well be having many more nightmares than they think they do, they just seem to forget some of them.

Who has nightmares?

There has been a research literature across decades looking at waking life correlates of idiopathic nightmare frequency. A high frequency of nightmares has been associated with psychoticism, neuroticism, depression and other psychopathology measures (Spoormaker et al, 2006). Tore Nielsen and colleagues (2000) found that adolescents at 13 years old with frequent disturbing dreams score higher on anxiety than those without frequent disturbing dreams, and found that they still had this anxiety three years later.

There is also the effect of stress. Wood and colleagues (1992) studied the effects of the 1989 San Francisco earthquake on the frequency and content of nightmares. Nightmare frequency was found to be twice as high among San Francisco Bay area students as among control students who lived in Arizona, far from the 1989 earthquake. They not only had more nightmares in general in the three-week period after the earthquake, but substantially more nightmares about earthquakes, with 40% of those in the San Francisco Bay area reporting one or more nightmares about an earthquake, as compared with only 5% of those in Arizona. However, the nightmares about earthquakes were not more emotionally intense than were the other nightmares, which brings in the idea that nightmares and dreams can often have the same emotion as was present in waking life, but with the dream or nightmare providing a different context or scenario for that emotion.

Nightmare distress

How bothered someone is by their nightmares is very different from nightmare frequency. The distress that people have from their nightmares can be measured by Belicki's (1992) Nightmare Distress questionnaire. It asks questions such as: 'when you awaken from a nightmare do you have difficulty putting it out of your mind?', 'do nightmares interfere with the quality of your sleep?', 'do nightmares affect your well-being?', and 'in the past, have you considered seeking professional help for your nightmares?' In general, the more nightmares people have, the higher their trait nightmare distress, but this is not a strong relationship and so there are some people with a lot of nightmares who are not bothered by them, and there are some people with only a very few nightmares who are extremely distressed by them. Interestingly older people have fewer nightmares than younger people but a very much lower level of nightmare distress (Salvio et al., 1992).

We have noted above that poor mental health is related to the number of nightmares that people have. Belicki (1992) showed that poor mental health is also related to the level of distress people have from their nightmares. Blagrove and colleagues therefore conducted the first study to measure waking life mental health, with measures of depression, anxiety, neuroticism and stress, diary assessed nightmare frequency and nightmare distress. Using a technique called partial correlations, they showed that poor mental health is related to the frequency of nightmares and also to nightmare distress (Blagrove et al., 2004). This suggests that low mental well-being in waking life causes one to have nightmares, and then causes a distressed reaction to the nightmares.

Theories of what causes nightmares

Levin and Nielsen (2007) put forward a theory for why nightmares occur. They stated that stressful and emotionally negative events can cause acquired fear memories. So, for example, bad experiences at work might cause one to have fear of the whole workplace. It is known that fear memory acquisition is rapid, but also very useful and adaptive for keeping us safe because it is good for people to respond to their environments with fear, where there is a basis to the fear. Such fear memories can extinguish in time, but can spontaneously recover and show themselves again.

Levin and Nielsen (2007) proposed their Affective Network Dysfunction model, in which fear memories are extinguished during dreams. The mechanism for this is that a fear memory might occur in a dream in a different context or different environment (e.g., the feared work office might be placed on a beach), or paired with some non-fearful content (e.g., a party in the office), or might even occur in a dream exactly as in real life, but without the experience of fear. This combination of a new factor with the fearful stimulus in dreams would cause the fear to diminish, and they proposed this to be the function of dreaming. The theory also specifies brain regions that underlie this process, there can be activation of the hippocampus (a memory area), so that we can think of new contexts, or the amygdala (an emotion area) may alter its activity so as to reduce the emotional component of fear associated memory. This theory explains why recurrent dreams are usually emotionally negative, and why people who have recurrent dreams score lower on well-being than do people who have never had recurrent dreams, or who in the past were recurrent dreamers (Gauchat et al., 2009). The theory holds that recurrent dreams occur because the fear reduction function has not yet succeeded, and there may be mental health problems as a result.

Levin and Nielsen then proposed that people differ in their predisposition for how much they react to stress and also how much they react to emotionally negative dreams. The latter predisposition overlaps with neuroticism and is, of course, very similar to the trait of nightmare distress. So, for some people, during a dream, the amygdala continues to express extremely negative emotions and the hippocampus is unable to produce sufficiently incompatible contexts for the fear memories. Nightmares thus result as a failure of this main function of dreams, and the person then continues to dream of their fears. Levin and Nielsen propose that the situation is worse in the case of post-traumatic nightmares, because these would be particularly resistant to being combined with other memories or to having reduced emotion in a dream, and the nightmares thus keep repeating the trauma that happened.

Unlike ordinary dreams, where we almost never copy what happens to us in waking life, in post-traumatic nightmares one repeats and replays what happened at the time of the trauma. It may even be that the disruption of sleep as a result of nightmares maintains their occurrence. In Walker and Van der Helm's (2009) Sleep to Remember and Sleep to Forget model, sleep has the function of reducing felt emotion in our memories of waking experiences, and reduces our emotional reactivity when awake: this processing in sleep would be adversely affected by awakenings due to nightmares.

A second theory also looks at the brain. Carr and colleagues (2018) replicated previous findings that individuals with frequent nightmares produce more errors than do control participants when asked to generate a list of words in a particular category or starting with a particular letter. They repeat words they have given already, showing impaired executive functions and difficulty in inhibiting their responses. It is as if their frontal lobes, which are involved in planning and inhibiting responses, cannot stop frightening imagery during the night.

A theory, however, that proposes that there is a benefit to nightmares is Revonsuo's (2000) threat simulation theory. This is an evolutionary view of why nightmares occur, and opposes the view that nightmares are a failure of dream function. It holds that dreams and nightmares are a selective simulation of the world, and are selective for what is negative in the world, including negative emotions, misfortunes, threats and aggression. This theory cites the findings of Hall and Van de Castle (1966) that misfortune is seven times as frequent as good fortune in dreams, and that 45% of dreams have at least one aggressive interaction. So, in this view, dreams provide a negatively toned environment in which the dreamer needs to overcome threats. The theory holds that we rehearse threat perception and threat avoidance in dreams, and that the default values for dreams are the simulation of violent encounters with animals and strangers, adverse natural forces and other threatening situations. The theory also highlights that children often have animal dreams, animals being a dangerous part of human pre-history. It also ties in with REM behaviour disorder, as mentioned in Chapter 4, which is a sleep disorder where actions are acted out when muscle atonia is lost during REM sleep. Many REM behaviour disorder actions are very negative and violent towards other people, and often the dreams associated with REM behaviour disorder are threatening.

Personality and susceptibility to nightmares

There is then a further evolutionary theory of the aetiology of nightmares which sees susceptibility to nightmares not as a negative trait but as due to heightened responsiveness to stimuli in general. Many illnesses are explained by a diathesis–stress model, where there is a predisposition to illness (the diathesis) from which illness results when a stimulus or stress occurs. Historically, nightmares have been explained in this way, with a predisposition, such as through adverse childhood circumstances (Nielsen, 2017), leading to an illness when adverse events occur. Susceptibility to nightmares has thus been seen as a psychopathology. The first alternative to this was put forward by Hartmann, who was finding in his clinical work that many nightmare sufferers were sensitive and creative, and he devised his thin boundary questionnaire to spot these sensitive creative people (Hartmann, 1991; Hartmann et al., 1991); scores on this questionnaire were related to nightmare frequency (Pietrowsky & Köthe, 2003). The predisposition was held, therefore, not to be a negative trait, but instead to be what is called a vantage trait, which is neither good nor bad, and which shows that the population has a range of people, diverse in their creativity and sensitivity.

A personality measure similar to thin boundaries was developed by Elaine Aron, who was working in clinical and personality psychology and investigating what she called Highly Sensitive Persons (HSPs). She identified these with the Highly Sensitive Person Scale (HSPS; Aron & Aron, 1997), which measures individuals' levels of Sensory Processing Sensitivity (SPS). As mentioned also in chapter 2, HSPs think deeply, are sensitive to the moods of other people, spot things that are subtle, are deeply moved by art and music, and although they are emotionally reactive they are also very cautious. They may become overwhelmed by too much stimulation, and so like quiet environments and to be alone if subjected to overwhelming circumstances. HSPs can have very adverse reactions to negative events in life, even to sudden noises, but in a positive environment, they can flourish even more than do non-HSPs. In positive environments, they can have curiosity, prosocial behaviour, empathy, hopefulness and excitement, whereas in negative environments they may feel threatened, have attentional narrowing, distress, anxiety and helplessness. Non-HSPs will also react differently to positive and negative environments, but HSPs react more extremely to both. Addressing these characteristics, Michelle Carr and Tore Nielsen (2017) devised the theory that SPS gives a predisposition to nightmares, with nightmares resulting more for HSPs when waking life conditions are adverse, whereas for non-HSPs, adverse conditions are not as likely to result in nightmares.

Jess Williams, an SPS researcher, Michelle Carr and Mark Blagrove tested this theory with 137 participants, whom they divided into high, medium and low SPS on the basis of their HSPS score (Williams et al., 2021). They assessed participants' levels of stress and how often they have nightmares. They computed the correlation between stress and nightmare frequency for each group separately, and found that HSPs have a larger correlation between stress and nightmare frequency than do non-HSPs. So, HSPs are more likely to produce a nightmare in response to stress than are non-HSPs. They also found that HSPs have a larger correlation between stress and trait nightmare distress, and so HSPs are more likely to be distressed by nightmares than are non-HSPs.

Treatments for nightmares

The main recognised treatment for nightmares is imagery rehearsal therapy (IRT), in which an individual imagines, or rehearses, across several days a recent nightmare but with part of the plot changed in any way they wish. They start the procedure again if there is a new nightmare. This has been found to reduce the number of nightmares (Neidhardt et al., 1992). However, even just writing down nightmares for a month can also decrease the occurrence of nightmares, as can relaxation and sleep hygiene advice, and so the relative benefit of IRT is a matter of debate (Gieselmann et al., 2019). Notably, though, the effects of IRT can be boosted by an associated sound stimulation during REM sleep (Schwartz et al., 2022).

Another option for treatment is lucid dreaming, which has the aim of increased feelings of mastery, both in the dream and when awake, so as to cause decreased fear of sleep and dreams, and to decrease nightmare frequency. However, there has been a concern that if people do not succeed in the training there is the possibility that this could make the nightmare disorder worse. Furthermore, the training method, such as requiring the person to wake up early and then later on go back to bed, might interfere with the person's normal sleep, and so the type of training needs to be considered so that sleep is not disrupted.

Holzinger et al. (2015) recruited participants who were having at least two nightmares per month, and were randomly assigned into a Gestalt therapy group and a Gestalt therapy and lucid dreaming training group. Over a period of 9 weeks, 75% of participants in the Gestalt therapy and lucid dream training group succeeded in having a lucid dream. However, although both groups had a significant decrease in nightmares, the groups did not differ in this. Interestingly, whereas Spoormaker and van den Bout (2006) also showed that training in lucid dreaming led to a significant decrease in nightmare frequency, lucid dreaming did not need to be achieved to obtain this effect. Research findings in this area are reviewed by Macêdo and colleagues (2019), who show inconsistencies between different studies, and a lack of clarity over the mechanisms by which lucidity training decreases nightmare frequency, in that the training may boost confidence and decrease fearfulness of sleep even if lucidity is not achieved.

Summary

Adverse life circumstances or mental health conditions such as anxiety are associated with having nightmares. Some people appear to be more predisposed to having nightmares as a reaction to waking life stresses. It is unclear whether nightmares occur due to a failure of some dream function, or are just reflective of current waking life experiences, or are part of the range of dreams that most people can have even under benign wake-life circumstances. IRT is a widely used treatment for nightmare disorder. The evidence for the efficacy of lucid dreaming, or of lucid dreaming training, for nightmare reduction is inconclusive.

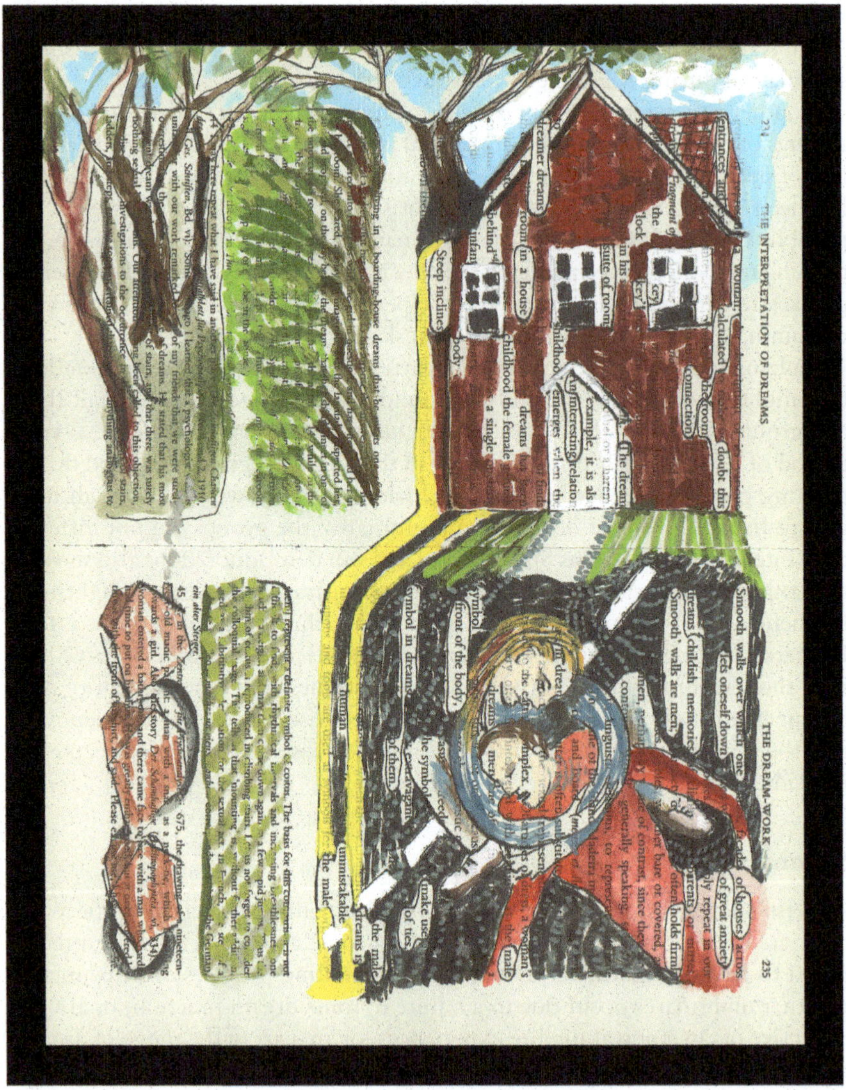

Figure 4.1 Dream of cradling my dying brother by the side of a road, 2019.

4 Sleep

This is a dream of BBC Science Correspondent Marnie Chesterton, told to us when making a programme at the Swansea University Sleep Laboratory.

DREAM NARRATIVE: *I am at my parents' large, reddish, Victorian house, our family home, which is at the edge of a village. It is a Spring afternoon, with a blue sky. My second youngest brother, aged about 17, is walking up the narrow lane by the house. It is a twisting, turning lane, which cars often whizz along. The lane has green trees and fields on both sides, and steep, brown, earth banks, 12–15 feet high, like a gully, so there is nowhere to escape. I have a sense that he has been hit by a car. I leave the house, run down the side steps, and run down the lane to find him. I see him, dead, covered in blood, with limbs at odd, irregular angles. Blood is on the tarmac. I hug him.*

DISCUSSION: The dreamer's brother is very much alive in waking life. The dreamer told us of her closeness to her brother, and that she would show him the painting and tell him about the dream.

JULIA: (Painting shown as Figure 4.1) I chose the pages because they had a white, negative space between the paragraphs when I turned the pages on their side. I used this to form the twisting, narrow lane, described as a gully, beside the house. I used the top paragraph to form the house, and highlighted in it Freud's words *in a house.*

As a visual colour device, I created double yellow lines dividing the page and demarcating the road. They also lead the eye to the enfolded figures of the dreamer and her brother. The brother is painted a distinctive red to symbolise blood, but this also acts as a device to draw the eye from the yellow road markings.

Under the dreamer's head, as she holds her brother, there are the words *front of the body.* In the body of the brother are the words *holds firmly.* And in the brother's arm, the word *male.*

The village is shown at the bottom of the road as a set of small houses and the fields are green to counterbalance the directional perspectival colours. Overall, the composition is formed in the shape of a cross.

DOI: 10.4324/9781003037552-4

Measuring sleep

For much of human history, sleep has been thought of as a lack of wakefulness. The Ancient Greeks saw sleep as like a temporary death, due to the body being motionless and unconscious, with a drop in body temperature that slows blood circulation in the brain, but with sleep also being related to health (Askitopoulou, 2015). For Aristotle, sleep occurs as a consequence of digestion causing exhalations to rise inside the body, and which take blood and vital heat from the brain as they cool and fall back down towards the heart. Without blood and vital heat in the upper parts of the body, the sense organs cease to function properly and the person falls asleep (Gregoric & Fink, 2022). This passive view of sleep was countered in the 19th century with the invention of the electroencephalograph (EEG), which showed the brain to be very active during sleep.

The basis of the EEG is that when two electrodes are placed on the head and their electrical outputs are compared, a brainwave is seen. In the 1920s the alpha wave was discovered, which has a rhythm of 8–12 Hertz (Hz). About 8–12 Hz means that in one second 8–12 waves occur, shown as 8–12 wave peaks on a centimetre of the moving EEG record. Different types of brainwaves were then discovered. These brainwaves are very recognisable to an expert reader of the EEG.

The electrical difference between two electrodes on the scalp is very small, thus EEG equipment has to amplify what is about 200 microvolts on the scalp so that it is seen onscreen, or, for much of the 20th century, sufficient to move an ink pen on a long stream of paper. Important are two electrodes on the left and right sides of the forehead, termed F3 and F4, and two central ones on either side of the top of the head, termed C3 and C4. The placement of these and other electrodes is shown in Diagram 4.1, and has to be measured very accurately, either with a tape measure or with a fabric cap with spaces on to mark where the electrodes go. Researchers are also interested in electrodes on the bone at the back of the ears, termed M1 and M2, so that we can compare each electrode on the scalp with the less active placement at the back of the opposite ear. In addition to electrodes across the scalp, there are electrooculography (EOG) electrodes to measure eye movements. One is placed at the upper right side of the right eye, and one at the lower left side of the left eye. These do not measure the actual movement of the muscles around the eye or the movement of the eye itself, but instead measure electromagnetic changes as the eye moves, which are caused by fluctuations in the cornea-retinal potential. This is the electrical potential difference between the cornea at the front of the eye and the retina at the back: as the eye moves, the electromagnetic change is picked up by the electrodes next to the eyes. The EOG signals are tested during wiring up at the start of the night by having the person look left and right rapidly before falling asleep.

There are also two or three electrodes positioned under the chin, for the electromyograph (EMG), which detects muscle tone. The muscle tone

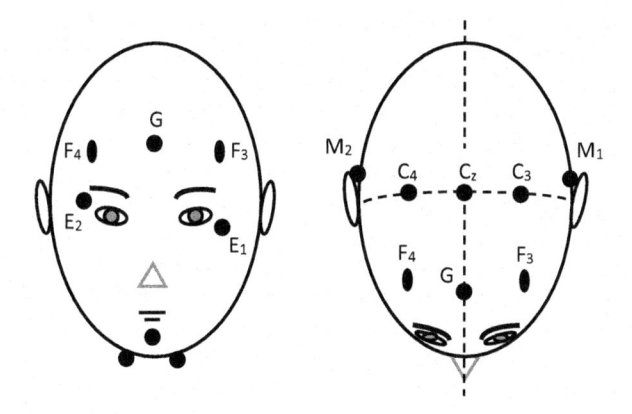

Diagram 4.1 Placement of electrodes on the head to measure sleep.

detected when the person is awake starts to diminish during sleep and then disappears almost entirely during REM sleep, when the only muscles remaining with normal levels of tone are the muscles of the eyes, heart and lungs. When we wire somebody up in the sleep lab we check the EMG by asking the person to grit their teeth, which increases their muscle tone; the trace of the EMG becomes very broad and fuzzy as a result of this.

A manual agreed upon by sleep researchers worldwide (Iber et al., 2007), published for the American Academy of Sleep Medicine, gives requirements and recommendations for the placement of electrodes and also for scoring sleep stages on the basis of EEG, EOG and EMG recordings. It is an updated and expanded version of the rules for scoring sleep stages that were published in 1968 by Allan Rechtschaffen and Anthony Kales.

Wakefulness is scored if EEG waves are small, that is, have low amplitude, and have very high frequency, that is, there are many wave peaks within each second of the onscreen record. This high frequency means that it is difficult to make out individual waves much of the time. Alpha waves then occur periodically as the person is becoming relaxed, each alpha wave lasts about one second. For most people, these disappear as they go into a light sleep. As people start to fall asleep their eyes may start to roll back and forth, these rolling eye movements are picked up by the EOG.

Non-rapid eye movement sleep

Within non-Rapid Eye Movement (NREM) sleep there are three sleep stages. The first stage of NREM sleep is termed N1 (N refers to non-Rapid Eye Movement sleep), which has a mixture of theta waves (3–8 Hz), and also the alpha (8–13Hz) and beta waves (above 12Hz) that are also

40 *Sleep*

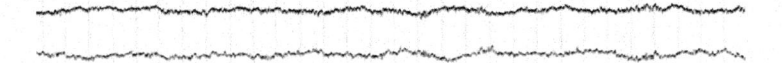

When a person is awake brain waves can be quite indistinct, it can be difficult to see individual waves. Here are traces from F3 and F4 soon after the person has laid down in the sleep lab.

As the person falls asleep, brain waves start to become more distinct. The waves have more amplitude and their wavelength increases, which means that their frequency decreases: it is as if the waking brain waves have been stretched out. Here the person has entered the first stage of non-REM sleep, termed N1.

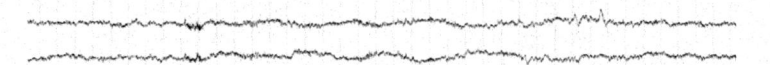

As the person falls asleep and goes into N1, the eyes can start to roll. The following is the record of the electrooculograph.

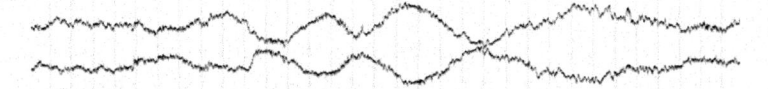

The eyes become still as the person goes into the next sleep stage, N2. Here the brain waves continue to become lower frequency, that is, longer wavelength, looking more stretched out. N2 is classed as starting when a K-complex or sleep spindle is seen.

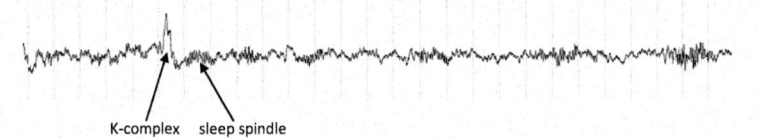

K-complex   sleep spindle

Next the person enters N3, otherwise called slow wave sleep, which has large slow waves, otherwise called delta waves.

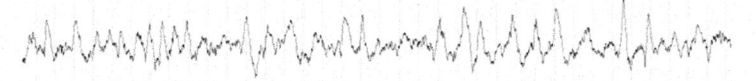

When the person enters Rapid Eye Movement sleep the brain waves look like a mixture of wake and N1.

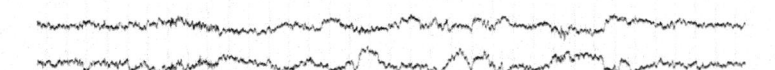

The eyes are still for some of REM sleep, but then have a series of sudden movements. In the following electrooculograph trace, the eyes are still for 4 seconds, and then start moving rapidly.

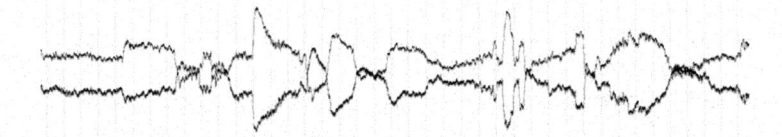

Diagram 4.2 Brain waves and eye movement traces found in wake and sleep stages.

seen in wake. The eyes roll slowly as sleep is entered but are then still. See Diagram 4.2 for the different brain waves and eye movement traces in wake, N1 and the other sleep stages.

N2 is the next stage of light sleep, marked by the presence of the theta waves seen in N1 but also by two types of sporadic events, sleep spindles and K-complexes. Spindles are bursts of 11–16 Hz activity, usually lasting between 0.5 and 2 seconds. Spindles were named because of their similarity to the shape of the spindle device for spinning wool. They are related to communications between the cortex and the thalamus, a sub-cortical area that is a relay for many incoming stimuli, and may inhibit incoming stimuli so that sleep is not disturbed. Spindles also have relationships to intelligence and memory consolidation during sleep (Fernandez & Lüthi, 2020).

K-complexes are very distinctive, with the wave going sharply positive and then negative, seen as a sudden up and then down movement on the EEG screen, and lasting at least half a second. K-complexes and sleep spindles occur spontaneously in N2 sleep, but are also seen in N2 if there is a noise in the sleep lab. This poses the question of whether they are a sign of arousal, or are they part of a neural process that is counteracting arousal with the aim of maintaining sleep. The latter seems to be true for K-complexes: when they occur they are followed by an increase in activity in the delta frequency band (showing deeper sleep) in good sleepers and individuals with insomnia (Forget et al., 2011). Also, K-complexes are less evident in people with sleep disorders such as sleep apnoea, where the sufferer repeatedly stops breathing while asleep, and narcolepsy, where the sufferer falls asleep frequently when they are awake and can sometimes go straight into REM sleep (Wauquier et al., 1995). If they were a sign of arousal they would be expected to be more frequent in these conditions in comparison to good sleepers.

N3, also termed deep sleep, or Slow Wave Sleep, has large, long, high amplitude waves termed delta waves. These waves are from 0.5 to 2 Hz, and so one whole wave from peak to peak could last two seconds. N3 is scored when at least 20% of a 30-second EEG epoch has slow waves. One of the biological effects of N3 is toxic metabolite clearance in the adult brain (Xie et al., 2013). These metabolites are proteins linked to neurodegenerative diseases. In tissues elsewhere in the body, but not in the brain, there are lymph vessels that remove excess proteins from the space between cells for degradation in the liver. Yet despite its high metabolic rate and the fragility of neurons in the brain to toxic waste products, the brain lacks a conventional lymphatic system. Instead, cerebrospinal fluid circulates in the brain and can remove proteins from the space between cells. During sleep that space, termed the interstitial space, increases by 60% compared to when awake, allowing the removal of the toxins.

Rapid eye movement sleep

Aserinsky and Kleitman in 1953 had been investigating the rolling eye movements present at the start of sleep and by accident found that during the night there were periods of rapid eye movements, which occurred periodically every 90 minutes. Oddly the brainwaves looked like the person was awake, but they were fast asleep, and this led to the term 'paradoxical sleep' to describe what is now called REM sleep. Although the brain waves in REM sleep have similarities to those present in wakefulness, including beta waves, they also include theta waves, and saw-tooth waves, which look like the teeth of a saw. While the REM sleep period continues, with this EEG activity, the eyes are sometimes still, and then have rapid bursts that can last up to a few seconds (See Diagram 4.2 for REM EEG and EOG traces.) Unlike in NREM sleep, breathing and heart rate can be irregular.

It is possible to see a person's eyes moving under their eyelids during REM sleep if you watch them, and there are some disturbing online videos where the eyelids of a sleeping person are rolled back and the eye can be seen moving backwards and forwards. These days people know to look for this, but in 1892 Ladd published a paper in the psychology and philosophy journal *Mind*, reporting that it is possible to see a person's eyes moving during sleep, and he proposed that sleepers may be watching their dream occurring. We now know that the rapid eye movements are physiologically based and are unrelated to dream content (with the exception of deliberate eye movements in lucid dreams, which we will address in Chapter 7). The interesting thing about Ladd's discovery was that it took another 60 years for the presence of rapid eye movements in sleep to become widely recognised, following the work of Aserinsky and Kleitman (1953).

Whereas the brain is very active in REM sleep, as can be seen on the EEG as well as on brain imaging, muscle tone disappears, having been decreasing in sleep from N1 to N3. Sleep talking and sleepwalking thus occur in NREM sleep, where some muscle tone remains. An exception to this lack of movement and lack of vocalisation in REM sleep is REM sleep behaviour disorder (RBD: Roguski et al., 2020), in which the usual muscle atonia of REM sleep no longer occurs and the sleeping person can act out motor actions, sometimes complex motor actions, and, in some cases, can possibly be acting out a dream. In some instances, aggressive actions can occur and may result in injury to others. After such acts courts of law may be required to decide whether the action was deliberate or involuntary. A further issue with RBD is that the neural changes involved in this sleep disorder can, in some cases, lead to Parkinson's disease (Tekriwal et al., 2017).

The stages of sleep, N1, N2, N3 and REM, as outlined above, occur in a cyclical manner across the night. This can be seen on a hypnogram, as shown in Diagram 4.3. The alternation between NREM sleep and REM sleep is called a sleep cycle. Most of the N3 occurs in the first half of the night

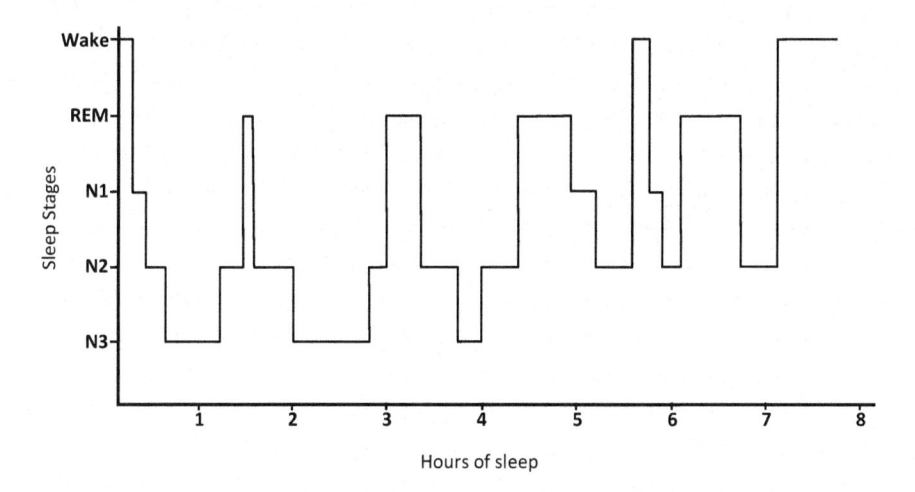

Diagram 4.3 Hypnogram showing the stages of sleep across the night.

whereas most REM occurs in the second half. The first REM period occurs 60–90 minutes after sleep onset, lasting 5–10 minutes, and REM periods get longer during the night, with the last REM period lasting up to 40 minutes. In humans there are four or five REM periods per night, and REM sleep accounts for about 20% of total sleep time in adults. N2 sleep occupies about 45–55% of total sleep time in adults. N3 occupies about 20% of sleep time, but this amount decreases with age.

There is a caution that if sleep is assessed in the lab rather than at home, there can be a 'first night effect'. This means that due to being in a new environment there is less REM sleep, more awakenings and a longer time to fall asleep than usual. So in studies of the physiology of sleep the first night's data are usually discarded as not representative of the person's usual sleep. The night is thus treated as an adaptation night. If the main aim, though, is to collect dreams, the first night effect does not really matter as dreams will still occur, even though the REM sleep is a little more fragile on that first night. There is a small effect on the dream content of being in the lab, however, as noted in Chapter 1.

All animal species have a drive for sleep which gets stronger the longer that the animal remains awake. Lack of sleep can be lethal for all species and there can be an intrusion of sleep into wakefulness (microsleeps) if sleep is deprived, as well as behavioural and cognitive impairment. When sleep is deprived, there is a partial catch-up of the lost sleep when sleep is finally allowed. And so sleep is absolutely necessary for all animals (Cirelli & Tononi, 2008).

Summary

Although humans and other animals may be very still during sleep, the brain is active and sleep is complex, comprising stages that are electrophysiologically and physiologically very different from each other. Aside from the biological function of neurotoxin clearance mentioned above, and other biological functions such as neurotransmitter resetting during sleep, there may also be memory processing that takes advantage of the sleep, or 'off-line', state. We now turn to this in the next chapter.

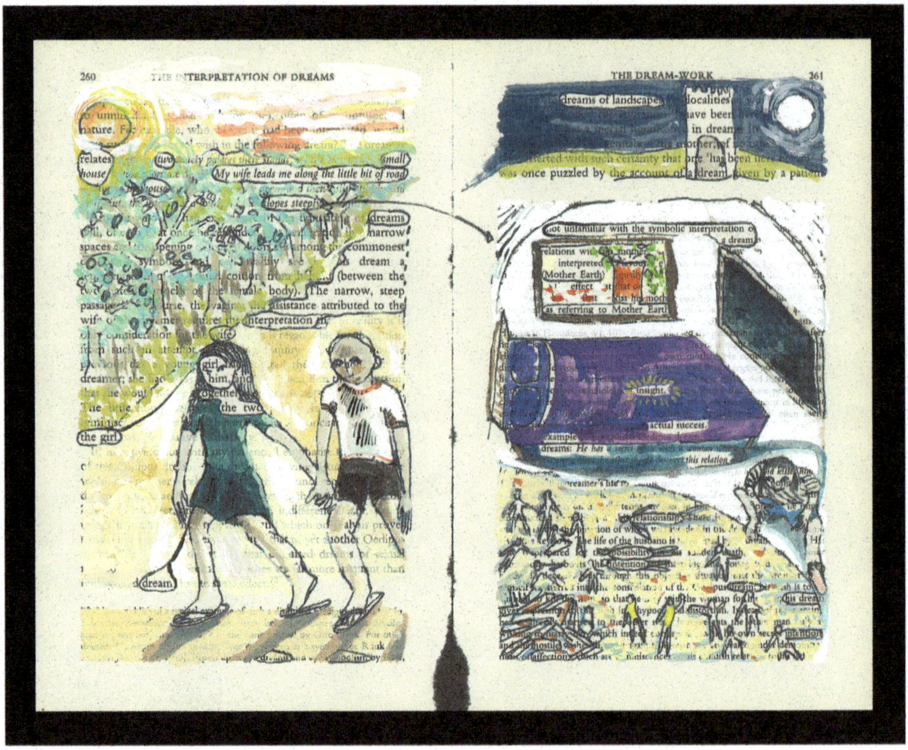

Figure 5.1 Dream of new life by a beach, 2020.

5 Sleep and memory

This is a dream of Tom, a recently qualified doctor, which combines images of a future responsible life with a memory from his previous time as a more care-free medical student. The dream was told to us and an audience as part of our Lockdown Dreams online performances in 2020.

DREAM NARRATIVE: *I am walking with my partner through a forest of low olive trees, which leads to a sunny and sandy beach. There are white cliffs at the edge of the beach, and on top of the cliffs is a castle, round, like a chess piece. We are looking for a place to live and are told by a man on the beach that on the cliffs there is a comfortable cave we could live in. We go there and it has a TV, purple bedding on the double bed, and paintings on the wall. We live in this lovely environment, and with a young boy, who in the dream is my son. But the beach starts to become full of holidaymakers, with some of them sunbathing, and others drinking and leaving rubbish. Security guards in yellow high-visibility jackets arrive, and the beach loses all the charm it had when we were there alone.*

DISCUSSION: Tom told us this dream in May 2020 during the first Covid-19 Lockdown. He had graduated early so as to care for Covid-19 patients. The dream has a theme of becoming more responsible, just as he had had to take on new responsibilities in waking life. In waking life he has no children, but in the dream he has a son. We realised during the discussion that the cave in the dream is based on a pub that is built into a cliff in his university town and which he would visit when he was a student.

JULIA: (Painting shown as Figure 5.1) I wanted to show a journey on one page and height on the other, so I chose two pages so as to have one with a large paragraph above a small paragraph, and one with a small paragraph above a large one. And so paragraphs of the same size were at opposing ends of each page. This allowed a mirroring effect of day/night, earth/sky, beach/sea, low/high, outside/inside. The following words are incorporated as a found poem into the area around the depiction of the couple walking together:

the girl, wife
girl had
him, and
together
the two
dream

DOI: 10.4324/9781003037552-5

The beneficial effect of sleep on memory

For many years, experiments have been conducted to investigate whether and how sleep aids learning. These have involved declarative learning, which is knowledge of information, such as lists of words, or arrays of photographs, or events on a film, and procedural learning, which refers to skills, such as a set of physical actions.

In 1924, Jenkins and Dallenbach found that if people learnt a series of nonsense syllables, there was better recall of the syllables after a period of sleep than after an equal period of wakefulness. This is known as the sleep effect. They also found, by testing memory 1, 2, 4 or 8 hours after learning, that, for much of a period of sleep, if the person is woken for recall, memory performance stays constant, whereas across the day memory slowly declines. At that time the behaviourist explanation for this effect was favoured; this held that, if one is asleep, what was learned before sleep is not interfered with by taking in new information from the outside world. The sleep effect is now known to be extremely robust, occurring for word lists, sets of photographs, stories, and motor and perceptual skills. There are three possible explanations for this effect:

– there is less forgetting because no new experiences or external stimuli are occurring during sleep; or
– metabolism is slower during sleep and therefore there is less forgetting; or
– there is some active process occurring during sleep, which acts on the memories in some way to consolidate them and make them more permanent.

Note that these explanations might all be true. For example, it may be that the lower metabolism and lower interference during sleep aid the active consolidation process, as they ensure that new memories remain temporarily strong enough for the active consolidation processes to occur.

Comparing sleep stages and wake for memory consolidation

Many sleep labs around the world investigate the sleep effect by using the 12/12 method. In this, one group of participants learn materials or a skill at 22.00 and are then tested at 10.00 the next day, having had a whole night of sleep, and another group learns at 10.00 and is then tested at 22.00 the same day. This method thus compares recall after a 12-hour period that includes sleep, with recall after a 12-hour period of wakefulness.

This design was used in a study of learning a finger-tapping task. Matt Walker and colleagues (2003) asked participants to repeatedly type 41324 41324 41324 on a keyboard for 30 seconds, followed by a 30-second break, then 30 seconds of typing, then 30 seconds break, this continuing for

10 minutes. The breaks occur so that the person is not fatigued when they are being trained. For each block of 30 seconds typing, the person gets faster and faster and makes fewer and fewer errors. If a break occurs, then performance does not improve across the break. Some participants were given a 12-hour break across a day, during which they remained awake, and no improvement occurred. However, if the break is for 12 hours overnight and includes sleep, improvement occurs even though there has been no practice in that time. A variation on this method is to have learning and testing during the day, but with one group having a nap between learning and testing, and a comparison group not having a nap: the sleep effect is seen here as well (Nishida & Walker, 2007).

A further variation on this method is to have learning before going to sleep at night with testing in the middle of the night, in comparison to a group which is woken in the middle of the night, who learn the material then, and are then tested in the morning. The length of the two time periods is the same, 3 hours for each, what differs is that the early half of sleep is slow-wave sleep (SWS) rich and the later part of sleep is REM sleep rich. This design compares the effects of those two different sleep stages on learning. It was first used by Ekstrand's team, who in 1971 showed that for learning pairs of words (a form of declarative learning), such as apple-beach, recall is better across early sleep than across late sleep (Yaroush et al., 1971). This led them to the conclusion that SWS seems to aid declarative memory. Gais and Born (2004) suggested that during SWS, low levels of the neurotransmitter acetylcholine enable this memory processing, whereas levels are high during wakefulness so as to enable the taking in ('encoding') of new learning.

The effect of sleep on procedural learning has been investigated with various skilled tasks, including the finger-tapping task mentioned earlier, and mirror tracing. Mirror tracing has been used in psychology for over 100 years: a person's hand holds a pencil above a piece of paper and has to trace around a shape, such as a star or track. But their hand is hidden by a screen and so the person has to look into a mirror so as to trace around the shape. This task is very difficult to do because, of course, the mirror reverses one's field of vision. Participants get better and better over time during training, but also do better if re-tested after a period of late sleep, in comparison to early sleep (Plihal & Born, 1997; Wagner & Born, 2008). It thus seems to be REM sleep that improves procedural memory.

Another procedural or skilled memory task is visual discrimination. In one version of this, a group of three forward slashes is hidden in a page of hyphens and must be found. The three slashes are either in a vertical or a horizontal line, and individuals have to respond to say there is a horizontal or a vertical group of slashes; this is repeated many times, with the slashes horizontal or vertical at random. Being able to find the group of slashes hidden in the array of hyphens is difficult, but the skill of spotting them improves with practice. Stickgold and colleagues (2001a) show that improvement in this visual discrimination task is correlated with the proportion of SWS in the first quarter of the night and the proportion of REM sleep in the last quarter of the night. This finding supports the sequential model of consolidation where SWS processing in the first half of the night is followed by REM sleep processing in the second half. This sequential model contrasts with the dual model of processing during sleep, which holds that there are different sleep stages consolidating different types of memory, as shown for the learning of pairs of words and mirror tracing, described earlier in this chapter.

Emotional memory and sleep

One form of declarative learning is memory for emotional episodes, and this is found to improve across sleep intervals with high amounts of Rapid Eye Movement (REM) sleep. In Wagner et al. (2001), participants were taught stories either at the start of the night, with testing in the middle of the night, or they learnt stories in the middle of the night and were then tested at the end of the night. Two stories that were very negative emotionally were used, as well as two that were emotionally neutral. The findings were that late, REM-rich sleep, aided memory for the emotional stories more than memory for the neutral stories. This and other studies that in general found that sleep benefited the learning of emotionally negative stories more than neutral stories led to the question of what is the effect of sleep on the learning of emotionally positive stories. This was addressed in a sleep lab study by Alex Reid and colleagues (2022).

In this study, negative, neutral and positive stories were learned by 61 healthy adults. They were tested for memory immediately, and then again after either a two-hour nap or after a two-hour period of wakefulness. The sleep group performed better than the wake group on recalling the negative and positive stories, but the groups did not differ on memory for the neutral text. Sleep thus consolidates memory for stories that are emotionally positive or negative, and this accords with the many findings that memory consolidation prioritises emotional memory.

Sleep and mood disorders

It has been known for a long time that the sleep of people with mood disorders is of poor quality and that such poor-quality sleep can last many years. Much research has addressed causes and cures for poor sleep arising from poor mood, such as, for example, the anxious rumination that can cause insomnia. However, Walker and Van der Helm (2009) brought forward a novel approach to the link between poor mood and poor sleep. Given the role that sleep has in processing our emotional memories, they suggested that mood disorders may be at least partly a result of poor sleep. This is now widely accepted. One of the implications now seen is that poor sleep, such as, for example, due to sleep apnoea, can be a predisposing factor for Post-Traumatic Stress Disorder for people who have a trauma (Krakow et al., 2002; Miller et al., 2020). In sleep apnoea the person stops breathing repeatedly in the night, often as much as 30 or 40 times per hour; this disruption of sleep had for many years been known to have an effect on memory processing as well as on alertness during the day, but seems also to have an effect on the processing of emotions.

Sleep, memory and motivation

For Stickgold and Walker (2013) there is 'memory triage', an evolution of memory items across time and selective processing such that the more important memories are processed during sleep. They point out that sleep-dependent memory consolidation is greater if participants are told that they will be tested on what they have learned, and sleep can selectively retain and consolidate memories if the person is told there will be a monetary reward at testing the next day, or if the person is told after learning different word lists that one list is the important one. Triage here means that some memories are given priority over others, a term taken from prioritisation in emergency medicine. This triage ensures that it is useful new knowledge that is consolidated.

In 2017 in Swansea, we did a study, led by Elaine van Rijn, in which we measured people's natural valuing of stimuli to see if that was related to memory consolidation (van Rijn et al., 2017). We studied 80 university students who were native English speakers and had recently arrived to study in Wales, and having no knowledge of the Welsh language. The participants learned Welsh translations of English words and were tested immediately afterwards by being given some of the Welsh words and being asked to respond with the corresponding English word. They were then tested again 12 hours later, using the 12/12 method described above. We found that recall was better across 12 hours that contained a full night of sleep compared to 12 daytime hours comprising wakefulness with no sleep. We had also asked participants to rate how much they value the Welsh language. We found that the higher the participants in the sleep group valued the Welsh language, the better was their memory recall across the period of sleep (measured as memory recall after sleep minus baseline memory recall before sleep), but this was not found for the wake group. For the sleep group, the level at which an individual valued the Welsh language was not related to their memory score on immediate (before sleep) or delayed (after sleep) recall, but only to the change in recall across sleep. We concluded, as did previous studies, that the amount that stimuli are valued affects their memory consolidation during sleep.

Theories of the mechanism of memory consolidation during sleep

Stickgold and Walker (2007) addressed the relationship of sleep to the three different components of learning and memory: acquisition, which almost always occurs when one is awake; stabilisation, whereby memories are made more stable, and so less likely to decay or to be interfered with by new learning; and enhancement, whereby stable memories are interconnected with each other and with older memories. As reviewed in the previous section, processes in sleep may be selective for certain memories. Indeed, sleep may preferentially bolster new memories that are incongruent, rather than congruent to current knowledge (Ashton et at., 2022). The interconnection of memories is a creative process that Stickgold and Walker (2007) and others link to REM sleep, because the high excitation, plasticity, and connectivity between brain areas that occurs in REM sleep would provide an ideal setting for forming novel, unexpected, and creative connections between memories (Lewis et al., 2018). Part of the evidence for this is from Walker and colleagues (2002), who found that there was better performance at solving anagrams when one was woken from REM sleep than when woken from non-Rapid Eye Movement (NREM) sleep. They thus proposed that cognitive flexibility is a characteristic of REM sleep, and that this may explain why sleeping on a problem sometimes results in sudden insight (Wagner et al., 2004).

However, the role of REM sleep has been de-emphasised in favour of SWS in a model put forward by Diekelmann and Born (2010). They suggest that there is a slow transfer of memories during sleep from the hippocampus to the cortex, aided by the replay of memories. While this transfer is going on there is also generalisation of the new memories, so that what is stored is not an exact copy of what occurred, but generalisation across experiences. Slowly the memory is lost from the hippocampus and is later stored only in the cortex. Importantly, this transfer of where memory is stored takes place off-line, in other words, during sleep. This is because during sleep no new encoding of stimuli from the outside world is occurring; one is shut off from the outside world and able to undertake this consolidation process without the interference of new experiences coming in. This transfer process is called system consolidation. However, Diekelmann and Born (2010) suggest that this occurs only during SWS. Their view of REM sleep is principally one in which the synapses in the cortex are changing to make the memories more robust. This is termed synaptic consolidation, and occurs at the current location of the memory. Diekelmann and Born are thus not supportive of the idea that REM sleep interconnects memories, rather they propose that this is done by SWS. This de-emphasis of the role of REM sleep in memory consolidation contrasts with Stickgold and Walker (2007), and was responded to by Walker and Stickgold (2010) as follows:

> Although the first stage of item memory consolidation might occur across a single night, or even during a single period of SWS, effective integration

of these memories probably takes several NREM–REM cycles or multiple nights before optimal representations are complete. Indeed, these memory-processing demands might be one evolutionary factor that has shaped the canonical human NREM–REM cycle, and within it, the shift from SWS to REM dominance across the night.

Memory Reactivation during sleep

There is general agreement amongst researchers that memory consolidation processes in sleep involve memories being reactivated, which enables interconnections between memories to be formed. A major advance in the field has been the discovery that such reactivations can also be induced experimentally, while the person is asleep, and this has been shown to have a beneficial effect on memory. This is done by presenting an incidental stimulus during learning, for example an odour, such as of roses. Then, during sleep, that odour is presented again. This is termed Targeted Memory Reactivation (TMR). So as to act as control conditions, some participants will not have an odour presented during learning, and for others, it is presented when learning but not presented during sleep. TMR was used by Rasch and colleagues (2007), who presented participants with an odour while they were learning card locations on a screen. Normally, for this task, performance across a period of sleep is better than across a period of wake. The experimenters found, however, that if the odour was presented again during SWS there was a significantly better performance in the morning than if the person slept without the odour being presented, or had the odour presented again during REM sleep. As a further control condition, the odour was also presented at re-testing in the morning when the person was awake; in this case, the odour was found to have no effect. This therefore seems to be a very specific effect of memory reactivation occurring during SWS.

There have been other variations of this design, including presenting puzzles before sleep with an accompanying sound. Performance on the puzzle task after sleep was better if the sound is played again during sleep versus not being played again (Sanders et al., 2019). These results show that we can boost creative problem-solving in sleep, and that ordinary sleep may be aiding creativity. In the first meta-analysis of the TMR field, Hu et al. (2020) brought together the results from 91 TMR experiments and showed that TMR is highly effective in NREM stages N2 and N3, but is not effective during REM sleep nor during wakefulness. They also showed that TMR is effective for declarative memory learning and for skill acquisition.

Neural replay during sleep

In the above research, it is hypothesised that reactivation of memories can occur during the night, and that we can experimentally increase that reactivation. Such reactivation of memories, in other words, their replay, has been shown directly in experiments on rats. Wilson and McNaughton (1994) monitored place cells in the hippocampus of rats. These cells fire when the rat is in a specific place. Wilson and McNaughton found that if a rat learned a maze, such that a series of place cells fire in sequence as the rat goes through the maze, then the place cells fire again in the same order during SWS. This has been termed neural replay, and it was found to occur at 6–20 times the speed at which the sequence was occurring when they were actually walking around the maze. The effect has been found in SWS by many studies (Gillespie et al., 2021). There have been reports of neural replay in REM sleep (Louie & Wilson, 2001), but although it is tempting to link this work on neural replay to the experiences of imagination and dreaming, those REM sleep findings are rarer than for SWS.

Sleep and the abstraction of schemas and gist from similar experiences

The replay of memories during sleep might also be more complex than just replaying a particular sequence. Replay has been proposed as a basis for the making of generalisations (Stickgold & Walker, 2013), which was mentioned above. It has also been proposed as the basis for the learning of complex sequences of events and choices across time and years, known as schemas, as put forward by Lewis and Durrant (2011) as one of the functions of sleep. The example they give of a schema is that of children's birthday parties, with arrivals, introductions, games, seating for food, a cake, candles and presents. They propose that sleep generalises from all our instances of children's birthday parties, or for other schemas, such as restaurant visits, to arrive at the abstracted prototype of the complex experience. They propose that replays of many memories during sleep results in the overlaps between events being learned. This repeated reactivation of overlapping memories in different combinations progressively builds schematic representations of the relationships between the components of these experiences.

So what we get from sleep is the gist of a large number of similar experiences, such as children's birthday parties, so that one might forget particular parties but still have the overall generalisation. Forming and storing such generalisations is adaptive, but can lead to problems, because emphasising the gist of several similar occurrences can produce false memories. In psychological experiments, a well-known method to investigate gist memory is the Deese-Roediger-McDermott (DRM) paradigm (Roediger & McDermott, 1995). In this, people are presented with lists of words. In each list, the words are all related to each other (e.g., ripe, citrus, cocktail, banana, bowl, cherry), and all are related to a particular major word (here, fruit), but that word is not on the list. That missing major word is called a lure. Participants are asked later to recall the words on each list. What is found is that people tend to recall the lure word as having been on the list. Some researchers have found that if participants sleep between learning and recall, then these false memories of a lure are even more likely to be created (e.g., Payne et al., 2009). So, in consolidating the list, the usually useful generalising function of sleep results in a gist of the list being created, and a false memory of a word that actually wasn't presented.

This process of generalisation and abstraction from different experiences during sleep has been linked to our dreams by some researchers, such as Walker and Stickgold (2010), Hartmann (2011) and Hoel (2021) because dreams often mix different but similar experiences together. However, Lewis and Durrant (2011) caution that there is limited evidence for memory reactivation during REM sleep, and that it thus seems unlikely that REM could contribute to abstraction, which they say is a function of SWS. Nevertheless, Walker and Stickgold (2010) propose that REM sleep is involved in 'overnight alchemy', and that SWS consolidates new episodic item memories while keeping individual memory representations separate and distinct. They propose that REM sleep integrates these new memories with old memories into rich associative networks, mapping our past to our present, and predicting possibilities for the future. It is this second stage of memory integration, that extracts, abstracts and generalises recently consolidated item memories, that Walker and Stickgold propose might be linked to the production of dreams.

Sleep, memory and dreaming

Like sleep, dreams seem to combine or integrate memories of different experiences, they also prioritise experiences that are emotional or important or valued in waking life. Because memory consolidation and dreaming are both linked to emotional memories, there has been the proposal from many researchers that dreaming may reflect or even have a role in memory consolidation during sleep (e.g., Perogamvros & Schwartz, 2012).

Wamsley et al. (2010a) studied the cognitive replay of a task in NREM sleep dreams. Participants were trained for many hours on the 'Alpine Racer' arcade skiing game, which involves visual and movement learning, with the player standing on a pair of skis and controlling an on-screen character through the use of leg movements. It is a very engaging activity of heading down the slope and along a path. They found that 30% of all verbal reports of sleep onset dreams were related to the task: 24% of the reports had related imagery, and 6% had related thoughts. This cognitive replay became more abstract from the original experience if the person slept for longer before the dream was collected. Thus direct references to the experience occur as the participant falls asleep, but further and further into sleep the relationship of the dream content to that experience becomes less direct.

This study found that there was an effect of the task on dream content, but it did not relate the dream content to performance change across sleep. This was therefore done in a second study, Wamsley et al. (2010b), titled 'Dreaming of a learning task is associated with enhanced sleep-dependent memory consolidation.' Here, participants were trained on a virtual navigation maze task, tested, and then re-tested five hours after initial training; this five hour period comprised only wakefulness for some participants, but included a two-hour nap for other participants. The nap group had better performance at re-testing than did the wake group, and so there was a sleep-dependent memory consolidation effect occurring. In addition, and importantly, the participants who dreamt of the task also had the greatest improvement across sleep. The paper is important as it is one of the first pieces of evidence relating dream content to memory consolidation.

However, there are two problems with the study which lead to a questioning of the often-cited results. One is that there were only four people who had a dream of the task, and so this is a small sample. The second is that dreaming of the task was not only associated with a large improvement in performance across the period of sleep, but was also associated with doing poorly on the task before sleep. This leads to an alternative explanation of this set of findings. Maybe these four participants dreamt of the task not because of their memory consolidation processes during sleep, but as a result of feelings and concerns about having performed poorly on the task before sleep. Perhaps the participants felt uncomfortable about that performance, and maybe thought of how the experimenters knew of that poor performance. So, although this study is frequently cited as evidence that the contents of dreams are related to memory consolidation during the night, the results can also be interpreted in terms of the dream referring back to how the person was feeling before they went to sleep. Nevertheless, this is an extremely highly cited and important paper and is referred to in the excellent Wamsley and Stickgold (2011) review paper, titled: 'Memory, sleep and dreaming: experiencing consolidation.' That review paper explains in detail the theory that dreaming is the experience of memory consolidation. It reviews arguments for and against this theory, including that dreams seem to have a tangential and abstract rather than direct or mimetic relationship to what was learned before sleep.

Wamsley and Stickgold (2019) replicated the dreaming and virtual maze navigation study, this time with a whole night of sleep rather than a nap. They showed again that dreaming of the task is related to memory improvement across sleep. But, again, they also found that those who dreamt of the task performed worse at baseline, and so it is still possible to argue that dreams reflect our previous waking life concerns, rather than our memory consolidation processes during sleep. A similar interpretation can be made of the findings of Ribeiro et al. (2020), where participants learned pairs of photographs before sleep and were tested for memory for the pairs of photographs before sleep and after sleep. The sleep group had better recall after sleep than did a control group who learned and were tested during a day, during which they remained awake. For the sleep group, those who dreamt of specific photographs had better recall for those photographs, which could be taken to mean that the dreams affected or strengthened these memories. However, as above, it may be that photos that were particularly interesting or salient to a participant were more memorable for the person, and hence better recalled the next morning, and were also incorporated into a dream due to their salience. It may thus be that the salience of the photo when learned causes incorporation into dreams, rather than that dreaming of the photo affects recall after sleep. We will return to the implications of these papers for possible functions of dreaming in Chapter 12.

Summary

Sleep helps to make recent memories more permanent and interconnects old and new memories. It also generalises our experiences so as to abstract common details from many memories. These processes occur more for emotional and important memories, and so some selection occurs between memories regarding which to consolidate during sleep. Some researchers think that dreaming is how we experience these brain processes of memory consolidation, and that dreaming might even have a role in memory consolidation during sleep.

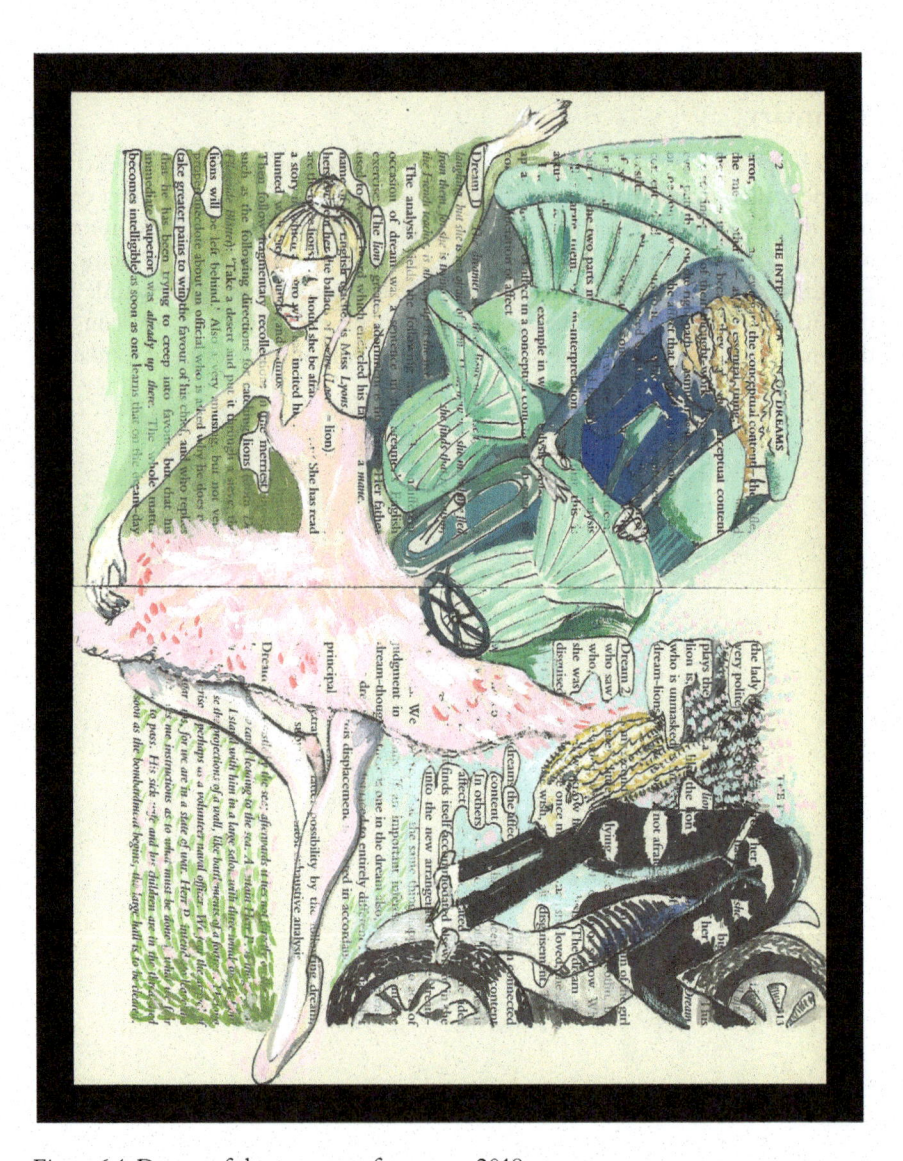

Figure 6.1 Dream of three stages of woman, 2018.

6 Dreaming and the brain

A debate in the study of how the brain creates dreams concerns why there are sudden scene changes in dreams, and addresses whether scene changes are the result of random brain stimulation or are motivated by alternative depictions or viewpoints of one background theme. This is a dream with three related but very separate scenes.

DREAM NARRATIVE: *I am in the back seat of a car, relaxed. Suddenly I am shocked to realise that no-one is driving and I have to take over the steering by reaching over from the back. I can't get to the pedals and I fear for myself and for others for what might happen, even though no one else is around outside. But I don't crash, I sense I manage the situation.*

I am next on a beautiful, large, black and chrome or gold motorcycle, like a Harley-Davidson or Triumph. I am wearing one-piece feminine black leathers, like cat woman. I am riding the bike fast, it is very large and I am astride it, leaning forward, no helmet. It feels fantastic, and not out of control. It is great, I feel a powerful woman.

I am then outside, I am a ballerina, pirouetting, beautiful, in a classical and pale pink leotard, with pale pink tights and pink ballet shoes. I do a high floating twirl, very graceful, like a musical box ballerina. I am very pleased with myself.

DISCUSSION: The dreamer, Amanda, was a confident mature student in a Gender and Culture MA course. We discussed how the three scenes depict different aspects of a strong, middle-aged woman, including controlling a dangerous situation, and of female life across the lifespan, including gracefulness and poise. The dream had sudden scene changes, but the three very different scenes produced a coherent whole.

JULIA: (Painting shown as Figure 6.1) I captured the tightly curled golden hair of the dreamer in the different scenes of the dream. However, it was not until the end stage of the performance, when I revealed the painting, that the dreamer pointed out the fortuitous incorporation of Freud's words, unnoticed by me when the pages were chosen for the particular dream. The dreamer told us that she had a nickname 'Lion' at school, because of her hair. We were all surprised and thrilled to see that the word *lion* recurs on these two pages of Freud's book. There is also

DOI: 10.4324/9781003037552-6

Miss Lyons, *dream-lion*, and *mane*. Although no doubt a chance effect, the incorporation of words, that Freud had written, into the artwork provides a personal link to Freud and to the history of the study of dreaming, and makes the artwork even more intriguing.

Dreaming and REM sleep

In 1953, the paper 'Regularly occurring periods of eye motility and concomitant phenomena during sleep' was published by Aserinsky and Kleitman. The authors started the paper by noting that slow rolling eye movements were known to occur during sleep and that they intended to study this. Instead, their major finding was of bursts of rapid jerky eye movements. It was a chance discovery that they had not expected. They realised that these eye movements were occurring in periods when the EEG had returned to being like a waking-life EEG. They found three or four of these periods in the night, and found that during these periods the heart rate and respiration rate were higher. On subsequent nights, they started to awaken people during what became known as Rapid Eye Movement (REM) sleep. Following 27 awakenings during ocular motility (the fast movement of the eyes), on 20 of these, there were reports of detailed dreams. In contrast, following 23 awakenings without ocular motility, a detailed dream was reported on only two occasions.

This research was followed in 1957 by a paper by Dement and Kleitman, who found that if the sleeper was woken from REM sleep they were far more likely to recall a dream than if woken from non-REM (NREM) sleep. Participants were studied across several nights and their ability to recall dreams did not change across the nights, so there was no learning effect for recall, but recall of a dream was more likely in REM periods in the second half of the night compared to the first half. For the vast majority of NREM awakenings, there was no recall of a dream. If, however, the person was woken up in NREM sleep but within eight minutes of REM sleep finishing, there was a greater chance of dream recall happening than there was for the rest of NREM sleep. At the time, this led to the theory that NREM dreams are the remnants of the memories of REM dreams. We now know that this is not true, that dreams do occur in all sleep stages. They also awakened people at different lengths of time into REM sleep periods and found that the longer the sleeper was in REM sleep, the longer was the reported dream, as measured by the number of words in the dream report. Furthermore, when repeatedly awoken 5 or 15 minutes into REM periods, participants were accurate in being able to categorise whether awakening occurred after 5 or 15 minutes on the basis of their estimates of dream duration. This showed that dreams progress during REM sleep at a rate comparable to a waking life experience of the same sort, and are not produced instantaneously, or with great rapidity, on waking.

Dreaming and the brain

These and other experiments that explored the association of dreaming with REM sleep led to the proposal by Hobson and McCarley in 1977 of the *activation-synthesis hypothesis* for dreaming. They proposed that there is a brainstem generator of dreaming, which is active in REM sleep. This is the pons area of the brainstem, which activates the vision-related geniculate area in the middle of the brain. When activated, the geniculate then causes rapid eye movements, and the activation of the occipital lobe (the visual area at the rear of the brain), and activates other areas of the cortex as well. Hobson and McCarley proposed that this PGO (pontine-geniculate-occipital) activation causes memories to be activated, and the brain then synthesises these chaotic memories together, resulting in a dream.

They also proposed that the bursts of PGO stimulation may cause changes of scene in dreams, and other discontinuities, such as of characters. The activation-synthesis hypothesis emphasises the link between REM sleep and dreaming, part of which also is that it is the activity in emotional areas of the brain during REM sleep that causes some intense emotions in dreams. However, on waking, the dream will often be forgotten very quickly, despite its vividness, and this Hobson and McCarley put down to differences in the physiology and neurochemistry of the brain during REM sleep compared to wake.

So, whereas for Freud, as we will see in Chapter 8, the driving force behind a dream is a wish, for Hobson and McCarley (1977) it is brainstem activation of memories during REM. And whereas for Freud there is a meaning behind the dream, which is then censored and hidden, the activation-synthesis hypothesis works the other way round: the contents of the dream start off as scrambled and are then given meaning through the process of the brain adding sense, reason, causality and plot to these disparate images.

There are other parallels between the physiology of the brain in sleep and the experience of the dream. For example, in sleep, external stimuli are blocked, and so the dream hallucination is believed to be real. This is like naturalistic explanations of *Out of Body Experiences* and *Near-Death Experiences*, which hold that the person may feel that they are floating up and looking down on their body because outside stimulation about the real environment is not being processed by the brain and so the person believes that a hallucinated imagined environment is real.

Added to this is a lack of critical awareness in dreams, so that one does not spot impossible or bizarre occurrences. This is tied by the activation-synthesis hypothesis to the deactivated dorsolateral prefrontal cortex, an area of the frontal lobe involved with critical thinking. As a result, for most dreams, we do not realise that we are in a dream, even when bizarre things happen. We also do not usually remark on discontinuities and changes of scenario in a dream, which for Hobson and McCarley (1977) are caused by the PGO stimulation. This is in contrast with Freud, for whom bizarreness can be interpreted, just as can other items in dream content, with bizarreness being part of the camouflaging aspect of the dream (Boag, 2017). For Hobson, PGO stimulation also explains his team's finding that bizarreness is twice as prevalent in dream reports than in daydreams (Williams et al., 1992).

The activation-synthesis hypothesis is based on the assumption that the physiology of REM sleep causes various psychological consequences. The emphasis on this specifically REM sleep activation differentiates Hobson and McCarley's (1977) hypothesis from the neurocognitive theory (Domhoff, 2001, 2019), which de-emphasises the role of sleep stages and their specific physiology. The neurocognitive theory instead sees dreaming as a developmental cognitive achievement that is an intensified form of daydreaming (Domhoff, 2018), supported by findings that approximately one in five daydreams are hallucinatory, and that approximately one in five daydreams feel involuntary rather than under the person's conscious control (Foulkes & Fleisher, 1975). On the neurocognitive view, dreams may thus result from the running of the default network during sleep (Fox et al., 2013). The default network is a network of connections between parts of the cortex that become active and connected when the person is very relaxed and is not undertaking tasks or focused attention, and it may be involved in daydreaming and imagination (Andrews-Hanna, 2012). Furthermore, stimulation of the default network causes an increase in divergent, or creative thinking (Shofty et al., 2022). General characteristics of dreams may thus be explainable in this way, rather than by prioritising the relationship with REM sleep.

However, testing the relationship between the brain and specific items of dream content is difficult because studies on this require an accurate measure of when in a dream an experience or action occurs. This was indeed achieved by Dresler and colleagues (2011) using lucid dreams. The authors recruited frequent lucid dreamers for a sleep lab study with brain imaging. Participants were instructed that if they had a lucid dream, they would signal this with their eyes; this method of signalling from a lucid dream is described in more detail in Chapter 7. They were instructed that once the signal was given, they would perform a particular sensory-motor action, hand clenching. The study found that there was activation in the same areas of sensorimotor cortex for these dreamt actions as there is for actual or imagined hand clenching in waking life.

Brain injury and dream recall

Mark Solms, in his 1997 book *The neuropsychology of dreams*, and summarised in Solms (2000), looked at case studies over the previous 100 years of individuals who had had brain damage, either due to accidents, disease or as a result of brain surgery. Where the case study reports mentioned dreaming, he divided them into cases where dreaming was stated as being present, versus those where it was stated as absent. He found that there were two areas of the brain where, if the brain was damaged, dream recall would cease. It is unclear whether dream cessation is a result of dreams no longer being produced, or whether they occur but are not recalled. Those processes are difficult to disentangle, but the importance of Mark Solms' work is to address the brain processes behind dreaming and/or recalling dreams.

Solms found that there is an area in the posterior part of the brain, the parieto-occipital junction, which is related to imagery, and if this site was damaged dreams were no longer reported by the person. Dream recall also ceased if there was damage to the medial frontal quadrant, an area of the frontal lobe. This area, Solms noted, is related to motivation and wishes. The process he proposed is thus that the content of dreams is produced in the frontal lobe and the information is passed to the posterior of the brain for the imagery of the dream to be produced. This mechanism has similarities to Freud's (1900/1997) proposal that wishes provide the emotional motive force to create a dream, with those cognitions and emotions feeding to imagery and visual areas of the brain. For Freud, this direction of information flow during dreams is in the opposite direction to when we are awake, as then our senses take in information and experiences and this is fed forward to memory and higher cognition areas at the front of the brain.

The major implication from Solms' (1997, 2000) work is that brainstem damage can impair REM sleep, but leave the person able to dream, whereas damage to the forebrain (the cortex and areas immediately below it) can eliminate dreaming but leave REM sleep intact. This leads to the conclusion that REM sleep and dreaming can be dissociated, contrary to the activation-synthesis hypothesis.

To extend Solms' work to take account of the severity of injury, Sam Fisher, Rodger Wood and Mark Blagrove (2004) studied some patients with traumatic brain injury, most as a result of road traffic accidents. The mean time since the injury for these patients was 49 months. They found that 30.8% of them were reporting at least one nightmare a month, which is a very high amount of nightmares and far in excess of the figure for the general adult population of 5%. Twenty-three per cent reported the occurrence of repetitive nightmares, which is again a high amount. Forty-six per cent reported dreaming at least once per month, which is similar to the general population, but 34% reported an absence of dreaming, which contrasts with the rate for non-reporting of dreams of 6.1% found by Pagel (2003).

These dream cessation results are supportive of Solms, although we did not have brain imaging data to confirm where the damage was, although much was known to be in frontal areas of the brain. We also found that the higher the patients' level of post-traumatic amnesia at the time of the accident, which is a measure of the severity of the brain damage, the lower was dream recall frequency at the time we assessed it.

Also supportive of Solms are the findings of Eichenlaub, Nicolas and colleagues (2014), reported in Chapter 2. Their results showed that participants who frequently recall dreams have a higher blood flow compared to low recallers in the temporal parietal junction during REM sleep, N3 and wakefulness, and in the medial prefrontal cortex during REM sleep and wakefulness. These two areas are similar to the ones found by Mark Solms (1997, 2000) to be supporting dreaming. Like Solms, they concluded that the prefrontal cortex area might facilitate the production of the story-like and social characteristics of dreams, including the creation of characters in the dream. Like Solms they also suggested that the temporal parietal junction has a role in mental imagery, hence creating the experience of the dream based on the information from the prefrontal cortex. They suggested that the temporal parietal junction might also be involved in the encoding of the dreams in memory, so that they are recalled when the sleeper wakes.

Dreaming in different stages of sleep

In the early days of dream research and as a result of popular understanding, dreaming was associated mainly with REM sleep. Yet as early as 1962, David Foulkes published a paper titled 'Dream reports from different stages of sleep.' He found that dream content was reported after 82% of awakenings from REM, and after 54% of awakenings from NREM sleep. Therefore, from the early view that NREM dreams might be the remembering of a REM dream, by 1962, the field had moved on considerably. Foulkes' findings showed the complexity of NREM dreams: in 50% of REM sleep dreams and 32% of NREM dreams the dreamer had an emotion; 90% of REM dreams and 66% of NREM dreams were visual; the dreamer had physical movement in 67% of REM dreams and 38% of NREM dreams; there were scene shifts in 63% of REM dreams and 33% of NREM dreams. Thus, there is complexity in NREM dreams, but on average REM dreams are more complex. Furthermore, if REM and NREM dream reports are shown to independent judges who do not know the stage of sleep they were obtained from, 10–30% of NREM dreams are indistinguishable from REM dreams (Solms, 2000). However, these generally have to be long NREM dreams and usually from later in the night, to be comparable to REM dreams.

Further comparisons and differences between REM and NREM dreams were shown by Stickgold and colleagues (2001b), who investigated the number of words in experience reports from REM sleep, NREM sleep, sleep onset, and alert and quiet wake. Individuals were cued many times across the day and night to state what had just been going through their mind. Participants gave reports with approximate median word length of 77 words in active wakefulness, 54 words in quiet wakefulness, 45 words at sleep onset and in NREM sleep, but 94 words for REM dream reports. This suggests participants are producing much more complex and longer dream reports from REM sleep than from NREM sleep and sleep onset.

They then looked at the sleep record of the person to work out how long the person was in the REM or NREM period before they woke or were awoken, and how this related to the length of a dream reported then. They found that as a REM sleep period lengthens the dream reports get longer and longer, but that after about 30 to 45 minutes of REM the reports do not get any longer, with a plateau of a median of 120 words. It is as if there is a limit to how much can be remembered of the dream. But for NREM dreams, the length of the NREM period is not related to the length of the dream. NREM dream length stays quite constant across the NREM period, at a median length of 40 words, which does suggest that NREM sleep seems to have an impoverished level of dream production. It is also possible, as proposed by Antrobus (1983), that attention and memory processes are deficient in NREM sleep, and hence many dreams produced in NREM sleep are not recalled or not recalled fully.

Fosse, Stickgold and Hobson(2004) woke participants during NREM and REM sleep and obtained dream reports. The reports were then scored by independent judges for the presence of hallucinations or images, and the presence of focused thinking, such as deliberation. The majority of REM reports across the night were classed as hallucinations or imagery, whereas NREM reports were more likely to be focused thinking in the first half of the night and more likely to be hallucinations in the second half. As the night progresses, therefore, NREM dreams become more similar to REM dreams. Fosse and colleagues concluded that hallucinations are more likely in REM than in NREM because brain areas involved in perception and attention during wake become reactivated in REM. This includes limbic, auditory and visual areas (Maquet et al., 1996; Nofzinger et al., 1997).

Why do dreams occur more often from REM sleep?

In a meta-analysis Nielsen (2000) showed that 82% of REM awakenings result in recall of a dream, versus 43% of NREM awakenings. Also, REM dreams are particularly vivid, and more likely to be a sensory experience than are NREM dreams. To explain these differences Nielsen proposed that REM sleep has many components, and he hypothesised that there are covert REM processes that operate at sleep onset and in a window 11 minutes before and after REM sleep. This is, he says, where most NREM dreams occur, and which he explained as REM sleep processes spilling over into NREM sleep.

To investigate this, Nielsen and colleagues (2005) had participants sleep in the sleep lab for three nights. The first night was to obtain baseline ratings of dreams or other mentation participants were having at sleep onset on a dream-like quality scale. This involved asking participants to answer the following question regarding any experience they were having before they were awoken: 'Apart from its length, how much like a real dream was the experience?' They would answer this dreamlike quality question on a scale from 1 = not at all, to 9 = very much. On the second night, half the participants were partially deprived of REM sleep by being woken after just 5 minutes of REM sleep in the third and subsequent REM periods. The other half of the participants had undisturbed sleep. On the third night, all the participants were awakened from sleep onset and were asked to rate any experiences they were having before being woken on the dream-like quality scale. The amount of REM sleep on the third night was slightly higher for the group who had been partially deprived of REM sleep, this is called REM rebound. Participants who had restricted REM sleep on the second night thus had a pressure for REM sleep on the following night. The important finding of the experiment was that the partial REM-deprived participants had a higher dreamlike quality for their sleep onset dream experiences, even though the sleep onset awakenings were from NREM sleep. According to Nielsen, this is because of a covert REM process that spills over into NREM sleep.

Suzuki and colleagues (2004) also addressed the hypothesised covert REM processes. They put participants on a 78-hour schedule which had repeated periods of 40 minutes awake, followed by 20 minutes nap, followed by 40 minutes awake, and 20 minutes nap. This protocol works to produce lots of naps because if a participant is allowed only 20 minutes to nap, and is then woken up, after the next 40 minutes of wakefulness the participant starts to get very sleep deprived. So people fall asleep very quickly when given the 20 minutes nap opportunity, and many naps occur, across the day and night, which can be of REM or NREM sleep, and reports of dreams occur in many of these naps. What was found was that if the participant went into a NREM nap, dreams were rarer than for a REM nap. And they were also shorter, less vivid and less pleasant.

The design of this experiment allowed the researchers to map dreaming onto the underlying biological rhythm. The main findings were that if a REM nap occurred, at any time of day or night, a dream was very likely. But the situation with NREM naps was different. If a participant had a NREM nap, dreams were more likely to occur if the nap was in the early morning, and a dream from a NREM nap was unlikely during the day or in the early part of the night. This meant that NREM naps were more likely to produce dreams if the NREM nap was occurring at a time of day when REM sleep would normally be more likely, that is, between 06:00 and 10:00. The conclusion was that this is the time of day when there would be most REM pressure, and that if a NREM nap occurred instead of a REM nap, this REM pressure would cause the NREM nap to produce a dream. As with Nielsen's covert REM theory, it appears that some REM sleep processes are intruding into NREM naps to produce a dream.

This chapter so far has addressed how sleep stages and areas of the brain are related to dreaming. But, of course, sometimes during sleep a person is dreaming, and sometimes they are not dreaming, and so the next question that arises is, how does a person's brain differ when dreams are occurring versus when they are not occurring?

Using multiple awakenings to study the neural basis of dreaming

To study the differences in a person's brain when dreams are occurring versus when they are not occurring, Francesca Siclari and colleagues (2017) used high-density electroencephalography on people who were sleeping, using 256 electrodes per participant so that very detailed information about activity in different parts of the brain was obtained. Participants were awakened many times throughout the night and were asked each time to report whether, just before awakening, they had been having a dreaming experience (termed DE), were experiencing something, but could not remember the content (termed dreaming experience without recall of content, or DWR), or not experiencing anything (termed no experience, or NE). Overall there were 240 awakenings conducted with 32 participants.

Siclari and colleagues found that brain activity in a small area at the back of the brain, which they termed the posterior 'hot zone', alters in activity between when a dream experience occurs and when no dream experience occurs, and that this was found for NREM and REM sleep. Dreaming was found to occur when brain activity in the hot zone becomes less like slow-wave sleep; so, as delta wave power decreases, the person starts to have a dream, and as delta wave power increases, there was less likelihood of a dream occurring. They also found that dream experience was associated with increased high-frequency EEG power in areas nearer the front of the brain, and having no dream experience was associated with decreased high-frequency power in that area. The high-frequency power in that frontal brain area during sleep has similarities to the EEG in wakefulness and in REM sleep.

In a further experiment, reported in the same paper, Siclari and colleagues then used the EEG outputs to predict whether a person was having a dream experience or not. Seven participants were awakened about 10 times each and the EEG outputs were used to predict the presence or absence of dreaming. Of 36 awakenings which were initiated by an algorithm that was predicting dream experience, 33 were accurate. There were also 26 instances where the algorithm was predicting that there would not be a dream experience, and of those, 21 were accurate. So the total prediction accuracy across repeated awakenings for predicting dream versus no dream was 87%.

However, Ruby (2020) reviews all of the literature using the multiple awakenings method across many authors and many experiments and shows that results have been inconsistent, with some researchers finding an association between dream recall and decreased delta wave power (e.g., Scarpelli et al., 2017), and some not doing so (e.g., Wong et al., 2020). Nevertheless, the work of Siclari and colleagues does accord with the findings of Solms and Eichenlaub on posterior and frontal areas that either produce dreams or allow them to be recalled.

Summary

We have dreams in all stages of sleep, but dreams are recalled more often from REM than from NREM sleep, and REM dreams on average are longer than NREM dreams. Researchers disagree about whether there is something special about REM sleep processes that leads to the creation of more complex dreams. But it appears that components of REM sleep might intrude into NREM sleep to produce dreams. In addition, in REM and NREM, some research shows neural mechanisms that turn dreaming on and off across the night, although there are inconsistencies in these findings.

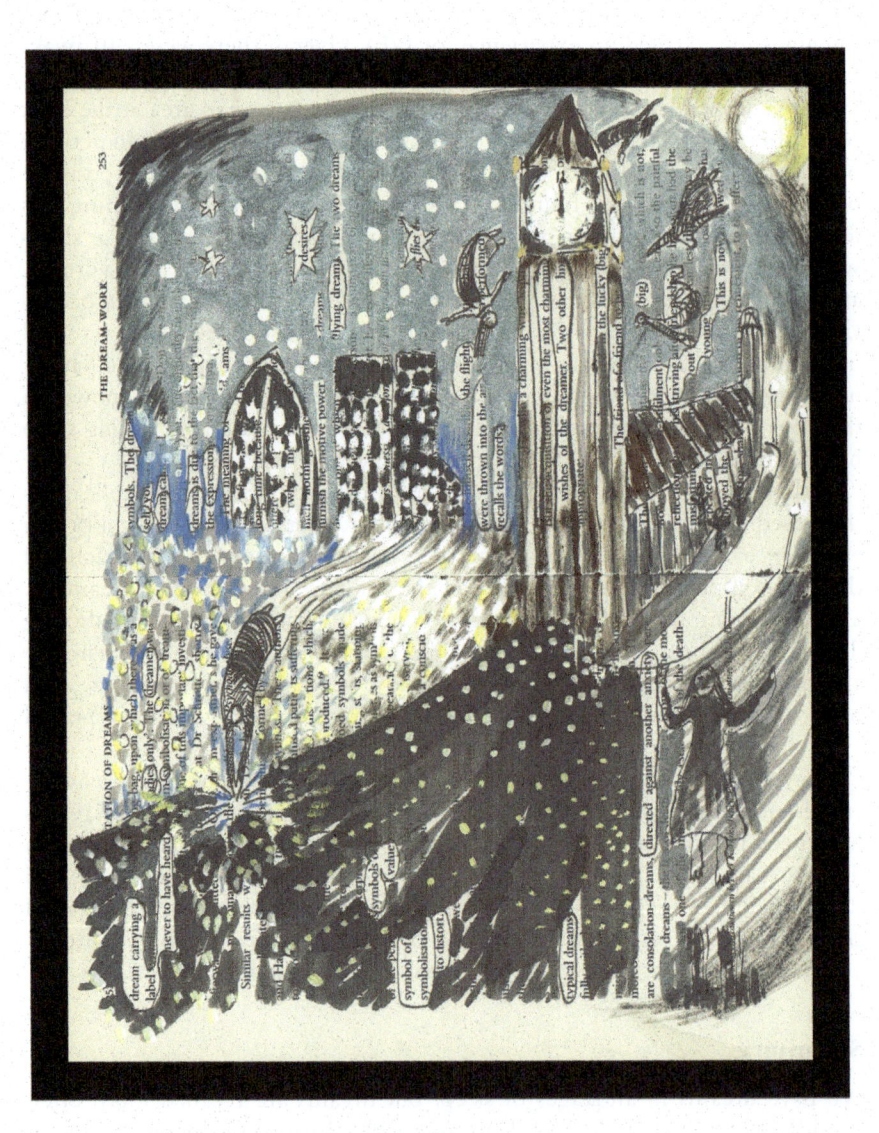

Figure 7.1 A flying dream with lucidity, 2018.

7 Lucid dreams

We were told this dream by Emi at an event at the University of California Los Angeles in October 2018. It includes themes of lucidity and control of the dream.

DREAM NARRATIVE: *It was night-time and I was in London. I was with my old high school friends, four, all girls, my closest friends, plus me. The city was really beautiful, really bright, in contrast to the blue, very dark sky. The bright lights were almost a little bit overwhelming. We were close to the Big Ben tower. We were talking about coffee, mainly the taste of it, which I don't like as it is bitter.*

Suddenly, it was like falling in a roller coaster, anti-gravity, where you feel your body lift up and feel strange. I looked around me and everyone started floating, their feet slowly coming off the ground. I then felt sort of lucid, where you can sort of control your body in your dream, and the first thing you want to do when you feel lucid is you want to fly around. I could control my movements. My friends could do the same. So everyone in the entire city, it was pretty crowded, started floating, slowly up, along with my friends. Some people were really scared and stopped, but I was thrilled with the fact that I could control everything now.

We were flying and spinning around Big Ben, like in the movie Peter Pan, the famous scene where they are flying around. It was like a picturesque version of that, swirling and doing loops with all my friends. I could look down at the whole world and city, the contrast of bright lights with the dark night sky. My vision was blurred black and yellow, with lots of noise. It was freezing cold, the wind was going really fast. I could feel how cold it was, but it was like an adrenaline rush. We kept going further out into the ocean, I could control everything.

I woke up but I didn't want the dream to end, I liked the dream so much I tried to go back to sleep and continue it. Miraculously the dream continued and I was flying again for a long time. My friends were no longer with me. I thought I have had my fun, so I flew straight down and dove into the ocean. It was completely black, and then I woke up.

DISCUSSION: The dreamer, Emi, had just finished her exams and was excited to be able to spend relaxation time with her friends. She had not been to London but had seen the film *Peter Pan* and her brother was living in London. The dream was a vivid depiction of freedom with friends.

DOI: 10.4324/9781003037552-7

JULIA: (Painting shown as Figure 7.1) Although I chose the pages because of the indented poem which I used to draw the clock tower for Big Ben, I then found the words *the flight, flies, flying dream* and *were thrown into the air,* which are all highlighted in the night sky. I drew the friends circling around the Big Ben tower, and highlighted the words *big* and *friendship* and *striving out young This is now.* The phrase *The friend of a friend* can be found on the clock tower. In a friendly but intrigued manner, an audience member asked for the numbers of the pages I had chosen because he wanted to see the original pages, and the words that happened to be on them, for himself!

Frequency and characteristics of lucid dreams

Lucid dreams are dreams in which the dreamer knows that they are dreaming. The term was first used to describe these dreams by Frederik van Eeden, a Dutch psychiatrist, in a paper in 1913, in which he reported the contents of some of his 352 lucid dreams, experienced between 1898 and 1912. He had correspondence with Freud at that time as Freud did not accept that such a cognitive ability could occur in a dream. It was indeed a prevalent scientific belief until the 1980s that lucid dreams were due to brief periods of wakefulness, with the person imagining that they are asleep and dreaming.

Keith Hearne in 1978, and Stephen LaBerge in 1981, showed that a person in REM sleep in the sleep laboratory could signal with their eyes that they had entered a lucid dream (LaBerge, 1990). This was termed the verification of lucid dreaming by volitional communication. It utilised the fact that eye muscles still work during sleep, and that moving one's eyes in a dream causes the body's eyes to also move. The signal that is now commonly used in sleep lab experiments is for the dreamer in the dream to make four left-right eye movements (LRLRLRLR), which are picked up by the EOG in the lab. In studies using this method, the sleeper is usually woken soon after the signal and a dream report is asked for. If the report is of a lucid dream and the eye movement signal also occurred, then this is termed a signal-verified lucid dream (SVLD).

Saunders and colleagues (2016) undertook a meta-analysis of studies from the period 1966 to 2016 and found that 55% of people have had at least one lucid dream (this is termed prevalence of lucid dreaming), and 23% of people are frequent lucid dreamers, that is, have one or more lucid dreams per month. The findings are consistent with earlier estimates of lucid dreaming prevalence and frequent lucid dreaming in the population. In the sleep lab, Purcell and colleagues (1986) found that 2.4% of Rapid Eye Movement (REM) dream reports are lucid, with non-Rapid Eye Movement (NREM) lucid dreams being very rare; however, the study did not use eye movements to verify these. The possibility of NREM lucid dreams was addressed by LaBerge and colleagues (1986), finding that 92% of a sample of 76 signal-verified lucid dreams were from unequivocal REM sleep.

Awareness of dreaming while dreaming is often associated with being able to control the dream and with making decisions and choices in the dream, and hence changing the plot. However, this is not a necessary characteristic of lucidity, in that a person in a lucid dream can simply watch the dream happening, rather than deliberately initiating actions in the dream or choosing the plot. Alarmingly, Schredl and Bulkeley (2020a) found that about a third of nightmares are lucid, with the dreamer aware that he or she is dreaming but being unable to change the terrifying plot of the dream, and/or being unable to deliberately wake up from it.

However, although a dreamer may be lucid about being in a dream, they might not be completely lucid about the consequences of that. In 1992, Deirdre Barrett published the paper 'Just how lucid are lucid dreams?' She examined the lucid dreams of 50 participants to discover whether they are fully lucid for corollaries of being in a dream. She listed four corollaries of knowing that something is a dream, including does the dreamer know that all dream characters are not real? and, does the dreamer know that dream objects are not real? She described a lucid dream report in which the dreamer broke off the bars on a window, threw the bars onto the roof underneath, but despite knowing it was a dream was then worried about having damaged the roof tiles and how much they would cost to replace. In this case, Barrett argues that the dreamer fails to realise a corollary of being in a dream, which is that there is actually no real object in the dream to break. Barrett found that less than a quarter of lucid dreams were lucid for all four corollaries, so even though the dreamer may know that they are dreaming, in most lucid dreams the full implications of that are not known.

A converse of Barrett's finding that not all lucid dreams are fully lucid is the finding by Kahan and LaBerge (1996) of metacognition being present in ordinary, non-lucid dreams. They asked participants who reported non-lucid dreams whether they had made a choice in the dream, and found that this occurs in 40% of dreams. They also found internal commentary in 53% of dreams. They then obtained reports from individuals about waking-life episodes, and found that levels of metacognition in waking-life episode reports were only a little higher than in dream reports. So, according to these authors, we do have metacognition occurring in our ordinary dreams, whereas dreams are often characterised as involuntary and as just happening to the dreamer, because the written or spoken dream report may omit or miss these instances of metacognition. Furthermore, although such metacognition may not reach the level of lucidity, it is still noteworthy that it may be present. Therefore, it is important in assessing this that the dreamer is asked specifically whether any metacognition was present in their dream. This is because if independent judges are asked to identify metacognition from dream reports, it may be absent if the dreamer had not been asked specifically to report it. This counters what has been termed the cognitive deficit view of dreaming, such as in Allan Rechtschaffen's (1978) paper 'The single-mindedness and isolation of dreams,' which sees the plot and events in dreams as happening to the dreamer without the dreamer having agency in the dream.

Personality and individual differences of lucid dreamers

Jayne Gackenbach (2006, and follow-up papers) has studied people who play large amounts of PC, video and online gaming, and found that they have a high level of lucid dreams. They also tend to have more dreams of gaming. She suggests that it may be the large amount of time spent on gaming that causes lucid dreaming, as the gaming is an alternate reality, or it may be that there is a personality feature common to lucid dreamers and high-level gamers. Mark has also looked at why some people are frequent lucid dreamers, and found they have a more internal Locus of Control than do people who have never had a lucid dream (Blagrove & Hartnell, 2000). Internal Locus of Control means that the person believes that they are responsible for events in their lives, and that people in general are responsible for their life circumstances, rather than life events being due to chance or powerful other people. It thus appears that this waking life personality characteristic continues during sleep. Blagrove and Hartnell also found that the personality trait Need for Cognition, which is the motivation to engage in and enjoy effortful cognitive tasks, is higher in frequent lucid dreamers, as if the self-questioning and monitoring needed for lucidity is a result of a general motivation for effortful cognition. People high in Need for Cognition might also be more likely to spot bizarreness in dreams, and then to question whether they are awake or dreaming.

That lucid dreams can occur when the dreamer spots an element of bizarreness in the dream led Mark to investigate whether frequent lucid dreamers have an advantage over non-lucid dreamers on a classic test of attention (Blagrove, Bell, & Wilkinson, 2010). The test used was the Stroop task. In this, participants are shown a word in a large capitalised font that spells out the name of a colour. The font of the word is also coloured, sometimes in the same colour as described by the word, sometimes in a different colour. The task for participants is to say out loud what the colour of the font is. This task is difficult because the colour spelled out by the letters has to be ignored, and some people are better at ignoring what is spelled out than are others. The time taken to correctly state the colours of the fonts is measured, and the researchers then subtract the average time each participant took to state the font colours when font and word are congruent from the average time taken to state font colours when font and word are incongruent. The longer this time is, the more the word interfered with recognition of the font colour for that participant. Blagrove and colleagues found that frequent lucid dreamers are faster at this task than are people who have never had a lucid dream. They speculated that as people who are fast at the Stroop task are able to ignore the distraction of the colour that each word spells out, they may also be able to ignore the distraction of the environment and events of a dream, and instead consider in the dream the question 'am I dreaming?' They concluded that this waking life ability of being able to ignore distraction carries over into sleep, and results in dreams in which metacognition and lucidity can occur. They also speculated that the ability to be self-critical and lucid in dreams might have been selected against by evolution because such lucidity might interfere with possible functions of dreaming. This would explain why lucid dreaming is so rare. But the evolutionary selection for self-awareness and attentional abilities in waking life would then partly counteract the selection for lack of self-awareness in dreaming, so, on the whole, self-awareness and lucidity only occur rarely in dreams, but can occur regularly for a minority of people.

Inducing lucid dreams

Although lucid dreaming is rare there have been methods devised to induce them. In Sheila Purcell's study with colleagues in 1986 on lucidity as a learned cognitive skill, a self-reflectiveness scale was used which ranged from the dreamer not being in the dream, to being part of a dream plot but with no other perspective, to being able to control the dream plot and even wake up deliberately, to being able to consciously reflect on the fact that one is dreaming. In one condition participants were given a bracelet to wear during the day. When the bracelet was noticed the person had to question whether they are awake or dreaming. This reality-checking method transferred into sleep and resulted in approximately 10% of dreams being lucid.

A systematic review by Stumbrys and colleagues (2012) concluded that most lucid dream induction methods have only a small effect, but that the most effective were methods to develop a reflective frame of mind during wake. As in the Purcell study, the person frequently reflects while awake on the question 'am I awake or am I asleep?', with the aim that this reflection will transfer to dreams. Another method is the mnemonic induction of lucid dreams (MILD), which involves having the intention to lucid dream just before you go to sleep. This can be combined with the wake-up-back-to-bed (WBTB) method, in which the sleeper goes to bed, wakes early, stays awake for up to two hours, and then goes back to bed with the aim of having a lucid dream. The WBTB method utilises the brain being in a more activated state as a result of the period of wakefulness. The rationale is that a greater level of activation enhances the cognition needed to realise that one is dreaming. In four studies, Erlacher and Stumbrys (2020) used a combination of a wake-up-back-to-bed (WBTB) sleep protocol and a mnemonic technique (MILD) to induce lucid dreams. On average participants were having a lucid dream once every three months at home. With the combined procedure 48% of participants reported a lucid dream during one night in the sleep lab, and 23% of participants had a signal-verified lucid dream.

Relevant to the WBTB method is the finding of Smith and Blagrove (2015) that lucid dreamers are more frequent users of alarm clock snooze buttons. There are several possible explanations for this. One is that during the industry standard snooze length of nine minutes the active brain of the sleeper enables lucidity, as with the WBTB method. Or it might be that lucid dreamers are more likely to use the snooze button, possibly as a result of being comfortable with going in and out of consciousness. Or maybe there is some personality trait in common between lucid dreamers and snooze button users.

It is also possible that eliciting lucid dreams might not occur solely as a result of deliberate practice. As more has become known about lucid dreams in the last 30 years, with books on them and films such as *Inception* (written and directed by Christopher Nolan, 2010), there is also the possibility that lucid dreams might increase in frequency simply because people know that they are possible.

Technological induction of lucid dreams

Relevant to the work by Jayne Gackenbach on high-level gamers and lucidity cited above is the finding of Gott and colleagues (2021) that a four-week dream-like Virtual Reality (VR) training course led to increases in lucid dreaming compared to a no-training condition. A more direct and widely used method, however, is to give people stimulation during sleep, with the aim of altering the dream environment so as to remind the dreamer that they may be in a dream. The first method devised for this was goggles that are worn during sleep and which can detect REM sleep and then flash red light at the eyes of the sleeper; these were Stephen LaBerge's *DreamLight* and *NovaDreamer* devices. The aim here was that the dreamer starts to see a red environment or red objects in their dream and recognises this reminder of being in a dream, so that they do a reality check of 'am I awake or am I dreaming?' LaBerge and Levitan (1995) found that, out of 14 participants using the *DreamLight* device at home and studied for 4 to 24 nights, 11 participants reported 32 lucid dreams, 22 of which were from nights with light cues and 10 from nights where the masks were worn but light cues were not presented. The non-light nights were included so as to control for a placebo effect. Red light was also seen in dreams significantly more often on cued nights than on non-cued nights, even if a lucid dream did not result. This and other devices that use the same or similar methods are described by Mota-Rolim and colleagues (2019).

Such stimulation has also been used in the sleep lab, which enables lucid dreams to also be verified by eye movements. In a study by Michelle Carr, Karen Konkoly and colleagues (2020), 41 participants were brought into the sleep lab at either 07.30 or 11.00. Participants were wired up for polysomnography and then would lie down on the bed and be given 'lucidity reactivation training'. In this, they would hear an electronic tune and also see flashing red lights, and at the same time be given mindfulness instructions to ask themselves 'am I awake or am I dreaming?' The lights and the sound were thus associated with the mindfulness training given before sleep, in which participants would consider what was happening in their current experience and whether it is different from their normal waking life experience.

The aim of the study thus was to go beyond the previous use of stimulation during sleep by training participants to link the cue of music and the flashing red lights to the metacognitive training. When REM sleep occurred the experimenters stimulated 28 of the sleeping participants with the electronic tune and red lights cue; 13 control participants were not stimulated during sleep. If a participant gave the four left-right eye movement signal, they were woken to see if they would report having been in a lucid dream. Independent judges later assessed whether the eye movements on the EOG trace showed the LRLRLRLR eye movements. Such signal-verified lucid dreams were achieved in 50% of REM periods for cued participants, which was the highest level achieved for any technique to date. Induction was also achieved in participants who had never previously had a lucid dream. This rate of induction was significantly higher than the rate of 17% found for the control participants, who were not cued during sleep.

Drug induction of lucid dreams

A further possibility is to use drugs to induce lucid dreams. The main drug used has been galantamine, which is a treatment for Alzheimer's disease and for various memory problems, but which has recently been made illegal in many countries for non-prescription use. In LaBerge and colleagues' (2018) double-blind, active placebo-controlled, crossover study, 121 participants were awoken approximately 4.5 hours after lights out, were given either 0, 4 or 8 mg of galantamine, stayed out of bed for at least 30 minutes, and then returned to bed and to practice the MILD technique. Participants were found to be four times more likely to have a lucid dream when on the 8 mg dose than on the placebo, and over twice as likely on the 4 mg dose as on placebo. The percentage of participants who reported a lucid dream was 27% for the 4 mg dose and 42% for the 8 mg dose, compared to 14% for those given the placebo.

What is happening in the brains of lucid dreamers?

As people who have had a lucid dream know, they are a very distinct type of dream, but are also fragile. Voss and colleagues (2009) studied the EEG of lucid versus non-lucid dreams in their paper 'Lucid dreaming: state of consciousness with features of both waking and non-lucid dreaming'. They obtained instances of signal-verified lucid dreams and found higher levels of frontolateral 40 Hz power in the EEG, which is a waveband associated with higher levels of cognition, but which is absent during REM sleep and present during wakefulness. They concluded that in lucid dreaming the brain is in a hybrid state that has a mixture of REM and wakefulness EEG characteristics. This ties in with the common feeling in lucid dreams that one could wake oneself up easily, or one could tip back into an ordinary dream and no longer know that one is in a dream. They concluded that lucidity occurs in a REM sleep state, but that this state has waking EEG characteristics. However, Baird et al. (2022b) countered that the apparent increase in frontolateral 40 Hz power in lucid REM sleep, used to justify the claim that lucid dreaming is a 'hybrid state', mixing sleep and wakefulness, is instead due to an eye movement artifact that can be mistaken for EEG waves. They concluded that lucid dreams occur due to high levels of physiological and cortical activation during REM sleep.

There has also been much speculation, and findings (e.g., Dresler et al., 2012), that the dorsolateral prefrontal cortex, an area at the front of the brain linked to metacognition, which is usually deactivated in REM sleep, is activated during lucid dreams. On this, when sleep lab subjects in REM sleep have transcranial Direct Current Stimulation applied to the skull just over the dorsolateral prefrontal cortex, higher ratings of lucidity and metacognition are found, but only in people who are already frequent lucid dreamers (Stumbry et al., 2013).

Another frontal area brain difference has been found by Baird and colleagues (2018), with frequent lucid dreamers having significantly increased resting-state functional connectivity between frontopolar cortex (the most forward area of the prefrontal cortex, and responsible for executive functions) and temporoparietal association areas, compared to non-lucid dreaming controls. These regions are normally deactivated during sleep.

Uses of lucid dreams

Spoormaker and others (see Chapter 3) have proposed that nightmare sufferers can change their nightmares or deliberately wake up from a nightmare through the use of lucid dreams, and this is now recognised medically as a treatment for nightmares. There are some problems with this, however. First, as stated above, there are occasionally lucid nightmares. These are nightmares in which one knows that one is having a nightmare, which one knows is not real, but the sleeper is unable to wake themselves from it. Another issue is that in attempting to be taught lucid dreams, many will fail to learn the skill and this can add to the stresses of their life. Although the Carr and colleagues (2020) study above found an induction rate of 50% it did require much technical effort to enable that to occur, and people having medical treatment for nightmares will not usually have that level of support. The findings and inconsistencies in research on the lucid dreaming training method for the treatment of nightmares are described in Chapter 3 and in the review paper by Macêdo and colleagues (2019).

A second use for lucid dreams is for experiments that require the induction of specific content in dreams. Dresler and colleagues (2011) gave participants instructions to perform motor actions, such as hand clenching, if they achieved a lucid dream. They were also instructed that if they started to lucid dream they should signal this with eye movements, this then showed exactly the start of a lucid dream, so that sensorimotor cortical activity could be measured by functional Magnetic Resonance Imaging (fMRI) and near InfraRed Spectroscopy and matched to the start of the lucid dream. Dresler's team found that brain activity in sensorimotor areas was related to the dreamt hand movements. This study could not have been done with an ordinary dream because if the participant woke up from an ordinary dream and reported having been clenching their hands, it would not be clear to the experimenters when exactly the hand clenching had occurred. This was the first evidence that specific contents of REM dreams can be related to brain activity. A second consequence of the paper is that there was a deliberate alteration of dream content, which is important if we are to achieve the random allocation to dream content conditions that are necessary for experiments on the effects and possible functions of dream content, as will be described in Chapter 12.

Communication between experimenters and lucid dreamers

A major paper in the journal *Current Biology* in 2021, with first author Karen Konkoly, was the first to show a real-time dialogue between experimenters and dreamers during REM sleep. The aim was to set problems for people in a lucid dream at sleep labs around the world, so as to investigate what cognitive abilities are possible in the dream. When participants gave a signal that verified they are in a lucid dream, they were stimulated by sound or touch, in some cases with morse code, so as to communicate questions, such as, 'what is 8 minus 6?', or questions about the biography of the person, such as 'can you speak Spanish?' or 'do you like chocolate?' Dreamers answered in real-time with volitional eye movements or facial muscle signals. There were usually several questions set for each lucid dreamer and such attempts at two-way communication were tried 158 times. What was found was, for 18% of the questions there was a correct response, for 3% of the questions there was an incorrect response, and for 18% of the questions there was an ambiguous response; in all other cases there was no response recorded. The significantly higher level of correct than incorrect responses meant that this was the first finding of two-way communication with a person who is dreaming.

There have been claims in the past of being able to communicate with sleep talkers, with questions asked of the sleep talker and then the sleep talker responding, but, of course, this is not the same as interaction with a person in a dream, as the sleep talker might not be dreaming of the communication. In the Konkoly study, the dreamer receives and experiences the question in the dream, and has to think in the dream of a response to the question, and then needs to communicate the answer back to the experimenters. This does suggest that a high level of cognition is possible in lucid dreams.

Possible adverse effects of lucid dreaming

Although there are scientific, health and recreational benefits of lucid dreams, there have been questions raised in the scientific literature on whether it is a good idea to cultivate lucid dreaming. Vallat and Ruby (2019) caution that lucid dream induction techniques might affect sleep quality, and correlational evidence for this was found by Aviram and Soffer-Dudek (2018). Furthermore, if dreaming does have one or more functions, as will be discussed in Chapter 12, then deliberately altering the plot or contents of a dream, or even just observing that one is dreaming, might adversely affect such functions.

Summary

Lucid dreams are a rare form of dream because the metacognition in them seems to be fragile and because the combination of personality, motivational and neural bases to them may also be rare. We may even have evolved to not be lucid in our dreams. But training oneself to lucid dream is possible, and it may even be that as more has become known about lucid dreams in the last 30 years, with books on them and films such as *Inception*, there is the possibility that lucid dreams might increase in frequency simply because people know that they are possible. However, although there are scientific, health and recreational benefits of lucid dreams, there have been questions raised in the scientific literature on whether it is a good idea to cultivate lucid dreaming, as lucid dream induction techniques might affect sleep quality, and deliberately altering the contents or plot of a dream might affect any functions it is performing.

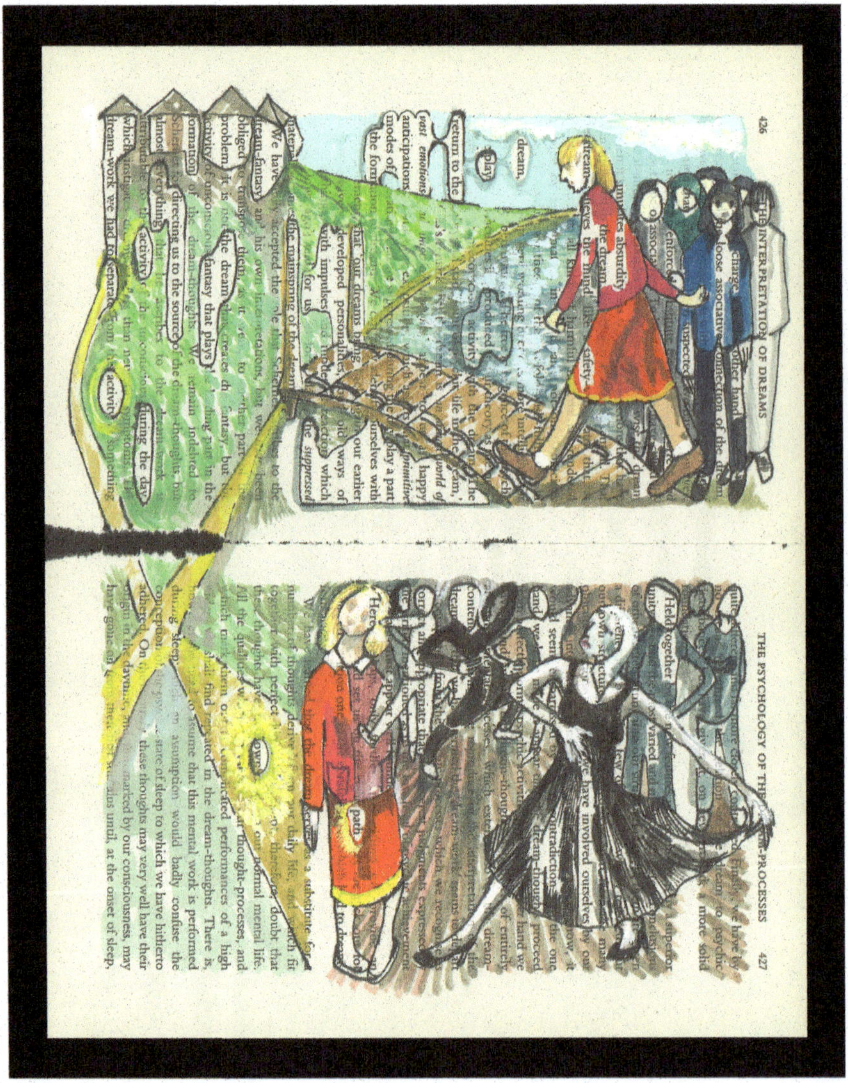

Figure 8.1 Dream of walking alone and then dancing with friends, 2020.

8 Freud, psychoanalysis and dreams

Although more nuanced in later years, Freud held that the motive force and conscious or unconscious meaning behind dreams lay in a wish. This wish-fulfilment dream of walking alone and then dancing with friends occurred at the end of the first Covid-19 Lockdown.

DREAM NARRATIVE: *I am walking alone in the country, trying to get to a village. I am wearing a red skirt and red jacket. It isn't possible to take the short route to the village as the sea is coming over the path. The longer route is difficult, and involves climbing and takes energy. I meet a group of people, who I do not know, and I ignore their advice to take the dangerous short route. Instead, I go across a thin rope-and-wood bridge. I am then alone and look at the remote village in the distance.*

I am then suddenly at my destination, in a big hall, the sort of venue that a wedding would be held in. My friend P is there, she is wearing a thin black dress and tells me that her favourite music is the waltz. She tells me that my friends are going to be there and a crowd of people start dancing to a waltz. I dance as well.

DISCUSSION: The dreamer, Alma, spoke of her life as an artist under Lockdown, and of how she could still go to her art studio. However, she said that as a result of the Lockdown she had had to put off a trip to see a friend in Paris, and that her plans with P for buying a house in France had also been put on hold. That hoped-for house would be a place for music. We and the dreamer and the online participants remarked on how the dream has two halves, one of being alone, even with a bridge for one person crossing at a time, and one of being with friends, dancing.

JULIA: (Painting shown as Figure 8.1) The composition is built around the two parts of the journey and the links between them. I painted a large yellow X to one side and there is also a zigzag running across the page to take the eye from one half to the other. The red dress acts as the motif for the dreamer and a focal point for the eye, while the brown bridge and black dress lead the eye into the composition. An objet trouvé, the word *safety*, can be seen in her red skirt as she crosses the bridge, and in the bottom half of the painting, the word *own* is found on the path, and the word *path* in her dress.

DOI: 10.4324/9781003037552-8

A small found poem is in the water below the bridge:

The free
produced
activity

And another found poem at the top left of the page:

directing us to the source of
everything
activity
during the day
activity

Sigmund Freud and the importance of dreams

The very detailed work of Sigmund Freud on dreams has resulted in dreams being taken seriously as a topic for scientific or therapeutic exploration, and as a topic for personal consideration and growth. There have been many criticisms of the wider work of Freud, but there is much plausibility to how he addressed dreams and dreaming, in terms of the presence of metaphors in dreams, and with his method of tracing back components of each dream to their waking life memory sources. Freud's work on dreams is described in his book *The Interpretation of Dreams* (1900/1997), and in part two of his *Introductory Lectures on Psychoanalysis* (ILP, 1916–17/1974), both of which are very readable.

Freud knew that the study of dreams is often criticised, and on this matter, he said 'an excess of criticism may make us suspicious'. (ILP, p.112.) He proposed that this criticism and dismissal of dreams is because dreams contain uncomfortable information about the self, and that people do not want to know that information. So, this is a quite typical Freudian comment, that he wants to address the possible motivation for people's criticism and dismissal of dreams and he asks about dreaming, 'why does mental life fail to go to sleep?' (ILP, p.112). In other words, why don't we just have blank minds during the night? His answer is 'probably because there is something that will not allow the mind any peace' (ILP, p.118). He concluded from the analysis of many dreams that what disturbs us during sleep are our unconscious wishes, and that dreams attempt to fulfil these wishes (1900/1997, chapter 3, pp.34–44), although he later qualified this and made it more nuanced, partly in recognition that nightmares could be difficult to interpret as wish-fulfilling. For the early Freud, though, dreams are similar to daydreams, in which we often imagine our wishes and desires being fulfilled.

The use of the free association method

In order to ascertain the meaning of a dream, Freud's patients were told that, without censoring their thoughts, they should state what comes to mind when thinking about each part of the dream. The aim of such 'free association' is to follow back from the parts of the dream to all the wishes and concerns and fears and possibly unconscious memories that created the dream in the first place. Important here is Freud's belief in psychic determinism, which means that even small and apparently unmotivated actions, such as slips of the tongue, or mistakes, or components of dreams, are caused by our conscious and unconscious motivations.

For Freud, an apparent mistake can be motivated, and many examples of these are told in his book *The Psychopathology of Everyday Life* (1901/1966). In one example, the speaker of the Parliament in Vienna at the opening of the new session of the legislature declared the Parliament closed, leading Freud to suggest that the Speaker indeed wished it so. Freud applied psychic determinism to the content of dreams, and to even apparently senseless or apparently random content. According to Freud, during the night our background wishes, concerns, fears and unconscious memories have created the dream imagery. This is a very natural science of dream content, claiming that apparently accidental actions of the person, and the contents of the mind, including dreams, are not the result of randomness, but are instead motivated. There is thus cause and effect, just as there is in a billiard ball view of the universe, with balls hitting and ricocheting off and hitting other balls, but all acting in a lawlike cause and effect manner. And so, for Freud, even bizarreness in dreams can be interpreted. Bizarreness is motivated rather than due to random or physiological processes, and individual instances of bizarreness might mean, for example, do not take this dream seriously, it is all senseless.

In order to see how this method is used in practice, we can take the analysis of a dream that Freud gives in the *Introductory Lectures on Psychoanalysis*. He gives this example (p.150, italics in original):

'As part of a longish dream, a patient dreamt that *several members of his family were sitting round a table of a peculiar shape.*'

He asked the patient to free associate to the separate items of the dream. Freud's method does not address the actual narrative of the dream, looking instead at the individual parts and where these components came from. Indeed, Freud held that the narrative of the dream might hide the sources of the components of the dream.

Regarding the peculiarly shaped table, the young man remembered that he had seen a table of that shape at the house of a family that he had recently visited.

The second free association he gave was that the family was called Tischler. Note that in German the word Tisch means table. He also remembered that he thought that the family was very odd.

Bringing together these associations, Freud surmised that the dream means that the young man is thinking that his own family is odd, like the Tischlers, and that the young man has depicted this by having his own family sitting around the Tischler's table.

Here is a longer dream (ILP, p.153; also in Freud, 1900/1997, chapter 6, section F, p.272, italics in original):

> A lady who, though she was still young, had been married for many years had the following dream: *She was at the theatre with her husband. One side of the stalls was completely empty. Her husband told her that Elise L. and her fiancé had wanted to go too, but had only been able to get bad seats - three for 1 florin 50 kreuzers - and of course they could not take those. She thought it would not really have done any harm if they had.*

The dreamer first free associated to her friend, Elise L. and said that she had just become engaged.

The second free association was that the previous week the lady herself had booked tickets in advance for the theatre, but it turned out that this had been unnecessary because there were plenty of tickets available. She had been teased about being in too much of a hurry to get the tickets.

The third association was that recently her sister-in-law had been in a hurry to take 150 florins to the jewellers. This is an association to the 1 florin 50 kreuzers in the dream.

The idea of hurry as a theme thus seems to recur in the free associations, which, according to Freud, are the thoughts that led to or created the dream. Freud concluded that the young lady had an underlying thought of it having been absurd of *her* to be so quick to get married. She had been teased about being in a hurry to get tickets for the theatre and so, according to Freud, what happened is that this waking life experience, which would usually be quite innocuous, provoked or excited the background and persisting thought that she had been in too much of a hurry to get married. This background thought is a long-term issue, maybe partially unconscious, but which can be activated by something innocuous that happens in waking life. For Freud, the activated idea then uses the innocuous occurrence to express or represent itself in the dream. Her long-standing concern about her marriage, thoughts of which were also provoked by the fact that her friend Elise L. had just got engaged, is also represented by having that friend incorporated into the dream as well.

To use terminology that Freud introduced for this, free association traces back from what he called the manifest dream, which is the dream as it is experienced and reported, to the latent dream thoughts. The latent thoughts are all the components from psychic life that produced the dream, including thoughts, wishes, concerns, beliefs and worries. Freud claims that free association follows in reverse the process that created the dream, a process that he terms the dream work. The dream work comprises various techniques (1900/1997, chapter 6; pp.169–266):

- Condensation, where two latent dream thoughts are represented by one dream item, such as the strange-shaped table seen in waking life and the

family name Tischler both being represented by the table in the first dream above.
- Displacement, where what is important in the latent dream thoughts is de-emphasised in the manifest dream, and what is prominent in the dream might really be unimportant in the latent thoughts.
- Representation, which considers how the latent thought might be represented in the dream, including by symbolism.
- Secondary revision, in which the dream is revised to make it a more sensible and rational narrative, providing explanations for events in the dream in terms of other events in the dream, and which hence disguises the latent thoughts which were the true causes of the manifest dream.

These processes result in what Freud terms regression (1900/1997, chapter 7, section B; pp.374–389). First, our thinking regresses from waking life rational thinking to the irrational and wishful thinking of the dream. Second, whereas in waking life our cognition follows the path of taking in information from perception to laying down memories, in the dream the path is in the opposite direction, our memories create perceptions that we see and hear and touch in the dream.

Although Freud held that dreams can refer to memories, concerns and fears, each of which can be conscious or unconscious, he concluded that it is our wishes that have the motive force to create the dream, and it is these wishes that might be taboo and so need to be disguised in the dream. He compared this to children's dreams, which he said often have very simple wishes occurring in them, which are undisguised. In one example, he refers to a family trip in the countryside with his three-year-old daughter, and a too-brief boat trip on a lake. 'The little girl had crossed the lake for the first time, and the trip had passed too quickly for her. She did not want to leave the boat at the landing, and cried bitterly. The next morning she told us: "Last night I was sailing on the lake." Let us hope that the duration of this dream-voyage was more satisfactory to her.' (Freud, 1900/1997, chapter 3, p.41.) In contrast, for adults, dreams will often have disguised wishes. The purpose of the disguise is so that the taboo wishes, or other mental content, do not wake the dreamer. Freud concluded that in expressing conscious, unconscious or somatic content, dreams 'serve the purpose of continuing to sleep instead of waking. The dream is the guardian of sleep, not its disturber.' (1900/1997, chapter 5, section C, p.130.) The dream thus represents disturbing internal or external sensations or materials that would otherwise wake us.

The interpretation of dreams enables the exploration and discovery of these various internal and external stimuli, including conscious and unconscious motivations. Freud (1900/1997, chapter 7, section E, p.441, italics in original) claimed that *'the interpretation of dreams is the* via regia [Royal road] *to a knowledge of the unconscious element in our psychic life.'* On this, there is some experimental support for 'dream rebound', in which dreams express thoughts that are suppressed during the day, in comparison to a control condition where these suppression instructions are not given (Bryant et al., 2011, Malinowski et al., 2019; Taylor & Bryant, 2007; Wegner et al., 2004).

The first full dream that Freud interpreted in *The Interpretation of Dreams* was his own 'dream of Irma's injection' (1900/1997, chapter 2, pp.20–21). Irma was a patient of Freud who had various physical and other ailments and Freud at the time of the dream was being blamed for her still being ill, despite his treatment of her. In the dream, there was Freud, Irma, and a large group of people, including colleagues of Freud. In the dream, a colleague gave her a harmful injection. Freud has many pages of his free associations to the dream, which he finally interpreted as showing his own wish that in waking life he was not to blame for Irma not yet being cured. The dream represented this wish by blaming her condition on a colleague of Freud injecting her with an unclean needle. Whereas for Freud, dream content usually represents libidinous content such as sexual and aggressive wishes, there can thus be other motives present, such as professional rivalry and response to professional criticism.

Evaluation of the free association method

The free association method has been used in a long programme of research by Italian researchers which has been summarised in a meta-analysis by Baylor and Cavallero (2001). The research programme investigated memory sources of dreams by waking participants in the sleep lab, and obtaining reports of dreams, which were then segmented by the researchers into thematic units. The thematic units were presented back to participants who were asked to identify memory sources for them or to associate to each segment. Memory sources were classified as a waking life episode, semantic knowledge, or abstract self-references or self-knowledge. The mean percentage of episodic memory sources was found to be significantly greater for non-Rapid Eye Movement (NREM) than for Rapid Eye Movement (REM) dreams, suggesting that NREM dreams have a more literal relationship to waking life experiences than do REM dreams. Another use of the free association method to investigate the memory sources of dreams is seen in Vallet et al. (2017a), which was reviewed in Chapter 1.

However, a problem with Freud's proposal for tracing back the components of a dream to waking life sources is detailed in Sebastiano Timpanaro's (1974) book *The Freudian Slip*. The book relates an account by Freud of a slip of the tongue made by a young man to whom Freud was talking, and who he met in a railway carriage. The young man missed out the word *aliquis* (Latin for someone) as part of a Latin quotation that he was telling Freud. In English, the full quotation is: *Let someone arise from my bones as an avenger.* Freud asked the man to free associate to the word *aliquis* and in a few steps arrived at the man's concern, which was that his fiancée was pregnant. Freud claimed that the worries about her being pregnant caused the young man to repress the word and forget it, and that the slip was therefore motivated and meaningful.

However, Timpanaro showed that other words of the quotation could also be free associated to, so as to arrive at the idea of pregnancy. Timpanaro concluded that it is therefore not possible to use the association as evidence that the slip of the tongue was motivated by worry about the pregnancy. For the study of dreaming the consequence of this would be that even if some meaning could be ascribed to a dream on the basis of free association, this would not be evidence that the dream content was caused by that meaning or latent thought, as other dreams of the person, or even the dreams of other people, might be able to be linked to that same meaning by free association. Indeed, even if a dreamer agrees with an interpretation, this would, by the same argument, still retain the problem that associations to another dream of the person, or to a dream of another person could similarly lead back in a confabulatory manner to that meaning.

Nevertheless, although these cautions regarding the interpretation of dreams and the use of free association are important, there is empirical work supporting the free association method. This work shows relationships can be identified between waking life experiences and literal, symbolic and metaphorical dream content through experiments, and it will be addressed in the next section.

Non-literal and metaphorical content in dreams

There is experimental evidence for the presence of non-literal metaphorical content in dreams, which supports the tracing back of dream content by free association to prior waking life experiences or concerns. In a study by Davidson and Lynch (2012), two films were played on different days to participants, one film about the September 11th attacks, and the other an education film. On the night after each film was played, each participant reported any dreams they had. The authors devised scales for associated and literal references to the content of the two films, and the content of the dreams under the two conditions was assessed against these criteria. So, for example, a literal reference for the 9/11 film would be President George Bush, as he was president at the time of the 9/11 attacks, another literal reference would be planes crashing into the Twin Towers, whereas a close association would be planes crashing into anything else. Judges were asked to indicate with a yes or no if each dream contained mention of a literal reference, a close association, or a distant association to either film. The findings were that dreams after the 9/11 film had more literal references and more closely and more distantly related imagery referring to 9/11 than did dreams reported after seeing the education film. These findings thus show that dreams may be creating novel or metaphorical references, as well as literal references to waking life experiences. For example, there were more dreams of being chased, attacked or threatened, or of falling or drowning, and vehicle and transportation accidents, after having seen the 9/11 film than after the education film. This is work that balances the caution that Timpanaro's work elicits, in that the waking life stimulus, unlike the fiancée's pregnancy, is presented before the dream as part of a controlled experiment, and so when judges link the dream to that prior stimulus, without knowing which of the two films was in fact presented, the results cannot be explained as solely due to confabulation.

Such distant associations that refer to a standardised stimulus were also found by Wamsley and colleagues in their (2010a) paper 'Cognitive replay of visuomotor learning at sleep onset: temporal dynamics and relationship to task performance.' Participants played the amusement arcade downhill skiing game *Alpine Racer II* across a period of one or more days. On the nights after playing it, the longer participants had been asleep, the more abstract were the representations of the skiing task in dreams.

Such findings of abstract references to waking life in dreams tie in with the wider cognitive literature on metaphor through the work of George Lakoff. For Lakoff, much of our waking life cognition is metaphorical, and is based upon concrete metaphors, which Lakoff and Johnson's (1980) book *Metaphors We Live By* terms conceptual metaphors. An example of one of these is: UP IS HAPPY: DOWN IS UNHAPPY, and this conceptual metaphor leads to thoughts such as 'I feel up', 'everything's looking up', 'I feel down' and 'down in the dumps'. Similarly, if people in a relationship say 'we have to go our separate ways', or 'we've gone through a bumpy patch', these follow from another conceptual metaphor, that LOVE IS A JOURNEY. So, we can talk about happiness, unhappiness, love, falling out of love with somebody, in these concrete metaphorical terms, and even understand them in these concrete ways.

These conceptual metaphors then appear in our dreams. And so, rather than talking or thinking about love being like a journey, or that 'we have to go our separate ways', the dreamer experiences these in the dream in a real environment. The metaphor thus becomes concrete, and in dreams we see the metaphors and physically experience them; the dream is thus a type of embodied cognition. This can occur in dreams even though we may not even know intellectually that, in everyday life, we use conceptual metaphors in everyday thinking and we experience and think about life in terms of these metaphors.

As a further example, if one has had an argument with a partner one might dream of standing on a volcano with them, everything being hot and dangerous, and so we physically experience this metaphor. In his (1993) paper, 'How metaphor structures dreams: the theory of the conceptual metaphor applied to dream analysis,' Lakoff applies to dream interpretation the theory of conceptual metaphor and of how we understand abstract concepts in concrete, everyday terms. He concludes that most dream symbolism makes use of our everyday metaphor system, and that familiarity with the system and with the life of the dreamer greatly facilitates dream interpretation. So as to consider further such metaphors in dreams, we will explore in the next chapter two famous dreams from one of Freud's early patients, Dora.

Summary

Freud had contentious theories on the function of dreams and on the types of knowledge that could be obtained from dreams. However, he devised the free association method, which claims to trace back from the components of dreams to the memory sources that created the dream during the night. This method does have experimental support and ties in with research on the cognitive science of metaphor. The free association method thus appears to have some validity, and the use of the method will be explored in the following chapters.

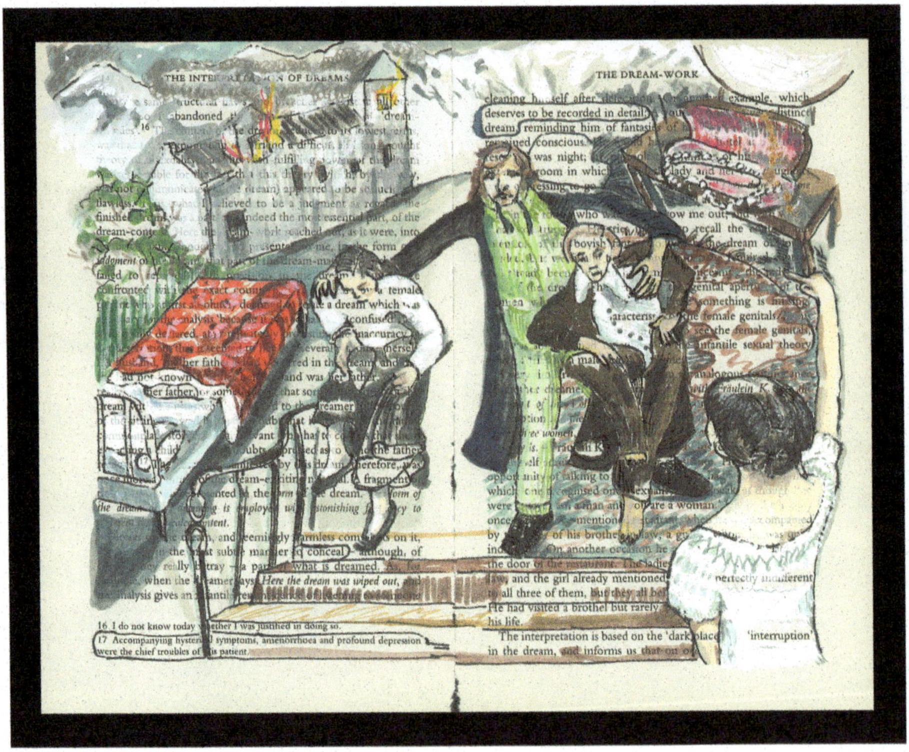

Figure 9.1 Dora's first dream, of escape from a burning house, 2020.

9 Freud and Dora

In 1900 Freud's patient Dora told him two dreams, which Freud published in a detailed and famous case study. This chapter details how the dreams poignantly depict her stressful and oppressive waking life circumstances. We present here the first of Dora's two dreams.

DREAM NARRATIVE: *A house was on fire. My father was standing beside my bed and woke me up. I dressed quickly. Mother wanted to stop and save her jewel-case; but Father said "I refuse to let myself and my two children be burnt for the sake of your jewel-case." We hurried downstairs, and as soon as I was outside I woke up.* (Freud, 1905/1977, p.99.)

DISCUSSION: Dora's free associations during psychoanalysis with Freud concerned the relationship of the dream to the sexual harassment she was being subjected to by Herr K., a friend of her father, and to her wish that her father would rescue her from this danger. Our discussion of the dream and Dora's associations with it are detailed in this chapter.

JULIA: (Painting shown as Figure 9.1) At the top left of the painting I depicted the spa town of Merano, where Dora lived with her family and where the K. family also lived. I chose two pages on which to paint the key scene, the escape from the burning house. The painting's composition brings together the father, Dora and her brother Otto, heading to the wide stairs at the bottom of the painting, and with Dora and Otto pulling on their clothes. Dora's mother frames the lower right corner, and she is pointing at her jewel-case, at top right. Note the words *female genitals* appearing twice under the jewel-case; *lady and her daughters* in the jewel-case; *perfectly indifferent* in the mother's dress; *boyish* in Dora's brother's head; *17*, at the bottom left, and also in the bed, which was Dora's age at starting to see Freud; the words *was night; room in which dressing to go*, next to her father's head; and, most eerie of all, *Fräulein K.*, in her mother's head! Although there is much argument about the case study and Freud's treatment of Dora, we are grateful that the dream was recorded by Freud after she discussed it with him: The words *deserves to be recorded in detail dream*, at the top right-hand side, are therefore very relevant and important, as part of the painting.

Background to the Dora case study

One of the most famous case histories from Sigmund Freud is that of 'Dora', a 17-year-old young woman, who saw Freud in the final months of 1900. Freud published the case study in 1905 as *Fragments of an Analysis of a Case of Hysteria ('Dora')*. The case study addressed two dreams of Dora and had a draft title *Dreams and Hysteria* (p.39: here and following, page numbers refer to Freud, 1905/1977). The case study is important because Freud started writing it in the aftermath of mixed reviews of his (1900) *The Interpretation of Dreams*, and for which the scientific reviews were generally negative (Kramer, 1994). The case study is also important because it provides one of the first instances of Freud publishing detailed examinations of full dream reports combined with considerable details of the life circumstances of the dreamer and of the dreamer's free associations to the dreams. In this case, so much so that, even with a change of name, the details allowed Dora to be identified later in life by her then-physician, Felix Deutsch (Deutsch, 1990).

This chapter argues that Dora's two dreams are poignant depictions of the distress, abuse and hopes in her life. The argument is that this can be seen clearly from Dora's free associations to her dreams. Unfortunately, these interpretations of her dreams, although present in Freud's account of the analysis, are overshadowed in the case study by the highly speculative further interpretations of the dreams by Freud, which derive from Freud's own associations. The interpretations are also obscured by the criticisms that are often made of Freud regarding this case (see Decker, 1991 and Bernheimer & Kahane, 1990, for further details).

Freud (1905), *Fragments of an Analysis of a Case of Hysteria ('Dora')*, was the first case study of Freud that involved the interpretation of dreams, and had a draft title *Dreams and Hysteria* (p.39). In Freud's (1900) *The Interpretation of Dreams,* the dreams are often excerpts, with only brief details given of the dreamer's life. In contrast, in the Dora case study, there is a much fuller description of Dora's background and experiences; indeed her life is documented not only by Freud in the case study itself, with some remarkable or unknowing honesty, but in historical (e.g., Decker, 1991) and feminist (e.g., Bernheimer & Kahane, 1990) accounts of the case that, to many, do not reflect well on Freud. This enables a contrast of instances where free association does seem to elucidate or find meaning in each dream, with instances that seem more contrived or motivated by other considerations.

Dora's life

The Dora case study is widely seen as reflecting very badly on Freud, and Dora has been acclaimed as a feminist hero (e.g., Moi, 1990) because she stopped her psychoanalysis with Freud after just 11 weeks, on 31 December 1900. She was, however, a hero who had two captivating dreams, told to Freud, who interpreted and recorded them. Dora was 17 years old when treatment started. She

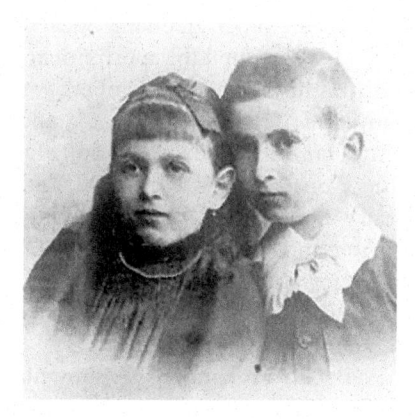

Figure 9.2 Ida Bauer, aged 6, and Otto Bauer, aged 7; photograph taken 1 January 1889, unknown photographer.

had developed in childhood possible hysterical symptoms of migraines, loss of voice and a chronic cough. Her father had arranged for her to see Freud due to her underlying health issues, but he also had a motive that, as he was having an affair with a family friend, Frau K., he wished Dora to cease her 'hatred' of Frau K. and of her husband Herr K. (Freud, 1905/1977, p.57).

Dora is now known to have been teenager Ida Bauer, who was living with her family in Vienna when she had psychoanalysis with Freud, and her biography has been pieced together by various authors despite Freud's aim to anonymise her (e.g., Bernheimer & Kahane, 1990; Decker, 1991; Ellis et al., 2015). (Ida Bauer is referred to as Dora for the majority of this chapter so as to be consistent with Freud, 1905.)

We now know that Dora was born on 1 November 1882 in an apartment on the Berggasse in Vienna, the same street on which Freud would later live and work. Her brother Otto was born one year later; he became a prominent Austrian socialist politician. Dora, who was Jewish, was able to go to the US in 1941 to be with her emigrant son, and died in the United States in 1945 (Decker, 1991).

Event held for commemorating and discussing Dora's first dream

So as to commemorate the first dream that Dora told Freud, we held an online event and performance as part of the Swansea Science Festival, on 24 October 2020. The event was timed for approximately 120 years after Dora told the dream to Freud. Our aim was to consider the Dora case study not as how it is often taken, as part of a critical debate about Freud, but to emphasise the first dream that Dora told Freud, her free associations to it and the historical events of Dora's life. This was so as to honour her strength and life, and to honour the poignant depiction of her teenage life in her dream. This was followed by an event on 31 January 2021 to discuss the second dream that Dora told Freud, also timed for approximately 120 years after she told it to Freud. Our distinguished panel members were: writer Katharina Adler, author of the novel *Ida* (2018), and great-grand-daughter of Dora/Ida; Dr Deirdre Barrett (Harvard Medical School); Dr Brigitte Holzinger (Institute for Dream and Consciousness Research, Vienna); Professor Dany Nobus (Brunel University London and the Freud Museum London); filmmaker Kate Novack (writer and director of the 2021 Oscar short-listed film *Hysterical Girl*, a documentary about Dora and the #metoo movement); Professor Sharon Sliwinski (author of *Dreaming in Dark Times*, 2017); and Zora Wessely (University of Vienna).

At the start of each event, Dr Holzinger was shown in a film reading the dream to the online attendees from Freud's apartment, where Dora first told Freud the dreams, in November 1900 for the first dream and the end of December 1900 for the second dream. The apartment is now the Sigmund Freud Museum, Vienna. Mark Blagrove chaired the discussions and read out contributions from attendees around the world. Simultaneous with hearing and discussing each dream, Julia Lockheart painted the dream onto two pages taken, with publisher's permission, from Freud's (1900/1997) *The Interpretation of Dreams*. The painting processes returned the dreams, existing for us as a text, to visual form, which aimed to honour the original dream experiences. The two pages were chosen by Julia while each dream was being read by Dr Holzinger. So as to emphasise solely the dream and Dora's free associations with it, the event followed the Ullman group dream appreciation technique (Ullman, 1996/2006), which is described in Chapter 10. The technique was adapted for the event as the dreamer was not present, with Brigitte Holzinger reading the published dream report and Zora Wessely reading the published free associations of Dora.

Dora's waking life circumstances, and free associations to the first dream

From Freud (1905/1977), we know that in 1895 Dora's father, Philipp, commenced an affair with a young married woman anonymised by Freud as Frau K. Her husband, Herr K., befriended Dora and started propositioning her. In June 1898, Dora and her father went to stay with the K.s at their house near a lake in the Alps. Herr K. propositioned Dora there in some woods after a boat trip on a lake, and she slapped him. After this, for the next four successive nights, until she could leave Herr and Frau K.s' house with her father, she had a recurring dream of being rescued by her father from a burning house. Her parents refused to believe her regarding what had happened on the lake, siding with Herr K., who denied it. Dora begged her father to break off the friendship with the K.s, seeing herself as 'handed over to Herr K. as the price of his tolerating the relations between her father and his wife'. (p.66.)

In October 1900, Philipp met with Freud and told him that Dora's 'phantasy' of the scene by the lake was causing her to be depressed and to have suicidal ideas, and that she was pressing him to break off relations with the K.s (p.56). He asked Freud to 'bring her to reason' (p.57). As a result of this, Dora started to see Freud in October 1900. Six weeks into the treatment, Dora again had her burning house dream. The text of the dream, from p.99 of the case study, is shown at the start of this chapter.

The case study gives details of Dora's free associations to the elements of the dream, which do give a very plausible understanding of what the dream was about.

For her first free association, Dora spoke about how recently her father and mother had been having a dispute, because her father did not want her mother to lock the dining room door at night, as her brother's room could only be reached through the dining-room. Her father said, 'something might happen in the night, so that it might be necessary to leave the room' (p.100), and this had made Dora think of the danger of fire.

She then free associated to the time in June 1898 when they arrived to stay with the K.s. Her father was afraid of fire in the K.s' small wooden house, because of a violent thunderstorm. She also said that the recurrent dream started after the scene by the lake. Freud concluded that the dream, when it first occurred, was an immediate effect of Dora's experience with Herr K. at the lake, which Freud, unlike her parents, believed to be real.

Dora gave another free association, that after returning with Herr K. from the lake, she had gone to lie down in her bedroom to have a short sleep, but suddenly awoke to see Herr K. standing beside her. Freud's reply was '... just as you saw your father standing beside your bed in the dream?' (p.101), to which Dora said 'yes', and that this episode with Herr K. had put her on her guard. The next morning she had locked herself in while dressing, but later that day the key to the room she was staying in was gone, and she believed that Herr K. had removed it. Freud observed that the theme of locking or not locking a room also appeared in the exciting cause of the recent recurrence of the dream.

Freud next asked about the *I dressed quickly* phrase in the dream. Dora replied that she had made up her mind not to remain at the K.s' without her father, as she felt afraid that Herr K. would surprise her while she was dressing, '*so I always dressed very quickly*' (p.102). Freud replied:

> I understand. On the afternoon of the day after the scene in the wood you formed your intention of escaping from his persecution, and during the second, third, and fourth nights you had time to repeat that intention in your sleep.
>
> (p.102)

Freud then asked about the jewel-case. Dora replied that a year before the dream first occurred, her father and mother had a great dispute about a piece of jewellery he had bought her, which she did not want: 'She was furious, and told him that as he had spent so much money on a present she did not like he had better give it to someone else' (p.104). Dora had stated that her father would indeed give jewellery to her mother and herself as cover for when he was giving jewellery to Frau K. (p.65). Dora also said that Herr K. had given her an expensive jewel-case a little time before. To this, Freud responded: 'Then a return-present would have been very appropriate', and that jewel-case 'is a favourite expression' for female genitals (p.105). Dora replied 'I knew *you* would say that'. Although Freud here alludes to his conclusion that Dora was unconsciously in love with Herr K., his speculation that the jewel-case, which is in danger in the dream, is a reference to Dora's genitals, is plausible. For in waking life she, indeed, was in danger.

Dora then added, at the next psychoanalytic session, a further free association regarding smoke, that 'Herr K. and her father were passionate smokers' (p.109), and that 'She herself had smoked during her stay by the lake, and Herr K. had rolled a cigarette for her before he began his unlucky proposal' (p.109). Whereas these recollections show additional reason to use fire in the dream to represent danger, Freud proceeds to speculate further, that the smell of smoke

> was probably related to the thoughts which were the most obscurely presented and the most successfully repressed in the dream, to the thoughts, that is, concerned with the temptation to show herself willing to yield to the man. If that were so, this addendum to the dream could scarcely mean anything else than the longing for a kiss, which, with a smoker, would necessarily smell of smoke.
>
> (pp.109–110)

Again, it is important to note that 'smell of smoke' is not part of the dream, yet Freud associates to it and speculates from it to arrive at the thought of Dora wishing to kiss Herr K.

Despite these extrapolations by Freud, Dora's free associations and Freud's initial interpretations of the dream do show how it is a poignant depiction of the situation Dora found herself in. Freud stated that the meaning of the dream was: 'This man is persecuting me, he wants to force his way into my room. My "jewel-case" is in danger…' (p.105), and that the dream 'presented as fulfilled the wish that her father should save her from the danger' (p.127). However, rather than relying only on Dora's free associations to the dream, Freud added extrapolations and claimed that there was also 'temptation to yield to the man [Herr K.], out of gratitude for the love and tenderness he had shown her during the last few years' (p.123), but based this on his own associations, which were in most cases not even to the dream, but to Dora's associations about the dream. This should serve as a warning to speculations becoming unbounded, and showing more relevance to the beliefs of the analyst/therapist rather than to the associations of the client/analysand.

The first event discussion

The online event provoked a fascinating and insightful discussion about the dream and Dora's life, and the relationship between these. Themes and questions from the discussion included:

- The surprising lack of overt emotion in the dream report, and that modern dream-work methods (see review in Ellis, 2020) include questioning of the dreamer about whether emotions were or were not present during the dream;
- Dora did not say whether anyone else escaped the fire;
- The oppressive and threatening situation that Dora was in, in waking life and in the dream;
- That her seeing Freud was arranged by her father rather than by Dora voluntarily, but that she was then able to confide in Freud for some of the issues with Herr K., and then was able to decide to leave psychoanalysis. It may be that other young female analysands were not able to halt treatment in that manner. In Dora's case, she then confronted the K.s and her father and mother soon afterwards and the truth of the events was admitted by Herr K. (p.163);
- The relationship between Dora's dream, with its metaphor of the need to escape from the danger of fire, and dreams more widely of trauma and abuse;
- The ethics of Dora's identity being named by authors after Freud, including the effects of this on the family. Her identity was first discovered by psychoanalyst Felix Deutsch in 1922, and published by him in Deutsch (1990). Deutsch was Ida's physician and had not mentioned to her that he would write about her, waiting until her death to do so. There are different standards of consent and anonymity now, but these are not universally agreed, for example, regarding what occurs to the need for consent in the case of psychosis, and what occurs if the person is deceased. Furthermore, regarding identities being discovered, Herr and Frau K. are now known to have been Hans and Peppina Zellenka, who died in 1929 and 1948, respectively (Ellis et al., 2015);
- The conundrum of why in the dream the jewel-case belongs to Dora's mother, whereas in waking life it is Dora (and her 'jewel-case') that are threatened. A possibility is that her father's dismissing of Dora's mother and her jewel-case in the dream refers to the lack of sexual relations in their unhappy marriage, her father having told Freud 'You know already that I get nothing out of my own wife' (p.57), and that, on occasions 'he tried to put the chief blame for Dora's impossible behaviour on her mother - whose peculiarities made the house unbearable for every one' (p.57). The dream may thus be expressing a wish of Dora that she would no longer be in danger 'for the sake of' her mother and her mother's 'jewel-case'. This is admittedly a patriarchal viewpoint and speculation in that it suggests that in the dream Dora was blaming her mother for

what happened with Herr K., and that it was her mother's 'jewel-case' putting her in danger;
- In contrast to the latter paragraph, it may be that, in the dream, Dora's mother's protection of her jewel-case can be interpreted as protective of Dora, rather than as putting Dora in danger from the fire;
- That the dream was used by Dora to show Freud the danger that she was in, and of her need for being rescued, and that the re-occurrence and telling of the dream may be seen as Dora challenging Freud with the dream;
- The risk of sexually transmitted disease for Dora and her mother;
- Dora's free associations may be influenced by Freud's presuppositions of female sexuality and infantile wishes;
- There is a question of whether Frau K. was punishing her philandering husband by having the affair with Dora's father;
- That Dora was closer to her father than her mother in waking life, and close to Frau K., whereas Otto was closer to his mother;
- The close relationship of Frau K. to Dora is especially interesting and important to explore, and continued into the 1930s.

During this first event participants and panellists did often refer to a narrative of abuse, and we are aware that we do not want to impose this, much as Freud imposed an infatuated and hysterical girl narrative. As we obviously did not have Dora present to respond, we accept that the narrative we discussed of this being a dream which metaphorically depicts Dora's experience of, and response to and struggle against sexual harassment is our own construction. Nevertheless, the dream does appear to be a poignant and metaphorical depiction of Dora's wish to be rescued by her father from the harassment she was subjected to.

Despite this wish of rescue, however, Freud correctly notes that in the first dream 'it was necessary to put on one side a certain thought which stood in the way; but it was her father himself who had brought her into the danger' and that 'this was, as we shall discover, one of the motive forces of the second dream' (p.127). This chapter thus now addresses the second dream, for which we must bear in mind that, after the four occurrences of the fire dream at Herr K.'s house, Dora had confronted her father about his affair and about Herr K.'s actions, and he had dismissed her concerns. Contrary to the wish expressed in the first dream, her father was thus not going to rescue her, and had instead sent her to see Freud, to 'bring her to reason' (p.57).

Dora's second dream, of travelling to her father's funeral

The following dream was told to Freud shortly before the end of December 1900. Dora and Freud discussed the dream for two sessions, and on the following session, Dora told Freud that this would be her final session with him. She told him that she had decided two weeks earlier to leave psychoanalysis by the end of the year.

The second dream (pp.133–134): *I was walking about in a town which I did not know. I saw streets and squares which were strange to me. Then I came into a house where I lived, went to my room, and found a letter from Mother lying there. She wrote saying that as I had left town without my parents' knowledge she had not wished to write to me to say that Father was ill. 'Now he is dead and if you like you can come.' I then went to the station and asked about a hundred times: 'Where is the station?' I always got the answer: 'Five minutes.' I then saw a thick wood before me which I went into and there I asked a man whom I met. He said to me: 'Two and a half hours more.' He offered to accompany me. But I refused and went alone. I saw the station in front of me and could not reach it. At the same time I had the usual feeling of anxiety that one has in dreams when one cannot move forward. Then I was at home. I must have been travelling in the meantime, but I know nothing about that. I walked into the porter's lodge, and enquired for our flat. The maidservant opened the door to me and replied that Mother and the others were already at the cemetery.*

In the next session Dora made two additions: '*I saw myself particularly distinctly going up the stairs*', and '*After she had answered I went to my room, but not the least sadly, and began reading a big book that lay on my writing-table.*' (footnote, p.134.)

Dora's associations to the second dream (pp.134–142)

- Strange town, streets, square and monument: At Christmas, a few days before, Dora had been sent an album of views of a German health-resort, including a square with a monument in it, and on the day before the dream she had shown it to relatives. It was from a young engineer she knew who had gone there to work 'so as to become sooner self-supporting' (p.135), and who wrote often to her;
- Wandering around a strange town: On the day before the dream, she had, 'with complete indifference', shown a visiting young cousin around Vienna. This visit reminded her of her own first brief visit to Dresden, where she wandered alone, including to the picture gallery, and declined a male cousin's offer to be her guide. At the gallery she remained two hours in front of a painting of the Madonna, 'rapt in silent admiration';
- She had seen her father look tired and ill at a family gathering the previous evening and wondered how long he would live;
- At the family gathering she had been impatient with her mother and had exclaimed that she had asked her '*a hundred times*' for the key for the drinks sideboard, to get brandy to help her father to sleep;
- The letter: She had once written a suicide letter to her parents. The letter in the dream had the same phrase ('if you like') that was in a letter from Frau K. inviting the family to their house by the lake;
- The thick wood and a man: The shore of the lake where she had had the scene with Herr K. had a wood like in the dream, and after the scene

with Herr K. she had spoken to a man there for directions to walk home round the lake. He said it would take 'Two and a half hours' and so she went back by boat with Herr K. She had also seen a painting with a thick wood and nymphs at the gallery the day before;

- Regarding arriving at her parent's house where 'she went calmly to her room, and began reading a big book that lay on her writing-table' (p.140), she said that the book was 'in encyclopaedia *format*', and she remembered that when a boy cousin of Dora's had fallen dangerously ill with appendicitis, 'Dora had thereupon looked up in the encyclopaedia to see what the symptoms of appendicitis were' (p.141). She said that later, when her aunt who she was fond of had died, she had pain in her abdomen like the symptoms of appendicitis she had read about. Freud's association to this was that Dora had read forbidden sexual matters in an encyclopaedia when young, and that in the dream she was asserting her freedom to do so on her father's death.

These associations seem to point to a wish or wondering of Dora about a life on her own, away from her family, but also to the dangers of being away from home, with association also to the K.s, and to her concern for her father's health.

The second event discussion

As with the first dream, we discussed how Dora's free associations do lead to plausible waking life causes and meaning of the dream:

- She was showing independence in waking life, including rejecting Herr K. and also leaving Freud, and showed independence in many actions in the dream, including in the town and in being alone in both rooms, and in rejecting the man in the woods;
- She had concerns for her father's health, and dreamt of his death. We speculated whether Dora's dreaming mind wondered that, if her father died, the pressure from Herr K. would stop;
- Unlike the first dream, there is emotion here, but it is anxiety and not grief;
- We questioned whether it may be victim blaming for Freud to say Dora was looking for sexual knowledge in the book.

Conclusions

We consider that the two dreams poignantly reveal Dora's hope of rescue by her father, and then her wish for an independent life in another town, and fears for her father. If these are plausible interpretations, the relationships of the dreams to Dora's waking life may have been so clear to her that it may explain why, after two hours of the second dream being 'elucidated' and Freud having expressed his 'satisfaction at the result', 'Dora replied in a depreciatory tone: "Why, has anything so very remarkable come out?"' (p.146.) The clarity and relevance of Dora's memory sources for the dreams may thus have been obscured in the case study, and in reviews and writings about the case study, by Freud's associations being given equal weight to Dora's associations, and with many of Freud's associations being not to the dream, but, one step removed, to Dora's associations.

Finally, though, a speculation, based on the similarity in age between Freud and Dora's father, due to which Freud wrote in the postscript to the case study that 'At the beginning it was clear that I was replacing her father in her imagination' (p.160). The first dream had first occurred after the scene by the lake and when Dora wanted her father to take her away from the K.s' house. After this, it was clear that her father would not rescue her from Herr K. The dream then recurred some weeks after Dora had started to see Freud. We note here that it is often remarked that dreams can indicate the progress of psychotherapy (Ellis, 2020). We suggest, therefore, that it may thus be that the first dream, of being rescued, and the second dream, of living independently in another city, away from the hoped-for rescuer who has now died, could depict the early and final state of Dora's relationship with Freud, as well as her changing relationship with her father.

The painting of the second dream

JULIA: (Painting shown as Figure 9.3) I chose two pages, each with two paragraphs, so as to create the visual narrative: the small town (top left); reading mother's letter about Dora's father's death before leaving (bottom left); the journey (top left); back in the family home, reading the big book (bottom right). Most notable, in terms of the palimpsest, is the section describing the journey to the train station where Dora meets an unknown man in the woods. This section contains the found poem:

return home
strange locality
home
the strange man in the dream
dead father
living in childhood
The dream
the dream of the girl
her ticket for
promised excursion

102 *Freud and Dora*

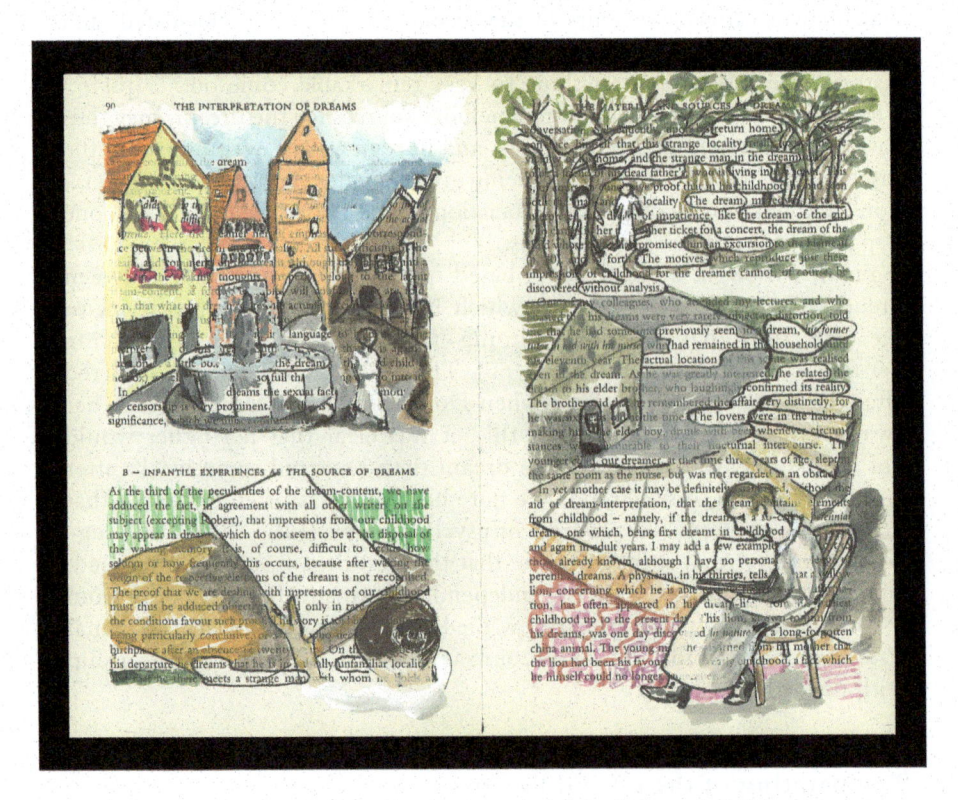

Figure 9.3 Dora's second dream, of travelling to her father's funeral, 2021.

And in the section beneath, depicting Dora's return to the family home:

> *previously seen*
> *had remained in the actual location*
> *former household*
> *he related*
> *confirmed its reality*
> *affair*
> *The lovers*
> *our dreamer*

And, in Dora's head, poignantly: *a so-called childhood*

At the end of the second event, the painting was discussed by the panellists and attendees. One observation was that painting the dream onto the pages of Freud, and with some of Freud's words taken from that context and incorporated into the emergent artwork, captured symbolically our prioritising of Dora and her life and dreams, above the often theoretical and conjectural record of the case study.

Summary

Although Freud did have oppressive and patriarchal judgements of Dora, he did believe that Dora was subjected to what he called 'persecution' by Herr K. We must credit Freud for that, and for recording, and interpreting the two dreams of Dora, on the basis of her free associations and her waking life, even though his own associations may overshadow that success and instead relate the dreams to unconfirmable unconscious processes. It does seem that the two dreams do depict, each in a vivid metaphorical way, Dora's life and circumstances at the time she had the dreams.

Note: The films of the two events and the films of the two dreams being read from the Sigmund Freud Museum, Vienna, can be seen on the DreamsID YouTube channel.

Acknowledgements: Some of this chapter was published by Lockheart et al. (2021) in the *International Journal of Dream Research*. We thank the journal for the helpful reviewer and editor comments. We also thank the authors of the paper, who at the two commemoration events contributed some of the ideas that we have included in this chapter. We also thank the Sigmund Freud Museum, Vienna, for their support for the two events.

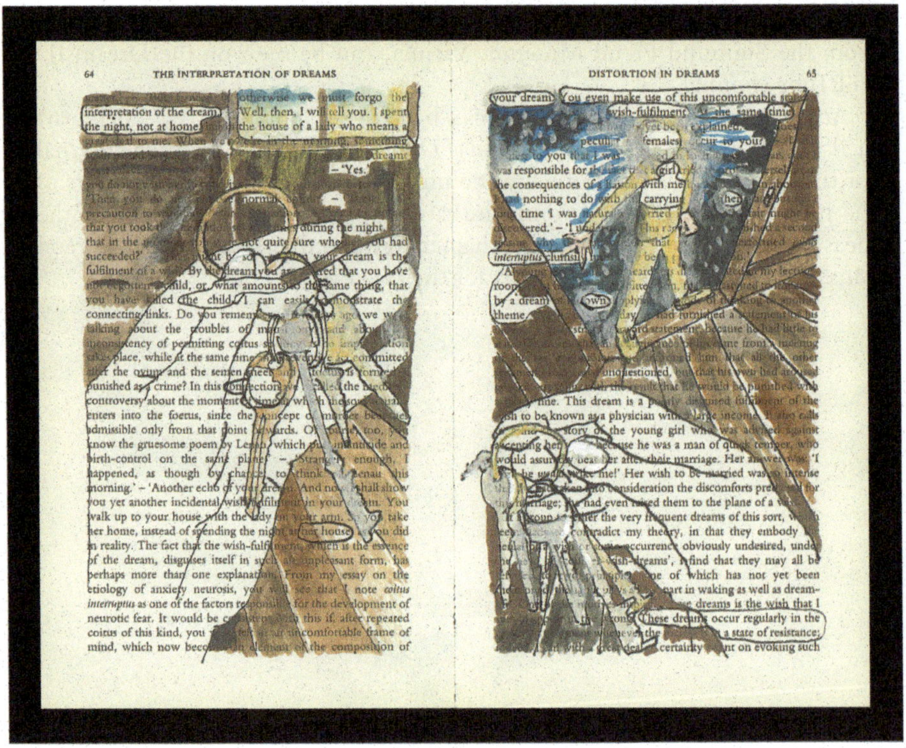

Figure 10.1 Dream of choosing between known and unknown keys, 2022.

10 How to find meaning in dreams

The Montague Ullman dream appreciation method

This dream of Lea Shaw, mezzo-soprano with Scottish Opera, was told to us in an online event organised by the company, which is the national opera company of Scotland. It illustrates the use of the Ullman method to obtain information about the dream and then about recent waking life experiences, so as to relate the dream to the dreamer's waking life.

DREAM NARRATIVE: *I am in a house with dark wood panelling and a wooden floor. There is a window that looks onto brightness outside. I know that the house is my home. I have two sets of keys, one in either hand. The set in my left-hand is familiar, the right-hand set is unfamiliar and has many more keys on it, some are small and some are large. I spend a minute trying to figure out which set of keys is for the big door I'm standing by, and I settle on the big unfamiliar ring of keys. I open the door, which leads onto space, with stars. At the door there's a little kid facing me, and I know it's me, but it has no features, it's just a small mass of light. It takes my hand and I step through, step out, and then I wake up.*

DISCUSSION: Lea had this dream when production and rehearsals were just starting for the opera *A Midsummer Night's Dream*, in which she was performing the role of Hermia. In the discussion, Lea spoke of the array of choices and possibilities that occur at the start of a production, and that this array might be depicted metaphorically in the dream by the set of unfamiliar keys. We also discussed the possibility that the metal lock keys might even be depicting the different musical keys of the opera. The wooden floor in the dream could thus be a reference to the operatic stage. Lea spoke of the interests she had as a child, including her interest in outer space, how she first went to performances at that age, and of how proud she as a child would be of her older self.

JULIA: (Painting shown as Figure 10.1) I chose two pages so that the left-hand page would have undivided text on which to represent the left hand and one set of keys, and the right-hand page would have a large bottom paragraph on which to paint the right hand and its keys, with a smaller paragraph above for the body and head of the child. The painting is composed so that the two hands curve together, and with the upwards side of the left hand following the left vertical edge of the text.

DOI: 10.4324/9781003037552-10

During the painting process words that I found on the page were incorporated into the artwork. Notable are two found poems.

In the window:

interpretation of the dream
the night, not at home
the house of a lady

And around and in the head and body of the child:

your dream
You even make use of this uncomfortable
time
wish-fulfilment
yet
females
girl
with me
carrying

From the last two chapters, we have shown the way in which tracing elements of a dream backwards to waking life experiences can provide or suggest meaning for the dream. For people in everyday life, there will often be the wish to consider a dream and its relationship to waking life, and so it is necessary to understand a method for doing this that explores a dream systematically and does not rely on using dream dictionaries that attempt to specify particular meanings for particular dream contents. Note that Freud opposed such dream dictionaries because they could not tailor a meaning of any part of a dream to the individual, a failing that results from not using the free association method.

The Ullman group dream discussion method

The method for dream appreciation and exploration described in this chapter is widely used worldwide, and was devised by psychoanalyst and psychiatrist Montague Ullman (1916–2008). It enables lay people to explore a dream in a group, or at least with one other person, because gentle questioning of the dreamer may lead to areas and topics that the dreamer had not thought of. Montague Ullman was president of the Society of Medical Psychoanalysts, and a Life Fellow of the American Psychiatric Association. Following his medical degree, he completed his psychoanalytic training at the New York Medical College, where he then served on the psychoanalytic faculty. However, as well as his professional practice, Montague held lay dream groups and wished to enable dream appreciation and the understanding of dreams to occur outside professional environments. He developed the technique described here over many years, resulting in the book *Appreciating Dreams: A Group Approach* (1996/2006). The book is very detailed, but accessible on the components of the method, the rationales behind it and on case studies that demonstrate its use.

The method is used for reasons of personal growth and self-understanding, rather than for therapeutic reasons, although therapeutic effects can no doubt occur. The method has two guiding principles:

> Safety – to ensure that the dreamer is happy or content in all that they are disclosing; and
> Curiosity – in which the group members gently and sensitively ask questions about the dream and about the dreamer's waking life.

The Ullman technique is structured with strictly defined stages so that information about the dream and about the dreamer's waking life is elicited separately. These two areas of experience are explored separately as fully as possible before they are compared and matched in the 'orchestration' stage (Stage 3B.3, described below). The theoretical basis for the method is that unresolved areas of recent emotional waking life, and especially from the day and evening before the dream, are the most likely to provide the content and motive force for the dream.

A note first on how to increase the chances of remembering a dream on waking up. We recommend making a voice recording of a dream on waking, with eyes shut, if possible, to remove all external stimuli. In line with the Ullman technique, this should be done without any considerations of a possible meaning of the dream or of trying to work out a meaning for the dream. It should also be done without consideration of whether the dream is even worth recording, it is important to put aside evaluations of the dream having an obvious meaning or no meaning at all, either of these evaluations can discourage the dreamer from making the effort to recall and record the dream. Instead, the aim should simply be to record the dream, and to then transcribe it.

The following is a summary of the technique that will then be applied to the dream. Page numbers are taken from the 2006 edition of *Appreciating Dreams: A Group Approach*. The technique can be done speedily, in about 20 minutes, if done with a partner or friend. Or it can take up to 60 minutes if the dream is long or is considered by a group that meets to discuss group members' dreams. If done in a group, it can be that more than one person wishes to share a dream. So as to decide which dream to explore each person can give a brief summary of their dream, and then the possible dream-sharers can be asked if they still have some urgency for their own dream to be explored, or if they would like one of the other dreams to be explored instead. The whole group can also be asked which of the dreams has more resonance for them, and a consensus or vote can decide which dream to choose. It can also be helpful to give preference to the dream that is the most

108   *How to find meaning in dreams*

recent, as the feelings of the dream, and the memory of the day before the dream, will be stronger.

Stages of the Ullman group dream discussion method

In the following, group can also refer to a partner or friend. Note that it can be helpful for those hearing the dream to write it down, as this can help to ensure that all components of the dream are paid attention to and addressed.

1: The dream is told by the dreamer as fully as possible, including what emotions were felt while the dream was happening, and the places, people and actions in the dream. The group members then ask clarifying questions, so as to make sure that the report is complete. Questions can include the setting of the dream, colours, time of day, weather, age of the characters, or emotions in the dream. It is important not to ask about any meaning or waking life referents of components of the dream, unless these are needed to help define the components.

2: The dreamer listens while the group members briefly treat the dream as if it were their own and generate their own projections onto it. Ullman calls this an 'exercise or game' (p.33). The friend or group members give their own views of the dream report and of how it would feel if they had had that dream, or what it would mean to them in terms of their own life if they had had the dream. Ullman suggests that the phrase 'If it were my dream …' can be used here so as to emphasise that the projections onto the dream by a friend or group members are their own projections coming from their own life, and are not to be taken as suggesting a meaning that may be true for the dream-sharer's life. To reinforce this, Ullman states that the group members should not look at the dream-sharer during this stage.

   This stage gets all the group members involved with the dream and often results in very different reactions to the dream from the different group members. This stage provides a pool of ideas that the dream-sharer might not have thought of in trying to make sense of the dream because other people will come up with different emphases and associations to the dream.

3A: The dream is returned to the dreamer so that they can respond to whatever was said in Stage 2. In some instances how a group member feels about or experiences the dream, or how they interpret the dream in terms of their own life, can be relevant to the dreamer. At other times the experience of the group member is not relevant, or is even opposite to how the dreamer sees the dream. The dreamer can agree with, disagree with, comment about, or not comment about, anything that was said.

3B.1: The dream-sharer tells of their recent thoughts and feelings prior to the dream, so as to provide or search for a waking life context for the dream. They then talk about what was on their mind in the days before the dream. The dream-sharer can talk about conversations, events, concerns or things they experienced, on the day before the dream and on the days before that, and, in particular on the evening before falling asleep. It is important at first that the dream-sharer does not think of the dream while relating what had been experienced over the days before the dream, these experiences might not be relevant to the dream but sometimes there is an inadvertent discovery of a source of the dream. The dream-sharer can also free associate to elements of the dream, stating what comes to mind in response to each item of the dream. It may help for a group member to ask 'When you consider the dream and the feelings in the dream, and you think back on what was on your mind the previous day, is there anything you'd like to say about that?'

3B.2 A group member reads back the dream report to the dream-sharer in the second person (e.g., 'You're at a dance. You walk to the centre of the room'). They should ensure to stop frequently to allow the dreamer to add any new details either about the dream or about what they remember had been happening to them in waking life in the days before the dream.

3B.3 The dream-sharer and group members should discuss any connections they can make between the dream report and the waking life background and recent events, experiences, conceptualisations and concerns of the dream-sharer. The purpose of this step is to discover any metaphorical or literal connections between the dream and the dream-sharer's recent waking life experiences and emotions. The dream-sharer and group members thus all attempt to connect 'image and reality' (p.90).

Note that the group can only discuss or comment on what the dream-sharer has said in reporting the dream, and anything the dream-sharer has said about their waking life, during the previous steps, unless new ideas come to mind for the dream-sharer in this stage. This restriction provides a constraint on the projections or conjectures being offered to the dream-sharer.

4: At a subsequent session, the dreamer can share further thoughts about the dream with the group, including whether any realisations have occurred about the meaning or significance of the dream.

To reiterate, it is very important that the above sequence and content of stages are adhered to because problems arise if the dream discussion becomes unstructured or amorphous. If that occurs, information about the dream or about the dreamer's waking life can be missed. The Ullman method can be seen as a systematic gathering of two types of information, about the dream and about waking life, and these two explorations need to be held distinct so as to ensure that each is thorough and focussed on its aim.

Relating characters in dreams to the dreamer's waking life

The Ullman method for appreciating dreams does not utilise any more extensive theorising derived from the many psychotherapeutic and psychoanalytic traditions and schools. However, one approach to considering the characters found in a dream, that of Jung (1948/2002a) in his *General aspects of dream psychology*, can be useful. Jung acknowledged that free associations can lead to memories of waking life individuals and their relationships to the dreamer, which he termed interpretation on the 'objective level', but he also posited that there can be interpretation on the subjective level, which 'conceives all the figures in the dream as personified features of the dreamer's own personality.' (p.54.) He proposed that objective interpretations are more likely if the character in the dream is connected to the dreamer in waking life by a 'vital interest', but a subjective level interpretation may be favoured 'if I dream of a person who is not important to me in reality' (p.55).

Initial assessment of dreamers' self-understanding following Ullman dream group sessions

As a result of taking part in dream groups at the conferences of the International Association for the Study of Dreams, Mark obtained training in the technique in 2009 and started to hold an Ullman dream group for students at Swansea University. In 2010, with Josie Henley-Einion, he published the following findings from a series of the dream groups. The groups discussed 22 dreams of 13 dream-sharers using the Ullman technique, each dream-sharer had a discussion lasting 45–75 minutes, for one or two dreams. Using a scale from 0 to 100, dream-sharers responded to the question 'Did the session for this dream give you new understanding or insight about yourself or about any aspect of your life?' On this measure the mean score was 57.0 (SD = 15.5) (Blagrove et al., 2010). The sessions were thus useful for increasing self-understanding of the dream-sharers, and indeed had led to wonderful and insightful discussions about dreams. More extensive and controlled studies on the insight and self-understanding that result from Ullman dream discussions are presented in the next chapter.

The relationship of the 'If It Were My Dream' stage to the other stages of the Ullman method

Unfortunately there is a common problem that can occur with the running of groups that claim to be following the Ullman method, or with groups that have adapted the method. This relates to Stage 2 of the method, which is the brief stage where members of the group treat the dream as if it were their own. What can occur is that this brief stage can sometimes expand to take up much of the allotted time, and group members might also use the technique of this stage during or instead of the other Ullman method stages. This means that the group members are then concentrating on themselves, and their own lives, rather than on the dream and life of the dreamer. Indeed, some dream group leaders advertise themselves as using what they call a 'If It Were My Dream' method, rather than this being seen as just one component of a more systematic method.

It is important to appreciate that the stage where group members imagine the dreamer's dream as if it were their own is very important in encouraging group members to fully engage with the dream as an experience, rather than solely as a dream to be interpreted. We will return to this phenomenological aspect of the method at the end of Chapter 16. However, although the stage is very beneficial for group members and for the overall process, issues can arise in how it is implemented.

In a symposium titled *Diverse Applications of Montague Ullman's Seminal Work* at the 26th Annual Conference of the International Association for the Study of Dreams, in June 2009, in Chicago, Gloria Sturzenacker presented a paper titled: 'The Ullman method: influential and often misunderstood' (Sturzenacker, 2009). In it she said:

> The Ullman Method is widely known in name, but not in essence. Its safety and discovery factors result from unfolding a dream in carefully delineated stages. Although the entire process follows the dreamer's lead, the familiar 'If this were my dream' is associated with a limited part of it.

From the point of hearing that paper, Mark began to wonder whether the 'carefully delineated stages' of Ullman's method might indeed be less well known than the minor, but frequently over-emphasised, 'If this were my dream' stage.

'If this were my dream' is used in Stage 2 of the Ullman method, but is used in some dream groups outside Stage 2, and Ullman warned that that should not occur. Stage 2 starts the process of associations for the group, it shows the dreamer that we can all make meaningful associations and that everyone is engaged with the dream they have just been told. The phrasing of the instructions for the stage also makes clear that group members are not seeking to impose interpretations of the dream onto the dreamer.

Ullman wrote of Stage 2 of his technique that the dreamer is told 'The group is going to make your dream its own. They are going to work with it as their dream' (p.32). The group is told

> You are now asked to try to make the dream your own. In some instances, you will find it relatively easy to superimpose your own past experience onto the dream and share the feelings and meanings that emerge. In other instances, this may not be easy. In that case, just use your imagination to see what you can do with the imagery.
>
> (pp.33–34)

Ullman then states:

'Throughout the time you are working with the dream as your own, it is imperative that you not address your thoughts to the dreamer. ... Make a conscious effort not to look at the dreamer as you offer your projections' (p.34). However, Ullman warns that in this stage group members might forget to talk about the dream as if it were their own,

> people will look at the dreamer and offer their remarks directly to him. Even though they may be using the first person, their intent is obviously to get something across to the dreamer. They are trespassing into the free space around the dreamer we spoke about.
>
> (p.39)

Ullman goes on to further warn that this stage can take up 'a disproportionate amount of time', that more important stages follow this stage, and that 'the group enjoys playing the game with someone else's dream and can go on and on with it' (p.40). In contrast, what should happen is that, when it becomes time to terminate this brief stage, 'we return the dream to the dreamer' (p.41), and there is then 'a change in mind-set on the part of the group members from being involved with their own thoughts to now listening' (p.53).

A concern arises, therefore, that in many supposed Ullman groups, the dream is not fully returned to the dreamer, and the group's enjoyment of the game of 'if this were my dream' carries on, even if intermittently, for the whole session. And Ullman alerts us to this. In his introduction to Stage 3, he states:

> The work in Stage 2 has stimulated many ideas in your mind about what the dream means. Fine! But keep them in the back of your mind – far back. ... Remember, the dream is coming out of the unique life experiences of the dreamer, not out of your life. If you are to be successful in helping the dreamer get at those experiences, your orientation has to be to the life of the dreamer.
>
> (p.59)

In the orchestration Stage 3B.3, the group members 'offer the connections they see between the images in the dream and those aspects of the dreamer's life that have been shared' (p.91). Ullman again cautions that here, unlike in Stage 2,

> You [the group members] are not being given free reign to express your ideas about the dream. You are being asked to help in fleshing out the metaphorical potential of someone else's dream, based on information you have been given by that person.
>
> (p.92)

He then proceeds to state:

> A common error is to continue to think of the dream as your own and to base your orchestrating projection not on what the dreamer has shared but on the continuing thoughts about your own life set off by the dreamer.
>
> (pp.92–93)

Ullman accepts that projections can occur during the orchestration, but these are given in a 'qualitatively different way than when the group members made the dream their own (Stage 2)' (p.96). Unlike in Stage 2, the projections now 'are offered directly to the dreamer and are built up on the basis of what the dreamer has told us' (p.98). He later states that a 'serious difficulty' can arise if a group member

> is still playing the game (Stage 2) and is talking about the dream as his or her own. It is difficult for some to realize that, *once we return the dream to the dreamer at the end of the second stage, it is no longer our dream*. They lose sight of the fact that they are to try to connect what the dreamer said to what the dream is saying.
>
> (p.101, our italics)

He then states clearly: 'The dream is no longer yours' (p.102).

The Ullman method has the aim of drawing links between the dream and the *dreamer's* waking life. The use of the 'If this were my dream…' phrase outside Stage 2 runs counter to that aim. Mark discussed some of this with fellow dream enthusiasts at a subsequent IASD conference, and was told that the 'If this were my dream…' phrase can be used so as not to make the dreamer feel pressured about accepting a particular view of the dream. But Mark's view was that the phrase, if used outside of Stage 2, can surely only diminish our concentration on the dreamer's life. Obviously, suggestions to the dreamer of how the dream may be connected to the dreamer's waking life must be done respectfully, gently and without the use of leading questions, and Ullman goes to great length in *Appreciating Dreams* to explain how this gentle non-leading questioning of the dreamer can be done. But using the phrase 'If this were my dream…' is not suggested as a way of gentle non-leading questioning. Ullman suggests that the Stage 2/Game part of his technique, although valuable and important, should last what is just one-sixth of the total time that the group examines a dream (p.41), and the use of the phrase 'If this were my dream…', should thus be only a minor part of the overall process, and used in only one part of it.

Other methods of finding meaning in dreams

Other methods for finding meaning in dreams are described in Ellis (2020), Hill (2004) and Leonard and Dawson (2018). Some of these methods are more appropriate within psychotherapy rather than lay use. The Leonard and Dawson paper also addresses why clinical psychology has deemphasised dreams, and examines the cultural-historical reasons for this, including the scientist-practitioner model, and the identification of psychology with behaviourism and the natural sciences.

Summary

The Ullman dream appreciation method allows the dreamer and individuals discussing the dream with the dreamer, to elicit as much detail as possible about the dream and about the dreamer's waking life, separately, so as to enable discussion about possible literal and metaphorical relationships between the dream and the dreamer's recent waking life. It is important that the stages of the method are carried out as Ullman designed them, including that the stage in which group members consider the dream as if it were their own is kept brief. We conducted initial work with positive findings on assessing self-understanding and insight that result from using the Ullman method to discuss dreams, and the extension of that research to controlled studies is described in the next chapter.

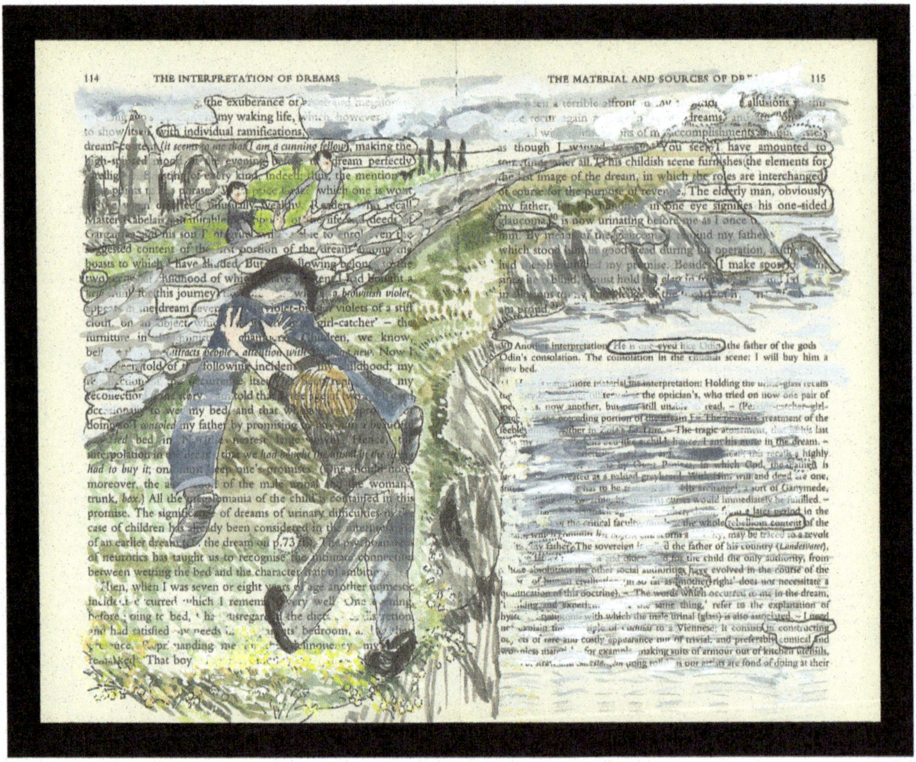

Figure 11.1 Dream of pulling through from Covid-19, 2021.

11 Dreaming and insight

This dream, of author and poet Michael Rosen, illustrates how dreams often depict waking life concerns and experiences in a metaphorical way.

DREAM NARRATIVE (Rosen, 2021, pp.231–232)

> We were at Land's End.
> We climbed over a stone wall.
> On the other side,
> I noticed that we were at the top of a cliff:
> sheer drop, hundreds of feet down.
> I said that I wanted to go back
> over the wall
> but I noticed a big hole in the wall.
> I squeezed into it so that I could get through
> but got stuck.
> I shouted to you: 'Push, Emma! Push!'
> You did.
> But I couldn't get through.
> Then I noticed that there were people
> walking around.
> It was a space like a ruined church
> made suitable for visitors
> with surfaced walkways.
> I called out to someone:
> 'Can you pull me through?'
> He tried but he couldn't.
> I felt so helpless
> and I was worried about you
> at the top of that cliff.
> You were still pushing.
> Then I called out to another person
> in the ruined church.
> He got hold of me
> and pulled me through.

DOI: 10.4324/9781003037552-11

118   *Dreaming and insight*

'Dream' from *Many Different Kinds of Love* by Michael Rosen published by Ebury Press. Copyright © Michael Rosen, 2021. Reprinted by permission of The Random House Group Limited and United Agents on behalf of Michael Rosen.

DISCUSSION: The dream was told to us at the Freud Museum London by author and poet Michael Rosen, with a worldwide online audience participating in the discussion. He had nearly died from Covid-19 during the early part of the pandemic and wrote a book about it, *Many Different Kinds of Love: A Story of Life, Death and the NHS*. The book tells of the care he received from the staff at the hospital and from his family. It also recounts several dreams he had during his recovery. We discussed the above dream and the metaphor of 'pulling through'. Michael stated that he was indeed physically stuck, motionless, on his bed at the hospital while he was recovering, but that he also 'pulled through' the illness, recovering with the help of many others. He also told us of having gone over a fence to get to cliffs when a boy, and that the church in the dream was similar to the coastal monastery ruins at Lindisfarne which he had previously visited with his family.

JULIA: (Painting shown as Figure 11.1) The painting depicts Michael Rosen's wife pushing him through the hole in the wall, the two men pulling him from the other side, and the church, coastline and cliffs.

As a result of his Covid-19 infection, Michael Rosen had glaucoma in one eye. My painting by chance has the following words near the cliffs, incorporated as a found poem:

The elderly man, obviously
one eye signifies his one-sided
glaucoma
He is one-eyed like Odin.

Also incorporated into the painting are the following words, relevant to Michael Rosen being famously lively and spritely:

the exuberance of my waking life

And, regarding the words:

I am a cunning fellow

Michael Rosen told us that in the dream he thought of himself as clever for deciding to go through the wall as opposed to over it, which may also be a reference to his famous book *We're Going on a Bear Hunt*.

The painting also incorporated near his and his wife's legs:

73

which was Michael Rosen's age at catching Covid-19.

Personal and group reactions to dreams

Although Mark's research since his PhD finished in 1989 had involved experiments on sleep, dreaming and memory, in 2008 he started to attend morning dream groups at the International Association for the Study of Dreams (IASD) annual conferences. He did this out of an interest in claims being made at the conferences that discussing dreams could result in personal insight for the dreamer, claims that went beyond the standard scientific questions of the relationship of dreams to the brain during sleep and to prior waking life experiences and variables. It was also because Mark had written a paper, with well-known sceptic Professor Chris French, on why some people believe in precognitive dreams (Blagrove et al., 2006). On the latter, Mark was interested in confabulation, how people can believe that any text, such as horoscopes and Tarot cards, is meaningful and specific to themselves. In that paper, 386 participants were interviewed about their experience of dreams that seem to predict an event in the future, and their belief about whether such dreams can be explained naturally or paranormally. Participants were also asked to answer three simple personal questions: whether they have a cat, whether they have a scar on their left knee, and whether they have back pain at the moment. They were each given a score for the number of affirmative answers they gave to the three questions.

It was found that experiencers of and believers in precognitive dreams were more likely to answer 'yes' to the three simple personal questions than were non-experiencers and non-believers. Blagrove and colleagues explained this in their 2006 paper as due to some people having an affirmative bias. In other words, if you are asked simple questions about your body that look objective, some people tend to agree with the questions, or, as that sounds a little like calling them suggestible, we can say they find ways of being cognitively flexible so as to define themselves as, say, owning a cat, or having back pain. This affirmative bias, or cognitive flexibility, also then occurs when they consider whether they have had a dream that has predicted the future, they find a way of relating the dream to a future event. These findings led Mark to be somewhat sceptical when people claim to have obtained some personal meaning from a dream, as ascribed meaning may have been due to how flexible they were in relating the dream to aspects of their life. Such scepticism regarding how people can confabulate or read into a dream, so that they construct a plausible interpretation and connection to themselves, is similar to the approach taken by Timpanaro, described in Chapter 8, and has parallels with the Barnum or Forer (1949) effect. In this effect, different people are each able to believe that the same text is an accurate description of themselves, an effect that Forer described as due to gullibility.

And so, at the 2008 IASD conference in Montreal, Mark attended a morning dream group run by Swiss psychotherapist Art Funkhouser, who combines Ullman and Jungian methods in a supportive and gentle manner. At one of the dream groups that week only Mark had had a dream that morning, but he thought it was too short and too bizarre to have any sense. However, he told it as no other dream was available. (As described in Chapter 10, the Ullman method has a preference for the 'freshest' dream available, as the feelings of the dream and the memory of the day before it are then strongest.)

In the dream Mark was being given a collection of CDs, with the top one having on it a Rembrandt-like (self-) portrait, with a big floppy hat, looking proud and calm. Written on the CD, either on the side or above the portrait, was the word Rembrandt or Rembrandts. In the dream, Mark wondered if this is the same Rembrandts as did the theme tune to *Friends*.

Mark and the group could find little sense in the dream until someone asked whether the hat was like a professor's hat. From there the dream became very meaningful and very poignant. Mark had just been promoted to Professor (hence the hat) and Head of Department at his University. There was also the realisation near the end of the dream group of the association of the portrait and the music group to REM, as in REMbrandt! There were many other poignant memory sources and family associations, which Mark reported in the article *Dreaming – motivated or meaningless?*, with the full text of the dream, in *The Psychologist*, professional magazine of the British Psychological Society (Blagrove, 2009).

Until these events, the aim at the Swansea University Sleep Laboratory had been to study dream content using the numerical coding of dreams, such as in quantifying emotions in dreams, or investigating how long dream reports are in the number of words, or why some people have more nightmares than others, or have more lucid dreams. As described in Chapter 1, other work addressed how incorporations of waking life experiences into dreams can be identified. Mark's experiences of dream groups, however, led to a different question. What if, after the dream is studied for an experiment, it is returned to the dreamer and discussed in an open-ended way, asking where its components might have come from, and what sense the dreamer could make of the dream. Making the transition from highly controlled, often physiologically based studies, of sleep and dreaming, to work on how the dreamer, with the help of others, makes sense of the dream, would not have occurred without the eclectic mixture of disciplines and people that gather at IASD conferences. There is a clinical literature on insight resulting from the consideration of dreams, but so as to address this experimentally, we developed a long research programme on the effects of the group discussion of dreams.

We used the Ullman technique in doing this, and then published papers (with PhD student Chris Edwards) on the outcomes of these Ullman discussions.

Outcomes were assessed by using Clara Hill's *Gains from Dream Interpretation* questionnaire (Heaton et al., 1998). After each discussion, the dream-sharer completed this 13-item questionnaire, which uses a nine-point scale for responses to each item, so as to assess whether the dream-sharer considers there have been benefits from the discussion of the dream. The questionnaire gives three scores: exploration-insight gains, action gains and experiential gains. The exploration-insight subscale combines scores for engagement in the exploration process, for having insight into the memory sources of the dream, and insight about the self, and it is this subscale that we were most interested in for the three experiments reported in this chapter. These are the items, numbered according to their position in the questionnaire:

1 I was able to explore my dream thoroughly during the session.
2 I learned more about what this dream meant for me personally during the session.
6 I learned more from the session about how past events influence my present behaviour.
7 I learned more about issues in my waking life from working with the dream.
8 I felt like I was very involved in working with the dream during the session.
12 I learned things that I would not have thought of on my own.
13 I was able to make some connections, that I had not previously considered, between images in my dream and issues in my waking life.

The experiential subscale comprises two items: 'During the session, I was able to re-experience the feelings I had in my dream' and 'I felt like I was actually reliving the dream during the session'. This subscale was used to test whether the dream-sharer had fully engaged with the dream during the discussion. We were less interested in the action gains score, as this is related to whether the dreamer will make changes to their life as a result of the discussion, and is more relevant to discussions about dreams that occur in psychotherapy rather than in a dream appreciation session designed by Ullman for laypeople.

Experiment 1 on home dreams and insight

In the first experiment we had 11 participants, all students, and each met separately with Mark and Chris Edwards to discuss a dream. Having only two people to discuss each dream was necessary so as to keep the group characteristics constant each time it met with a new dreamer. Before sharing the dream, at the start of the session, the dream-sharer completed Cernovsky's (1984) *Attitude toward Dreams* questionnaire. This has 16 items that participants rate their level of agreement or disagreement with, such as 'there is something strange about people who tell their dreams', or 'listening to people's dreams is 'interesting' or 'I would like to learn more about my dreams'. This questionnaire measures whether people have a positive or negative attitude towards dreams.

The dreamer would then read out loud their dream and the Ullman group procedure was followed for about 50 minutes. They then completed the Gains from Dream Interpretation questionnaire.

The results were that the participants gave high ratings for the exploration-insight gains from participating in the dream appreciation group, and these were comparable to gain scores obtained when psychotherapy clients discuss a dream with a therapist, such as in the research of Clara Hill (2004), using her cognitive-experiential therapeutic method for working with dreams. These ratings showed the Ullman method to be an effective procedure for establishing connections between waking life and dream experiences. We also found that the relationship between one's own attitude towards dreams assessed before the group was significantly correlated with exploration-insight gains (with a very strong relationship of Spearman's rho = 0.68), so people with a more positive view towards dreams had higher exploration-insight scores as a result of the discussion.

Many of the participants had an 'aha' experience when discussing their dream. We realised that there is a distinction between having an 'aha' insight about the sources in recent waking life of an item of dream content and having an 'aha' insight about oneself. The latter, for example, could be a realisation that something is really on one's mind, or a realisation that the dream is giving a new metaphor about waking life that provides restructuring of waking life knowledge. But we were finding that this may require a lengthy examination of a dream for such emotional insight to be obtained, and that sometimes the dreamer only spots that something in a dream is connected to waking life when somebody else asks a question, or makes a suggestion about the dream content.

Although this study, published as Edwards and colleagues (2013), found a high level of exploration-insight as a result of discussions of dreams, there was no control condition in the study, there was instead a comparison with scores obtained from therapeutic studies by Hill. This is important because we need control conditions to show that there is something specific about discussing dreams for obtaining such insight, as opposed to, say, discussing a reading of tarot cards. Tarot cards can cue personal discussions, and so sceptics could claim that dreams do nothing more than tarot cards can do, in eliciting conversations and self-disclosure.

Experiment 2 on home dreams, waking life events and insight

We therefore did a further study (Edwards et al., 2015) in which we again had people coming to the psychology department to talk about a recent dream using the Ullman technique. But we also asked them to report a recent personally important waking life event, and the Ullman procedure was used for the separate discussion of that event as well. So as to conduct the experiment rigorously, half the participants discussed an event before discussing a dream, and half discussed a dream and then discussed an event: this is termed counterbalancing.

We found that the discussion of a dream led to greater exploration-insight scores than did the discussion of the recent personally important event, where both were discussed using the Ullman technique. Very importantly, we also used a measure of personal insight, defined as the total of the scores on items of the Gains from Dream Interpretation questionnaire relevant to getting ideas for changing aspects of one's life, learning a new way of thinking about oneself, learning how past events influence current behaviour, learning about issues in one's life and intending to use what was learned in the discussion in one's life.

This measure of personal insight was significantly higher after discussing a dream than after discussing a recent personally significant event. It is as if during sleep our brains and our dreams filter our waking life experiences and concerns so as to create dreams based on what is emotionally important to us during the day (see Chapter 1), and so discussion of the usually metaphorical representation of these distilled experiences in dreams results in more personal insight than the discussion of a recent meaningful event. There is obviously a problem, however, in that these studies cannot be done double-blind, which is the gold standard for an experiment, and requires neither the participant nor the experimenter to know what experimental condition the participant is in. In this study, the experimenters did know whether a dream or an important event was being discussed, and also, the dream-sharer knows they are telling and discussing a dream, and they may have cultural beliefs that dreams are an important source of self-knowledge. That such cultural beliefs about dreams are widespread has been shown by Morewedge and Norton (2009). They investigated laypeople's interpretation of their dreams, finding that participants in both Eastern and Western cultures believe that dreams contain hidden truths and that dreams provide meaningful information about the world.

Experiment 3 on REM and NREM dreams, daydreams and insight

The dreams that were shared in the 2013 and 2015 experiments occurred to participants sleeping at home. It is likely that most such dreams were Rapid Eye Movement (REM) dreams, but our next question was whether the discussion of REM dreams would result in a different exploration-insight score than would the discussion of Non-Rapid Eye Movement (NREM) dreams. A reason to think they would differ is the role of REM sleep in processing emotional events, which would suggest an advantage for discussing REM dreams in comparison to NREM dreams. REM dreams also tend to be longer than NREM dreams, and so might provide more material from which to elicit personal insights. Conversely, Domhoff's (2001, 2019) neurocognitive view downplays such sleep stage differences, and so would predict little difference in outcomes from discussing REM and NREM dreams, at least when reports are of similar length.

We therefore undertook a sleep lab study, reported in Blagrove et al. (2019a), in which people would be woken from REM sleep and from N2 sleep, the main light form of NREM sleep (see Chapter 4), and the dreams from each stage would later be discussed. Using a counterbalanced method, we woke up half our participants for a dream report after ten minutes of N2 sleep, let them go back to sleep, and then woke them ten minutes into a REM sleep period for a dream report; the other half of participants would be woken in the order REM sleep and then NREM sleep. As well as knowing the stage of sleep that each dream was from, doing the study in the sleep lab also had another advantage, because we were able to collect daydream reports from participants before they fell asleep for the night. We did this as follows. As usual, we wired up each participant and had them lie down in one of the bedrooms. We asked them to remain awake while we checked the wires and connections and then told them that we would practice the protocol for the night, which would involve playing a buzzer and then asking them to report what was going through their minds before the buzzer. We asked them to do this as a practice session, for using the intercom and recording devices. We then let them lie awake for ten minutes in the dark, and at the end of this period played the buzzer, and hence obtained a daydream report following the ten minutes of EEG recorded wakefulness, just as we would later in the night get REM and NREM dream reports after ten minutes in each sleep stage. The EEG recording also ensured that for the daydream condition they were in fact awake for the whole ten minutes.

Thirty-one participants were cued in the sleep laboratory for a daydream report and then awakened from REM and N2 sleep for dream reports. Participants subsequently discussed each of their dream and daydream reports for approximately 40 min each with Chris Edwards and Mark Blagrove, following the Ullman procedure. After each discussion session, participants responded to the following question: 'Did you experience any realisation, or realisations, about yourself, or other people, or your life during the session you have just had? If "yes," please can you describe the realisation(s) and when and how the realisation(s) happened?' Realisations about the self or the dream or the relationship of the dream to waking life occurred in approximately two-thirds of the discussions of REM dreams, which was higher than for N2 dreams and daydreams, although this difference was not statistically significant.

To illustrate a realisation and its relationship to the dream report and discussion, the following is an example of a participant's dream report from this study, a summary of the discussion, and the participant's realisation report. The participant had recently moved from the family home to start being a student at Swansea University.

Dream report: *I was at home and found my dog in a chair. My dog was scared because it was thunder and lightning, I held my dog's mouth to stop her barking. I was carrying my dog around trying to calm her down and then I found the half-eaten bacon sandwich in my room, fed that to my dog and then she wasn't shaking anymore. I walked downstairs. It was like a grand staircase with like marble stairs. There were two people in my [university residence] hallway, next to the front door, talking, but one of them was someone who lives in the flat opposite, who was smoking and then I didn't know who the other one was, he smiled at me.*

In the discussion, we asked about grand staircases, marble staircases and marble, and elicited the following responses from the dreamer:

> I don't remember seeing any grand staircases during the week.
> I think it was like a marble-topped table, I think that comes from when we were on holiday [last family holiday before university] … there was a table [for the family meals] and it was, it was wooden on the inside but it had like kind of marble on the sides and on top.

The following is the participant's description of the realisation, written after the session:

> Linking the dream to be about family life and the change of home to University has made me realise that the nostalgia of my family back home has had a greater influence on me than I'd first thought.

It appeared that the marble-topped table at the final family holiday may have been incorporated into the dream as the marble stairs that connect home to university.

As well as the question of whether participants had obtained any insight from each discussion we also obtained scores on the Gains from Dream Interpretation questionnaire, with the phrasing of items amended to allow responses for the daydream discussions. On the exploration-insight subscale, we found no difference between REM and N2 dream discussions. We thus combined the REM and N2 scores together and compared them to the daydream discussion scores. Importantly, the dream and daydream discussions did not differ significantly on the participants' ratings of whether they explored the dream or daydream thoroughly during the session (item 1), or on the participants' ratings of having been very involved in working with the dream or daydream (item 8), and so the dream and daydream conditions were treated equally in the experiment. The important findings here were that dream discussions were scored higher on exploration-insight than were day-dream discussions, and that dream discussions were scored higher than daydream discussions on the following individual items, with effect size of the difference stated after each item:

> 'I learned more about what this (day)dream meant for me personally during the session', with a large effect size,

'I learned more about issues in my waking life from working with the (day)dream', with a small to medium effect size, and

'I learned things that I would not have thought of on my own', with a large effect size.

Dream discussions were also scored higher than daydream discussions, but not significantly so, on 'I was able to make some connections, that I had not previously considered, between images in my (day)dream and issues in my waking life'.

These findings of high ratings of exploration-insight after discussing dreams occurred even though participants did not select the dreams to discuss, as we had woken them for the dream report in the sleep lab. It may be that higher scores on exploration-insight or the presence of a realisation could be obtained if people choose which dream to discuss.

Relevant to this is the distinction made by Jung between little dreams and big dreams. He wrote in his paper 'On the nature of dreams' (1948/2002b, p.78) that 'not all dreams are of equal importance', and he distinguished 'little' and 'big' dreams; the little ones are less significant, easily forgotten, and their 'meaning is limited to the affairs of everyday'. Also of relevance is that only one or two dreams were discussed for each person: higher levels of exploration-insight or realisation may have been obtained from the discussion of a series of dreams. On this, Jung makes the point in his paper 'The practical use of dream analysis' (1931/2002, p.98) that 'I attach little importance to the interpretation of single dreams. ... the basic ideas and themes can be recognized much better in a dream-series'.

Insight and metaphor

We consider that as dreams are more metaphorical and non-literal than daydreams this may explain the higher exploration-insight scores for the dreams than for the daydreams. As part of the last study, independent judges were given the dream and daydream reports and rated the dream reports as having more movement and being more visual than were daydream reports, and we suggest that it is this physical environment that allows for metaphors to be experienced in an embodied and emotional manner in the dream.

Malinowski and Horton (2015) expand on the idea of dreams containing metaphors to claim that we assimilate emotions from the day into our wider and previous memory through such dream metaphors, in that we connect current events and concerns to similar events and concerns in the past through the 'hyper-associativity' of dreams. Waking life events and concerns and conceptualisations can thus be reframed in dreams in terms of metaphors or through connection to earlier memories. Dreams might thus indeed give us what Freud termed knowledge of unconscious processes, as they might enlighten us as to metaphors we are inadvertently following in waking life. It may even be that the dream gives the dreamer a new metaphor, which will provide some restructuring of waking life knowledge, and inspires a way to move forward and grow, even if the waking life issues that are referred to are quite well known, and already well considered in waking life.

The following is an example of this self-knowledge that can result from a dream metaphor. A dreamer reported that he had dreamt that he was typing a tweet, but in the second half of the tweet, he used all capital letters. He was told by a character in the dream that 'you shouldn't send tweets with capital letters because it sounds like shouting'. The person who had the dream had indeed in waking life been shouting at some family members during the previous day and so the dream acted as a reminder not to shout at people, as shouting is like sending a tweet with capital letters, something that is widely known to be inappropriate. The importance of this concrete metaphor is that the dreamer might have known about the need not to shout in waking life, but was now provided with a reminder in the metaphor of what that behaviour is like, and a vivid picture of its unacceptability that could come to mind or be brought to mind on future occasions.

Summary

The work reviewed here suggests that dreams can be a source of insight about the self. The work here also supports Ullman's contention that dreams are provoked by the emotional events and issues of recent days. Dreams do seem to act as pointers to implicit cognitions that we sometimes are not fully aware of, and seem to depict metaphorically our waking life conceptualisations and concerns. Given these characteristics of dreams, we address in the next chapter whether dreaming might have some adaptive function.

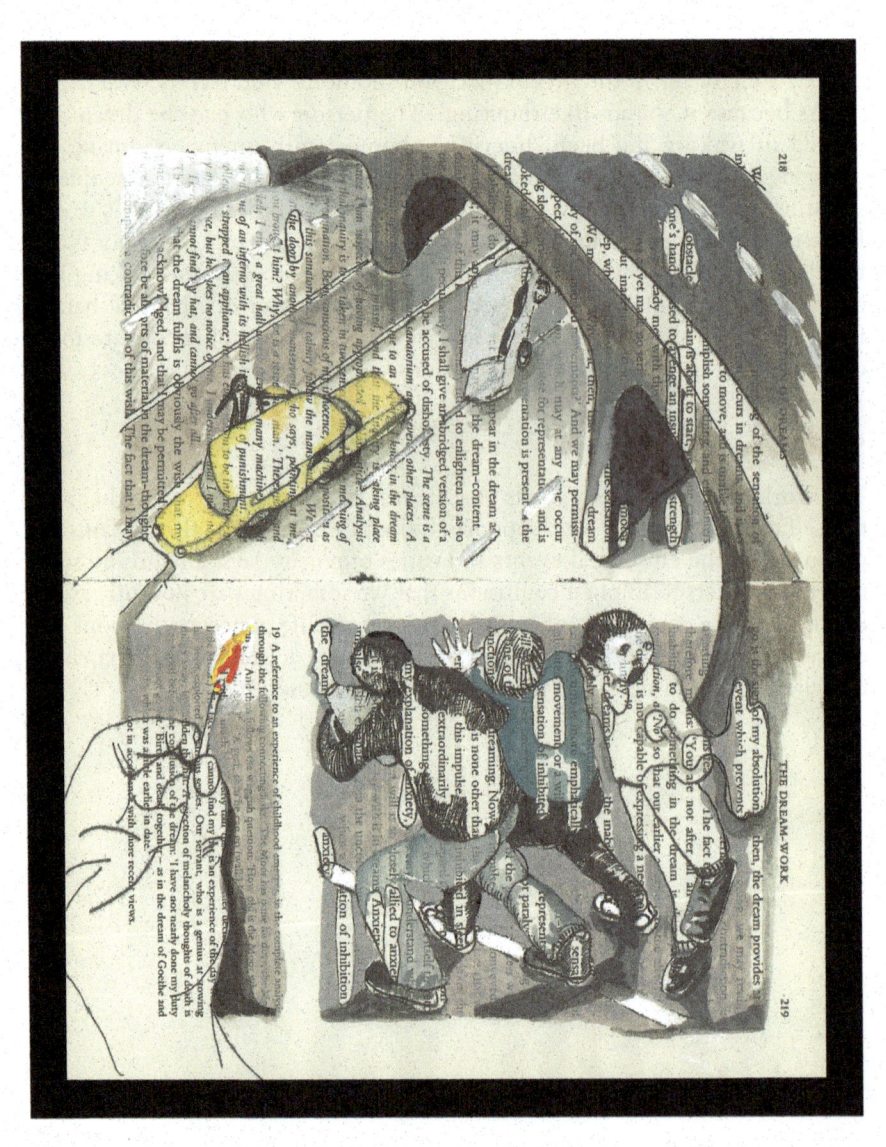

Figure 12.1 Dream of mother and daughter attacked on freeway, 2019.

12 Functions and theories of dreams

One proposed function of dreams is that in dreams we simulate and practise overcoming physical threats. This dream illustrates the Threat Simulation Theory.

DREAM NARRATIVE: *I am driving on a motorway or American freeway, with lots of lanes. All is grey. My daughter is in the passenger seat on the left. There is a grey bridge ahead and under it the road is blocked by some cars. I stop before getting to them and get out of my car, going round to the passenger side. There is a group of young men, who are from the city where I live. One man sprays petrol on my car, and strikes a match to set fire to it. I try to stop him, saying he will kill my daughter. They say they are doing this as she wouldn't go out or be friends with one of them.*

DISCUSSION: The dreamer, Laura, had recently driven her teenage daughter to start university in London and had concerns for her daughter's safety, having heard of an assault in her home city. The dreamer recalled living in Los Angeles when her daughter was a baby and worrying about freeway bridges falling down onto her car when her daughter was strapped in the baby seat.

JULIA: (Painting shown as Figure 12.1) I turned the two pages to create a portrait composition in which the bridge could occupy the topmost point and act as a compositional link that draws the eye across the two parts of the image. In the mainly grey composition, the yellow car draws the eye, as does the yellow and red flame of the match. The hand has its own separate footnoted section and I positioned the aggressive boys together in the main, central paragraph of that page. The following found poem is in the body of one of the boys:

Dreaming. Now
is none other than
this impulse
extraordinarily
something
my explanation of anxiety

And at the bottom of that panel:

*The dream
allied to anxiety
Anxiety
action of inhibition
anxiety*

Theories of dream function

The chapters of this book so far have introduced various theories that hold that dreaming has some function. This chapter will critically examine those theories.

The threat simulation theory of dreams was described in Chapter 3, on nightmares, and is one of the virtual reality theories of dreaming. It was first put forward in 2000 by Antti Revonsuo, who hypothesised that individuals who practise overcoming threats in the dream environment will have an evolutionary fitness benefit in waking life. To provide further evidence for the theory, Valli, Revonsuo and colleagues (2005) investigated the dreams of Kurdish children who live in an environment in which their physical and psychological well-being is constantly threatened, and found that they reported a significantly greater number of dreams with threatening content than do children not living in such circumstances. The threats in their dreams were usually aimed at the self or significant others, rather than on resources or personal property, and realistic responses to the threats were made in the dreams. The threat simulation theory has now been extended by Revonsuo and colleagues (2016) to include dreaming being a simulation of social reality, as well as simulation of physical threats, with the simulation of the social skills, bonds, interactions and networks that occur during our waking lives. This is called the Social Simulation Theory. To test this theory they investigated the frequency and quality of interactions in late versus early REM and NREM dreams, and found that dreams had a higher representation of social events than do waking life reports, but with no effect of time of night or sleep stage (Tuominen et al., 2019).

In contrast to such virtual reality theories, Wamsley and Stickgold (2011) put forward the theory that dreams are the experience of the brain undertaking the consolidation of memories, so that dreaming reflects, or is part of, functional neural processes during sleep. This is supported by Eichenlaub and colleagues (2018), who built on the work of previous researchers who had shown that REM sleep and frontal EEG theta wave power are related to the processing of recent emotional memories. They found that the number of references to recent waking-life experiences in REM dreams was positively correlated with frontal theta activity in the REM sleep period. This effect seems to be specific to REM sleep and recent memories, because the number of older memories incorporated into dreams was not related to REM theta power, and the number of recent memories in non-REM N3 dreams was not related to theta, or to delta power, in the N3 sleep period (for an understanding of these sleep stages, see Chapter 4). These findings accord with theories that dreaming reflects emotional memory processing taking place in REM sleep.

However, dream content often has only a very abstract or metaphorical relationship to waking life experiences. Stickgold and colleagues (2001a) had suggested that during REM sleep, the emotional limbic forebrain and amygdala areas are activated while lower activity in the Dorsolateral Prefrontal Cortex inhibits the ability of the dreamer to spot bizarre incongruities in dreams. They reviewed how REM dreams are constructed largely from the weak memory associations that are prioritised during REM sleep. Wamsley and Stickgold (2019) expanded this to the idea that dreams do not copy previous experience but link specific recent experiences with subjects' pre-existing knowledge structures, and that this allows for the extraction of generalisations, and integration of new information with past experience. Sleep and dreaming would thus enable the generalisation of memories, a point explored at length by Hoel (2021).

Stickgold further extended this approach in his book with Antonio Zadra, *When Brains Dream: Exploring the science and mystery of sleep*, by proposing their NEXTUP theory of dreaming (Zadra & Stickgold, 2021). This holds that in REM dreams 'weakly associated networks are being explored to understand possibilities' (p.111), and that the brain combines memories 'into a dream narrative that explores associations the brain would never normally consider' (p.109). A similar proposal from a psychoanalytic standpoint is made by Blechner (2001), in his theory of oneiric Darwinism, in which dreams produce 'thought mutations', from which we can select those that are most useful or fit for waking life.

The notion that REM sleep, and dreaming, produce novel associations and combinations of recent and past memories has been proposed by many researchers over the years. An early version was by Ernest Hartmann, who, in 1995, wrote the paper 'Making connections in a safe place: is dreaming psychotherapy?' He proposed that dreaming and psychotherapy involve the freeing of associations in a safe place without acting out behaviours. For Hartmann, the clearest case for the associative function of dreams is in the associations made between recent memories of a trauma and previous memories that are already in long-term memory. Thus dreaming (like psychotherapy), makes connections between trauma and other relevant memories, which first involves the dream replaying the trauma, but then the content changing to include related material using metaphors, hence connecting the traumatic memories to previous memories in order to process them. Hartmann says that when dreams and psychotherapy produce such metaphorical connections, the same dominant emotion remains, but it is given a new context. The trauma and its associated disturbing emotions are thus eventually integrated into the patient's life.

According to Hartmann (1995), dreaming thus makes broader and more peripheral connections than does waking thought. In 2011 he put forward a theory on the nature and functions of dreaming, in which he proposed that dreaming is 'hyper-connective', in that it elicits a larger number of connections between memories, and with a greater spread of excitations, than occurs with the more focussed thinking of waking life. This results in dreams 'contextualising' emotions, in other words, they take an emotion from waking life and give it a new context, thus explaining metaphorically the emotional state of the dreamer.

Hartmann (2011) gives the example of the dream of a new mother that 'my children are lost in a storm and I can't find them'. This is her way of depicting her concerns and worries, he says. He characterises dreaming as a 'thin boundaried state', so that whereas people differ in their level of boundariness, everyone becomes more thin boundaried during dreams. (The thin/thick boundariness personality measure was described in Chapter 2.) He acknowledges that most dreams are forgotten, but states that cross connections can be made during unremembered dreams. This view thus has similarities to memory consolidation views of dreams, although Hartmann is cautious here, stating that the process is 'probably' functional.

Most of the theories that dreaming has a function hold that dreams that we do not recall when we wake are still held to be beneficial for us. And so we dream of fears so as to diminish fear memories (see Chapter 3), or we dream of threats so as to practise overcoming them, or we dream of combined memories so as to make new connections between memories, and these functions occur even as we sleep, and can occur for dreams that we do not recall. Applying the Hebbian maxim that 'neurons wire together, if they fire together' (Krupic, 2017), or, more formally, that when neurons fire together consistently, then neural connections become stronger, then that firing together during sleep would thus make the neural connections stronger during sleep, whether or not the dream was subsequently recalled. We will now examine this characterisation that dreams cause changes to memory during the night and that they do not need to be recalled in order to serve that function.

The correlational issue in studies on functions of dreams

The first issue for proposed within-sleep functions of dreams is that there is, as yet, no experimental (as opposed to correlational) evidence that dream content alters the brain during sleep and thus causes a change in waking life behaviour. For example, in Wamsley et al. (2010b) and Wamsley and Stickgold (2019), as described in Chapter 5, improvement in learning task performance across sleep is associated with dreaming of the learning task. This leads to the implication that the dream content caused the change in memory performance after sleep. However, these are associational findings, which fall under the well-known caution that correlation does not mean causation. In correlational studies, two variables are measured and their relationship is calculated statistically, neither variable is altered by the researchers. In contrast, in experimental studies, the levels of one variable are determined by the researchers and the effect of that variable (the independent variable) on another variable (the dependent variable) is calculated. But what could be causing a correlation between dream content and change in memory across sleep? It may indeed be that dreaming of the task is somehow involved with neural processes in sleep that cause better learning of the task and better performance after waking. But, importantly, as discussed in Chapter 5, dreaming of the task in both these studies was also found to be related to poor performance before sleep. Task-related dream content in these studies may thus be emotional residues of a waking life concern of having shown, before sleep, poor performance on a task set by the experimenters.

These studies, and, for example, Cartwright's (1991) study on dreaming and response to divorce, can be classed as correlational, rather than showing a cause-and-effect relationship. Ros Cartwright's work is often cited as evidence of a functional role of dreams. She had been working on major studies of the dreams of people undergoing divorce, and found that the incorporation of the spouse in dreams was associated with later on having less depression about the divorce. This has been interpreted as the dreams being involved in some emotional processing during sleep that helps people get over the divorce. However, this is a correlational study, and it is possible that those who are better able to later recover from the divorce, those who are more resilient, were more able to dream of the spouse while the divorce was happening. So it could be that the causality works in a different direction, from pre-sleep factors to the dream, rather than from the dream and sleep to subsequent waking life. But note that in this case it can still be said that Cartwright was finding dreams are meaningful, in that they give an indication about how the person will respond to the divorce, even if the dream is not functional. A similar issue arises with Sterpenich and colleagues (2020), who found that a higher incidence of fear in dreams is associated with reduced emotional arousal, behaviourally and in the brain, to fear-eliciting stimuli when the person is awake. This research aimed to test the theory that emotions experienced in dreams contribute to the resolution when awake of emotional distress and to preparation for future emotional reactions. The study is intriguing, in that it is plausible that activity in the brain when asleep affects the brain and behaviour the next day, but the possibility remains, as with Cartwright's study, that individuals with reduced reactivity to fear when awake have, for some reason, more fearful dreams.

The difficulty here is that all studies to date of the relationship between dream content and any subsequent waking life behaviour are correlational, and cannot show causation. A similar argument was made in chapter 5 concerning the intriguing results of Ribeiro and colleagues (2020). To show causation what is needed is to assign participants randomly to dream content conditions. So, in Cartwright's design, we would have to alter participants' dreams so that the spouse appears in some people's dreams, but not in others, and we would have to randomly allocate people to those conditions to then see if the presence of the spouse in the dream causes a better adaptation to the divorce. Or in the Wamsley et al. (2010b) design, we would have to cause some participants to dream of the maze, and some to not do so, and to allocate them to these conditions at random. But such methods of altering dream content are not yet on the horizon, although Horowitz and colleagues (2020) have designed a novel device and protocol for the targeted modification of dreams through the playing of auditory stimuli at sleep onset. Experimental studies have shown psychomotor performance benefits of mental simulation when awake and during lucid dreams (Stumbrys et al., 2016), but in these cases, there is awareness of the simulation occurring, and an intention to undertake the mental simulation, which would not be true for dreams in general.

Dreaming and higher social memory

As described in Chapter 5 and above, in the Wamsley and colleagues (2010b) and Wamsley and Stickgold (2019) papers, those who had poor task performance at baseline, and who might thus have been concerned about that, dreamt of the task. Similarly, De Koninck et al. (2012) found, in a study on learning French, that participants dreamt of making mistakes in language learning, mistakes which would not be cognitively helpful, but which could depict the waking life concerns of the person as they learn French. A related finding is by De Koninck et al. (1996), in which participants were given lenses to wear in the day which inverted their field of vision by 180°. The participants made mistakes in their dreams, which could be seen as practising the new waking life skill, or alternatively as depicting concerns about having to wear the inverted lenses. Here indeed the authors concluded that 'the changes in dreams are consistent with the notion of continuity between waking and dreaming since they appear to reflect the waking preoccupation and psychological state associated with visual inversion'.

That dreaming may thus be related to waking life preoccupations can lead to the view that dreaming is an epiphenomenon, a by-product of neural processes, which, like the noise from a factory, itself has no function. We will address the epiphenomenal view in the next section. But we can ask now, though, given these findings, is there still a possibility of dreaming having a function? One possibility is that maybe higher level learning or restructuring of information about the self, or interpersonal emotional learning, or social cognitive memory, is occurring in REM sleep, and it is this that is reflected in dream content. In the Wamsley et al. (2010b) and Wamsley and Stickgold (2019) papers, maybe the dreams are related to the processing during sleep of the experiencing of interpersonal events and the resulting social cognitive learning and memory, such as is involved in processing the emotions and questions of 'why was I being tested?', 'how was I treated?', 'do I feel vulnerable or even feel judged?' In these instances, dreams could still be reflecting or even be part of functional brain processes during sleep, but brain processes to do with learning about the self and about one's often very complex social circumstances and interpersonal emotional reactions. This would also accord with the Social Simulation Theory of dreams (Revonsuo et al., 2016).

Although speculative, this higher-level interpersonal learning proposal may be connected to the default network running during sleep, as described in Chapter 6. However, although the default network and daydreams can be functional when awake, Domhoff (2018) cautions that dreams produced by the system running during sleep might not have a function, even if the dreams refer to conceptualisations and concerns that the person has in waking life. This therefore brings us to the question, why propose a function for dreams anyway?

The epiphenomenal view: why propose a function for dreams?

For all the hypotheses of dreaming having a function, there remains the alterative, which is the *null hypothesis,* that there is no purpose or function to our dreams, even when they are very meaningful and related to waking life fears, threats and memories. For Domhoff (2011), we dream of our waking life conceptualisations, and there is continuity between our waking life cognition and dream cognition, but he concludes that this continuity has no function. Now, this null hypothesis does not mean that dreams are a scrambled version of waking life memories, as in Hobson and McCarley's (1977) *activation-synthesis theory,* with dreaming being a type of delirium. Rather, the null hypothesis proposes that dreams can still have some meaning, in that they refer to our individual waking life experiences, and they thus do differ between people, just as cognitions or memories or personalities differ between people, but they might have no function when doing so.

Owen Flanagan's (2000) book *Dreaming Souls* supports the null hypothesis that dreams do not have a function, and he describes dreams as decorative 'spandrels'. The term spandrel is used in evolutionary theory to describe a functionless feature of an organism. The term was originally derived from architecture, where a spandrel is the triangular space at the two corners of an arch, these triangular spaces often then being decorated. The corner of the arch occurs as a side-effect of the overall structure, but itself, and its decoration, would have no architectural function. In evolution, such by-products might not in themselves be harmful, and so would not be selected out or removed by evolution, just as, if our dreams are functionless, evolution might not have acted to stop us from having them, although it may have acted to make them more difficult to remember.

The epiphenomenal view is that claims to tie the general characteristics of dreaming (for example, their mixing of memories, and their emotionality) to possible functions of sleep, and in particular REM sleep, such as in Perogamvros et al. (2013), Perogamvros and Schwartz (2012), and Stickgold et al. (2001a), or to tie dreams to virtual reality simulation, such as in Valli et al. (2005), are speculative and lack experimental evidence. Also speculative is the proposal to link dreams to neural replay during sleep (e.g., Wamsley & Stickgold, 2011). Neural replay is reviewed in Chapter 5; it refers to how sequences of neurons that are activated in waking life then replay during sleep, and this has been found for rats after following a path or maze when awake (Gillespie et al., 2021; Louie & Wilson, 2001). However, neural replay has not been shown empirically to be related to dream content, and neural replay is mostly found in non-Rapid Eye Movement (NREM) sleep and wake rather than in REM sleep (Findlay et al., 2020).

Dreams might thus take their initial content from the memories that are being processed during sleep, but then utilise those memories for other purposes, or for no purpose (Blagrove, 1992, 2011; Flanagan, 2000). A similar point is made by Wamsley (2014).

Other possibilities for testing for a function of dreams

Intriguingly, the NEXTUP theory from Zadra and Stickgold (2021) proposes that the subjective experience of emotions in dreams is necessary for the dream function of within-sleep evaluation of the novel associations that are created in dreams, as the emotional response is a signal that a novel association might be adaptive. This is indeed an interesting possibility, but cannot currently be tested empirically.

One other possibility that may also in time be empirically testable comes from Siclari et al.'s (2017) work on the neural correlates of dreaming, which found the posterior 'hot zone' which is activated when dreams occur. As was said in Chapter 6, future work can investigate why the hot zone, or other neural correlates of dreaming, become activated. Maybe the hot zone is turned on for some function and the dreaming that results is an epiphenomenon. Or maybe there is a deliberate turning on of dreaming by the hot zone periodically during the night, in REM and NREM sleep, so that after all the non-conscious processing that is going on in the brain of what we've learnt during the day, a virtual simulation of the world occurs to complete or enhance that memory or emotional processing. Much processing in sleep would thus occur without consciousness, but sometimes consciousness may be needed, such as for the processing of emotions or for taking into account the feeling of emotions. This possibility would overcome an objection to the functional view, that much declarative memory processing occurs in slow-wave sleep when dreaming is rarer, because dreaming would be turned on only when the processing required it.

As the evidence is not yet in, we don't know whether dreaming has a function. But then we do not even know whether waking consciousness has a function either. There are claims that waking consciousness is an epiphenomenon, and that all of consciousness, including apparent free choices and free will, are a result of neural processing and that consciousness follows after that processing (Libet, 2005). Jeffrey Gray (2006) considered that waking consciousness is a way for us to scan for incongruities or unexpected events in the environment, and that consciousness has the function of drawing our attention to things that we did not expect to be happening. It could indeed be that dreaming has a similar role of alerting us to incongruities, or things we have not quite fully noticed yet in waking life. But the epiphenomenal view, that dreams have no lasting effect on the brain during sleep, remains very plausible. This would mean that dreams, unless attended to and recalled on waking, might be simply ephemeral, and we now turn to this possibility.

The ephemerality of dreams

A final critique of proposed functions of dreams is the view that dreams are ephemeral. It may be that, unless attention is paid to them on waking, dreams are no more permanent than short-term or even sensory memories. Sensory memories are the fleeting impressions of stimuli that impinge on each of the senses, and that need to be paid attention to so as to be transferred to short-term memory (Sperling, 1960). We must therefore be alert to the possibility that unrecalled dreams might have no effects lasting longer than the duration of the dream itself, except for some residual and diminishing felt or bodily emotion. Although only suggestive of whether lasting neural effects occur, it is well known that recall of dreams on awakening in the morning is indeed fragile, and requiring the dream to be attended to and rehearsed, an effect partly resulting from the different brain states between sleep and wake (Koulack & Goodenough, 1976). There are reports of people remembering dreams later in the day, having seen some accidental cue or cue in an experiment (Montangero et al., 2003), but arguably this does not count against an ephemeral view of unrecalled dreams, given that it is very rare for people to suddenly recall for the first time a dream from previous days or weeks in this manner. Nevertheless, if remembered, dreams do sometimes seem to have an effect on us after we wake, and we now turn to this.

Dreaming, creativity and insight

There are many claims of personal insight from dreams, and also literary (Epel, 1993) and scientific insight (Barrett, 2001). For example, the claim by the chemist August Kekulé, that he had realised the circular shape of the benzene ring after dreaming in 1854 or 1855 of atoms dancing, and in 1861 or 1862 of a snake biting its own tail. Regarding this, it had been known at the time that benzene has six carbon atoms and only six hydrogen atoms, and possible solutions for the shape of the molecule had been explored by many chemists, until the eventual solution of six carbon atoms in a ring, with one hydrogen atom attached to each carbon atom, was proposed by Kekulé in 1865. There is an argument about Kekulé's claim, however, in that some historians assert that many people were working on the problem of the arrangement of the carbon molecules in benzene and that Kekulé reported this dream as a way of giving himself priority for the solution (Rudofsky & Wotiz, 1988). In contrast, Strunz (1993) supports the counterargument that this instance of creativity was indeed instigated by a dream.

An example of artistic creativity comes from the German composer Karlheinz Stockhausen, who was a very major figure in 20th- and early

21st-century classical and electronic music. The following is taken from Stockhausen (1999), describing how in 1991 he was commissioned to compose a string quartet. He reports a dream in which:

I heard and saw the four string players in four helicopters flying in the air and playing. At the same time, I saw people on the ground seated in an audio-visual hall, others were standing outdoors on a large public plaza. In front of them, four towers of television screens and loudspeakers had been set up: at the left, half-left, half-right, right. At each of the four positions, one of the four string players could be heard and seen in close-up.

As a result of the dream, the quartet was written as a confluence of the sounds of the string instruments with the sounds of helicopter rotor blades. It is hence called the *Helicopter Quartet*. Some recordings are made with helicopters and string players and no audience, but the full public version has helicopters flying above the people in the concert hall. Unlike some claims of scientific discovery, an issue here is how to assess the novelty and validity of insight or creativity in artistic fields, and in this case, the value of the novel combination of music and rotor blades is in some respects a matter of taste, even though Stockhausen is greatly lauded and praised. So we now proceed to discuss whether the presence of scientific, artistic and personal insight from dreams has a relationship with suggestions for dreams to have a function.

Insight and function of dreams

Whether dreams are sources of insight, and whether they are functional, are two separate questions. As reviewed in Chapter 11, dreams might give personal insight because of their metaphorical content (Malinowski & Horton, 2015), but, as pointed out by Antrobus (1977), apparent metaphors in dreams might just result from dreams partially depicting waking life experiences, causing the dream to be a metaphor by default, rather than by design. We have shown in Chapter 11 that by using the Ullman dream appreciation technique there can be greater personal insight from discussing dreams than from discussing recent events or daydreams. But obtaining insight from dreams is a different issue from whether dreaming or REM sleep is functional during sleep. To illustrate this we can examine Table 12.1, which categorises theories of dreaming on two dimensions: function and insight.

Table 12.1 Theories of dreaming categorised as functional or not functional, and as eliciting or not eliciting insight

	Function	No function
Insight	Hartmann; Freud; Zadra & Stickgold: NEXTUP theory.	
No insight	Revonsuo: Threat Simulation Theory	Flanagan; Domhoff; Hobson & McCarley: Activation-Synthesis theory

The first dimension is whether there is some adaptive function of dreams that might have been selected for in evolution as conferring a benefit on the individual and the species. (The role of evolution for characteristics of dreams is reviewed in Valli & Revonsuo, 2007.) The second dimension is whether dreams can be a source of insight.

No function / no insight

For Hobson and McCarley's (1977) activation synthesis theory, there is no evolutionary function of dreams, and dreams are not a source of insight either. As stated by Hobson: 'I never learned anything from a client's dreams that I did not already know' (Hobson & Schredl, 2011). Similarly, for Flanagan (2000) and Domhoff (2018), dreaming is an epiphenomenon, a by-product of sleep, albeit a complicated and cognitively complex by-product. So, for Domhoff (2011), dreams are embodied simulations that dramatise our conceptions and concerns, but individuals do not get insight from dreams even though the dreams have a statistical and lawlike relationship with dreamers' waking lives. For Domhoff, there is not any information obtainable from dreams that is not already known to the person in waking life.

Function / No insight

Revonsuo's (2000) theory of threat simulation is an evolutionary theory, holding that dreams have a function of enabling us to overcome waking life threats, but the dreams would not be a source of insight because one would certainly know that one is threatened by those situations.

Function / insight

For Ernest Hartmann, as dreams are involved in the making of novel connections between memories, they can be sources of insight and he says that arguably they also have a function during sleep. Similarly, for Freud, the function of dreams is to keep the dreamer asleep, and of course, Freud is very much in favour of dreams being a source of insight. Zadra and Stickgold's NEXTUP theory would fall into this category, as the unlikely associations produced by dreams may well provide insights to the dreamer if recalled on waking.

No function / insight

It is unclear whether any current theory of dreams holds that dreams are functionless but can provide insight.

Summary

Many proposals have been made for possible functions of dreams. Almost all such proposals state that the function of dreams occurs during sleep and does not require the dream to be recalled when awake for the function to have its effect. However, these theories are not currently testable and dream content might be explainable as an epiphenomenon with the dream content based on conceptualisations, and pre-sleep emotional events and concerns of the dreamer. Given these issues, Blagrove, Lockheart and colleagues proposed that functional consequences of dreaming and dream content could instead occur after sleep, as a result of the sharing of dreams. That work, on the empathy theory of dreaming, is described in the next chapter.

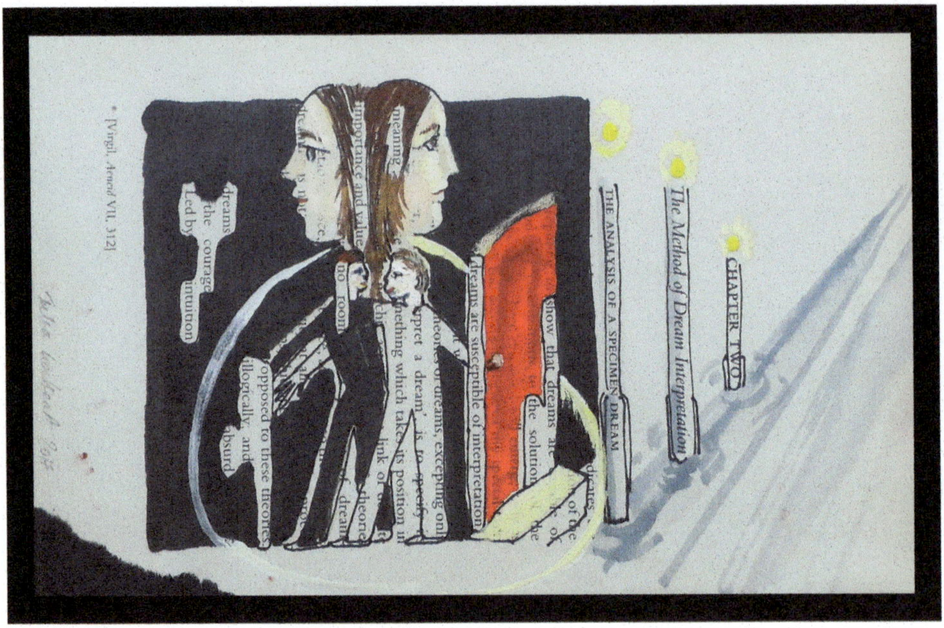

Figure 13.1 Dream of 'where is my home?', 2017.

13 Dream-sharing and empathy, a new theory of dream function

Having aimed, in our DreamsID dream discussion and painting events, to enable dream-sharers to achieve some personal insight from considering and discussing their dreams, the dream below was the first dream told to us in which we both felt considerable empathy towards the dream-sharer. As a result of this dream, we started working on the empathy theory of dreaming. This dream was told in one of the 30-minute sessions we held in the early years of our collaboration; the collaboration is detailed in chapter 14.

DREAM NARRATIVE: *I am walking up a street in the evening. I walk past street lights running down the street and come to stop beside a red door. My daughter is beside me with her boyfriend and I realise this is her new home. She can enter the house through the door with her boyfriend and they step over the threshold. I stand outside the house and turn away thinking 'where is my home?'*

DISCUSSION: We discussed the relationship of the dream to the current situation of the dreamer, whose daughter was soon going to leave home.

JULIA: (Painting shown as Figure 13.1) I chose a page with chapter headings and subtitles so that when turned on its side these could be used for the lamp-posts, and provide perspective for the street scene. The red door was a significant colour symbol, as was the head of the dreamer looking in two directions to ask 'where is my home?'

Noticing the empathic effect of sharing dreams

As a result of the use by Mark over many years of the Ullman dream discussion method, described in Chapter 10, and his research on dreams and insight, presented in Chapter 11, we started to undertake public discussions of dreams with the aim of eliciting insight in the dreamer, with an artwork produced simultaneously by Julia. The artwork would be given to the dreamer, so that they could revisit the dream and discuss it and the painting with family and friends. (More details on these public discussions of dreams and our DreamsID science art collaboration are given in Chapter 14.) However, whereas the DreamsID project was devised so as to elicit insights for the dreamer from the discussion and artwork, we started to realise the effect that

DOI: 10.4324/9781003037552-13

the discussions about dreams can have on us, and on others who were taking part in the discussion. The first dream for which we noticed this is reported at the start of this chapter. We therefore decided to address this issue by testing in experiments whether there is a relationship between dream-sharing and empathy. Before we describe the experiments, we will first review what is known about the social effects of sharing dreams.

Frequency, motivations and social effects of sharing dreams

Dream sharing is a frequent activity: Schredl et al. (2014) found that 35% of respondents representing the general population share dreams at least monthly, and about 10% weekly or several times per week; in a sample of teenagers, recruited in a study of library users, average frequency of dream telling was just under once per month, and dream listening was twice per month (Georgi et al., 2012); in Schredl and Bulkeley's (2019) diverse sociodemographic and ethnic background online survey, 23% of the sample reported sharing dreams at least once per week. Schredl et al. (2015a), with a sample most of whom were psychology students, found that two-thirds of participants reported that they had, in the previous month, told a dream to someone else, and two-thirds had listened to a dream of someone else. Furthermore, one-third of participants had told a dream to someone else in the previous week, and one-third had listened to someone else's dream in the previous week. Regarding the last situation in which the participant had told one of his/her own dreams to another person the three main motives for dream telling were that the dream topic was relevant for the interaction between the dreamer and the listener, that it was an extraordinary dream, or that the dreamer wished to understand the dream better. Similarly, Olsen et al. (2013) found that the main motivations for sharing dreams were, in order to importance, 'Entertainment', 'I want to understand what the dreams mean', and 'To let the other person know what is happening in my mind'.

In a sample of undergraduates, Vann and Alperstein (2010) found 97.9% had told a dream to someone else at least once, and that dreams were told in order to entertain, or to elicit a reaction, or to share the content. They concluded that dream-sharing is a means to bring people closer together. Likewise, Ijams and Miller (2000) found that disclosing dreams enhances feelings of intimacy and trust within established relationships, provided the other person's response was supportive and non-judgmental. Dream-sharing can also enhance marital relationships through providing a forum for self-awareness and self-disclosure (Duffey et al., 2004). Similarly, Schredl and Schawinski (2010) found that dreams are shared mainly with romantic partners, friends and relatives, and that the sharing is often associated with the enhancement of relational intimacy, and stress relief, such as in the case of sharing nightmares.

Relevant here, although not addressing the sharing of dreams, are the findings of Selterman and colleagues (2014), that participants felt more love and closeness to romantic partners on days subsequent to dreaming about them, although dreams of infidelity resulted in less intimacy on subsequent days. There may even be a biological or neural basis for some of these effects of dreams. McNamara (1996) reviews evidence that REM sleep has a role in promoting social bonding, and that it may reactivate the systems utilised by infants to attach to a care-giver, and he proposes that this may be reflected in dream content showing 'bonding themes', especially in individuals not currently closely attached.

It is clear then that the sharing of dreams is common, and that positive effects occur between people as a result of such sharing. It is thus plausible that dream-sharing could elicit or be associated with empathy as part of these interpersonal effects. Dreams would be able to have this relationship with empathy because of their high level of social content, as shown in the Social Simulation Theory of Revonsuo et al. (2016), and detailed in Chapter 12. Domhoff and Schneider (2018) similarly characterise dream content as the embodied enactment of waking-life conceptualisations and concerns, and report that only 6.5% of dream reports are not social simulations. It is important to appreciate, however, that Domhoff and Schneider have a non-functional view of dreaming and of this social content, as they point to the presence of long-term concerns in dreams, and social interactions with deceased loved ones across years and decades, and past misfortunes, all of which they say are not characteristic of Social Simulation Theory's proposal that dreams involve beneficial 'forward-looking social rehearsal'. The observations here of Domhoff and Schneider may be seen as more fitting to a view that dreams can elicit uncomfortable self-disclosure, which we will return to after describing the experiments on dream-sharing and empathy.

Testing the association between dream-sharing and trait empathy

In Blagrove et al. (2019b), we first tested whether trait empathy is correlated with dream-telling frequency, with the frequency of listening to others' dreams and with a positive attitude towards dreams. Trait empathy was measured by the Toronto Empathy Questionnaire (TEQ; Spreng et al., 2009), which has 16 items, each scored on a 5-point scale, anchored at Never (0) and Always (4), with half the items reverse scored. Example items are:

It upsets me to see someone being treated disrespectfully.
I become irritated when someone cries.
The total score is the sum of all item scores and can vary between 0 and 64; the second example here is reverse scored.

We also used the Mannheim Dream Questionnaire (MADRE; Schredl et al., 2014). The items used from the MADRE were:

> How often have you recalled your dreams recently (in the past several months)? Participants responded on a 7-point scale, with points ranging from 'never' (0) to 'almost every morning' (6).
>
> How often do you tell your dreams to others? Participants responded on a 8-point scale, with points ranging from 'never' (0) to 'several times per week' (7).

Attitude towards Dreams, in which high scores mean that the person has a positive attitude towards dreams, was measured with the following items, each responded to on a 5-point scale, ranging from 'not at all' (0) to 'totally' (4):

> How much meaning do you attribute to your dreams?
> How strong is your interest in dreams?
> I think that dreams are meaningful.
> I want to know more about dreams.
> If somebody can recall and interpret his/her dreams, his/her life will be enriched.
> I think that dreaming is in general a very interesting phenomenon.
> A person who reflects on her/his dreams is certainly able to learn more about her/himself.
> Do you have the impression that dreams provide impulses or pointers for your waking life?

We also added an item that was not present on the MADRE, responded to using the 8-point scale above:

> How often do you listen to others telling their dreams to you?

We recruited 160 participants (average age = 21.3 years; 40 males and 120 females) and found that females scored significantly higher on all the variables, except for the frequency of listening to the dreams of others, where females scored only marginally higher than males. This sex difference was taken into account in the statistical analyses. In those analyses, we found significant correlations between trait empathy and each of attitude towards dreams ($r = 0.29$), frequency of telling dreams ($r = 0.32$), frequency of listening to dreams ($r = 0.14$) and dream recall frequency ($r = 0.19$).

There are different possible explanations for these relationships between sharing dreams and empathy. First, it may be that individuals high in empathy, due to their connectedness to others, wish to share their own dreams, and hear and consider the dreams of others. Second, it may be that there is a trait or individual difference that is correlated with empathy and with these dream variables, such as, for example, thin boundariness (Hartmann et al., 1991) or sensory processing sensitivity (Aron & Aron, 1997). Usually, there is a third explanation for a correlation, which would have causality in the opposite direction to the first explanation above, that is, here, the sharing of dreams affecting trait empathy. However, as there will be many factors leading to trait empathy, this causal relationship would be expected to only be minor. It does though raise the issue of whether dream-sharing might increase empathy between people involved in dream-sharing. We therefore investigated this experimentally.

First experiment on dream-sharing and empathy

Whereas the correlational study above concerned empathy as a trait, which for a person is their long-standing level of empathy towards people in general, we now addressed state empathy, which is the level of empathy that someone feels towards someone else at a particular time. In this, we differentiated between the empathy of a dream-sharer towards the person discussing the dream with them, and the empathy of the discusser towards the dream-sharer. The primary hypothesis was that the discusser will have increased empathy towards the dream-sharer. A second hypothesis was that the dream-sharer will have increased empathy towards the discusser.

We thus recruited 27 pairs of participants (average age = 21.0 years; 22 males and 31 females). Each pair applied to take part together, as friends or in a relationship, knowing that one would be sharing dreams and the other of the pair would discuss the dreams with them. The sharer was identified as the member of the pair who was recalling dreams the most often. At the start of the study each participant completed online an adapted version of the 12-item Shen (2010) state empathy scale (see below), regarding their empathy towards the other member of the pair, this was their baseline empathy score. The items on the scale were scored on an 11-point scale, from 'not at all' (0) to 'completely' (10), and items included:

> My friend's / partner's emotions are genuine;
> I can feel my friend's / partner's emotions;
> I can see my friend's / partner's point of view;
> I can understand what my friend / partner goes through;
> My friend's / partner's reactions are understandable;
> When I talk to my friend / partner, I am fully absorbed;
> I can relate to what my friend / partner goes through.

Upon having a dream, the dream-sharer arranged to meet the other member of the pair as soon as possible to discuss the dream with them. Due to the need for untrained participants to quickly learn and apply a dream exploration method, we taught them the technique devised by Montague Ullman (1996/2006), described in Chapter 10. The discussion duration was set at 15–30 minutes. Each participant then completed the state empathy scale after the dream discussion. During the study, the majority of participants had one dream discussion, but some had from two to five dreams and discussions. The empathy score of each participant following the last or only dream discussion was used as their post-intervention measure, and was compared to their empathy score measured at baseline.

As hypothesised, the dream discussers had an increase in empathy towards the dream-sharers from baseline as a result of discussing dreams, with medium effect size of $d_z = 0.34$. The dream-sharers had a non-significant decrease in empathy towards the discusser. The latter finding can be understood in that the dream-sharer is addressing their own dream and own life during the discussion process, and so would not necessarily have a significant change in empathy towards the discusser. An increase in empathy for both members of a pair would thus need them to take turns in sharing and discussing.

Second experiment on dream-sharing and empathy

We then replicated the dream-sharing and empathy effect in our paper 'Dream sharing and the enhancement of empathy: theoretical and applied implications' (Blagrove et al., 2021, including co-authors Michelle Carr and Katja Valli). Again, participants were recruited in pairs who already knew each other, and were assigned dream-sharer and discusser roles. We again used the Ullman dream appreciation technique to explore the relationship of the sharer's dreams to recent experiences in the sharer's life, with an aim of having four dream discussions per pair within a two-week period. The mean length of dreams discussed was 140.15 words, and the mean discussion length was 23.72 minutes. Forty-four participants (average age = 26.7 years; 26 females, 18 males) provided empathy scores at baseline and after each dream discussion. Our findings were that the discussers had significantly increased empathy towards dream-sharers, with a medium effect size, except where empathy scores at baseline were already high, in which case the high empathy was maintained. These results occurred even though the aim to share four dreams may have resulted in sub-optimal dreams being examined. In naturalistic circumstances, the main predictor of sharing for both negative and positive dreams is the emotional intensity of the dream (Curci & Rimé, 2008). The dreams shared for this current experiment might not have had such emotional intensity and apart from being in an experiment the dreamer might not have had any urgency or reason for sharing the dream, and yet the hypothesised increase in empathy for discussers towards dream-sharers still occurred.

Individuals' reactions to listening to dreams

This chapter earlier reviewed findings showing that dream-sharing occurs frequently, that people are motivated to share dreams, and that there are beneficial effects of the sharing: it is thus plausible that the results of the two experiments reported above can be generalised to the population in general. However, there is a further issue that may temper the claim that empathy can be elicited by dream-sharing in the general population, this is the often repeated sceptical admonishment that 'There is nothing more boring than listening to someone else's dream!' This would imply that in the real world, and even when dream telling does occur, individuals might not be as welcoming or enthusiastic about listening to the dreams of another person as occurred in our experiments.

Individuals' reactions to the telling of dreams have indeed been studied, and can be reviewed here to reply to this sceptical view. Regarding the last time participants shared a dream, Schredl et al. (2015a) asked them what was the perceived reaction of the person they shared a dream with. Participants reported that laughter/amusement and sympathy are the most common reactions to dream telling, together accounting for about 57% of responses, with only 10% of reactions being neutral or there being no response to the dream, and with no reporting of the other person showing boredom. Indeed the most common emotion associated with the last time participants listened to a dream of another person was joy, mentioned by 62% of participants, with anxiety, and the dream being seen as strange, as the next most common reactions.

Further data on how listeners respond to dream-sharing also show that boredom is not a common reaction. In Schredl and Göritz (2018), 21% of respondents reported enjoying listening to dreams very much, and 35% much, with just 6% responding with 'not at all'. Regarding the last-remembered situation in which a dream was told to the participant, the emotional reaction was most often positive (49.2%), with 45% of the participants rating the last listening experience as neutral, and only 2.1% as negative. Although this online sample may have been biased towards people who are interested in dreams, the sample was of 935 women and 655 men, with a mean age of 51 years, and was representative of the general population and with heterogenic demographic backgrounds. It is thus plausible that listeners are not uninterested in other people's dreams, nor emotionally indifferent. This is also supported by Schredl and Göritz's (2018) findings that after the most recent instance of listening to a dream, the responses were (with percentage giving that response): 'I thought about the dream' (19%); 'I talked again with the person about the dream' (20%); 'I feel more close to the person who shared the dream' (13%); 'I talked with others about the dream' (5%); and 'I learned something about myself' (1.6%), these being overall marginally more frequent reactions than 'I did not do anything more with the dream' after listening to it (45%). In summary, the findings reviewed here support a view that in general listening to the dreams of other people is a positive experience emotionally and in terms of social interaction.

How to explain the empathy effect: dreaming and fiction

Dream-sharing may increase empathy because the dream acts as a piece of fiction, which is explored by the dreamer and others as part of the sharing process. Dreams would thus be like literary fiction, which has itself been shown to elicit or be associated with empathy (Oatley, 1999; 2011; Schrage-Früh, 2016). In the Mind in the Eyes test (Baron-Cohen et al., 2001), participants view 36 photographs, each showing only a person's eyes, and choose from four adjectives to indicate what each photographed person was thinking and feeling. This is a behavioural test of empathy. Mar and colleagues (2006), using the Mind in the Eyes test, showed a correlation between the amount of reading fiction the person does and trait empathy. Furthermore, Matthijs Bal and Veltkamp (2013) showed that empathy was increased over a period of one week for people who read a fictional story, in comparison to a non-fictional piece. They concluded that the emotional response to fiction is greater than with non-fiction because of the reader's involvement with the characters and story, and because 'the focus of fiction is primarily on eliciting emotions, rather than on presenting factual information', and that the reader sympathises with the characters in the story, through taking the perspective of the characters, and experiences the events as if they are the reader's own experience.

On the question of what is a literary narrative, Mar and Oatley (2008) include in this category novels, films, TV dramas and theatre. They state that these narratives are 'carefully crafted, written, and rewritten by authors intending their products for public consumption', and that they offer 'a form of cognitive simulation of the social world with absorbing emotional consequences for the reader'. Some of these characteristics of literary narrative obviously do not hold for dreams, but for the present chapter, the crucial characteristic that they have in common is that literary narratives and dreams are simulations of the waking social world, and that both can elicit engagement and emotion when told. This similarity between dreams and fictional stories is explored by States (1993), who concludes that a dream does

> much the same thing as the fiction writer who makes models of the world that carry the imprint and structure of our deepest concerns. And it does this by using real people, or scraps of real people, as the instruments of hypothetical acts. (p.114)

In their chapter, 'The function of fiction is the abstraction and simulation of social experience,' Mar and Oatley (2008) state that 'engaging in the simulative experiences of fiction literature can facilitate the understanding of others who are different from ourselves, and can augment our capacity for empathy and social inference.' They conclude that 'In much of literature, the author challenges readers to empathize with individuals who differ drastically from the self', and they propose that narrative fiction represents 'learning through experience'. We emphasise that the functional Social Simulation Theory and Domhoff's non-functional view of dreaming both see the dream as fiction. Dreams are fictional because they feature events that only very rarely copy waking life episodes (Fosse et al., 2003). Furthermore, in Vallat et al. (2017a), an unknown dream environment occurs in 47% of dreams, and this is significantly more frequent than the dream environment being wholly (26% of dreams) or partly (27% of dreams) taken from waking life. (In contrast, characters in dreams are more likely to be known than to be unknown or mixed.) Having an unknown environment tilts the dream further to be fictional. Another characteristic of dreams that could support their being fictional is the incorporation of non-recent memories, and this provides an alternative explanation for the dream-lag effect that was described in Chapter 1. There we saw the common conclusion that the dream-lag has a role in or is a consequence of memory processing during sleep. However, we can speculate instead that the mixture of recent and delayed incorporation of waking life events in dreams is part of the production of fiction, rather than part of any neural processing of memories during the night. In Chapter 17, we will return to this proposal that dreams have a function through the production and telling of fiction.

Implications for psychotherapy and other relationships

Pesant and Zadra (2004) and Ellis (2020) describe how the consideration of dreams increases psychotherapy clients' self-knowledge and insight, increases clients' commitment to and engagement in therapy, due to the emotional valence of the material, and can result in the revelation of information or emotions that the client is unable or unwilling to acknowledge. Changes in dream content can also indicate the progress of therapy. However, these authors note that the use of dreams is now rarely taught to new clinicians. The findings described in this chapter and in Chapter 11 support the use of the Ullman technique, as a systematic way of detailing and cross-mapping a dream and its waking life context, and the technique may thus be found useful by therapists and by the wider lay population. The technique can also be used in the training of psychotherapists, so as to provide hands-on experience in the skills of exploring dream content and the relationships of dream content to recent waking life.

A second implication of the current findings is that clients can be advised that, in addition to dreams being usefully addressed in therapy, they can also be told and discussed with significant others, and that this can result in closer understanding and empathy towards the client, outside the therapeutic environment, and also result in increased empathy from the client towards a dream-sharing significant other. Clients and the wider population may be receptive to this advice of practising dream-sharing. Relevant here are the findings of Grant and colleagues (2020) that there is a positive influence on the grief process for people whose loved ones shared end-of-life dreams and visions (ELDVs) compared to those who did not, as measured by accepting the reality of loss, working through the pain of grief, adjusting to the new environment and continuing bonds.

Dream-sharing may also be beneficial in professional circumstances. The public telling and performing of dreams have been undertaken in the training and rehearsals of actors by playwright and director Jon Lipsky. In his (2008) book *Dreaming Together: Exploring Your Dreams by Acting Them Out*, drawing parallels between dreams and drama, and between dream telling and theatre, he writes:

> 'Most dream work is self-referential. We explore our dreams to find out more about our inner lives. ... By performing our dreams with and for others, we make a commitment to share what we've discovered. ... We are doing the work first and foremost to let others into our world. ... It is often thought that the therapeutic benefit of art comes from the artists' release of their pent-up emotions. While undoubtedly there is some truth in this, it pales beside the therapeutic benefit of moving other people.' (p.27)

Future research on dream-sharing and empathy

The main limitation of the studies reviewed here was that there was no comparison condition in which some narrative material other than a dream report is used to elicit a meaningful discussion. Comparison conditions in future work could be the discussion of a recent significant event in the life of the dreamer, as in Edwards et al. (2015), the dream-sharer telling and discussing someone else's dream as if it were their own, as in Hill et al. (1993), or having the dreamer tell and discuss a story based on an ambiguous photograph or drawing. Whatever the results of such comparison conditions, dreams may still anyway be valid and useful stimuli for discussion even if the outcomes and benefits from dream discussions are no higher than for other objects of discussion. This is because the discussion of dreams may be expected to be at least as fruitful as the discussion of other narrative stimuli given that the brain is sifting memories for consolidation during sleep on the basis of their emotional relevance (van Rijn et al., 2017), and dreaming may reflect or be part of this filtering process (Eichenlaub et al., 2018; Malinowski & Horton, 2014; Wamsley & Stickgold, 2011; Zadra & Stickgold, 2021). Furthermore, whatever the outcomes for sharing dreams are, in comparison to outcomes for sharing other narrative reports, such as of a favourite film, it must be remembered that people often wake with a dream in mind that they want to tell. The personal and social benefits of such dream-sharing thus do need to be investigated further, albeit with comparison conditions that present or generate narratives other than dreams as the basis for discussion. This is also important because of the finding by Schredl and colleagues (2015b) that frequency of sharing dreams is highly correlated with the frequency of sharing personal experiences.

We conclude optimistically that increased dream telling across society might counteract current societal decreases in empathic concern and perspective taking, the main two components of empathy (Konrath et al., 2011), and may be useful in countries with lower empathic concern and perspective taking (Chopik et al., 2017). Research on this would be difficult, and require large samples of participants, but would be useful in investigating whether there can be a wider social impact of the findings reported in this chapter.

Summary

The sharing of dreams leads to increased empathy towards the dreamer from those with whom the dream is shared. This may be due to the dream being a fictional story that is explored and linked to the dreamer's waking life. We will return to the empathy effect, and a possible function for dreams that follows from it, in Chapter 17. But first, we look in detail at our science art collaboration DreamsID, which led to this work on empathy and dream-sharing.

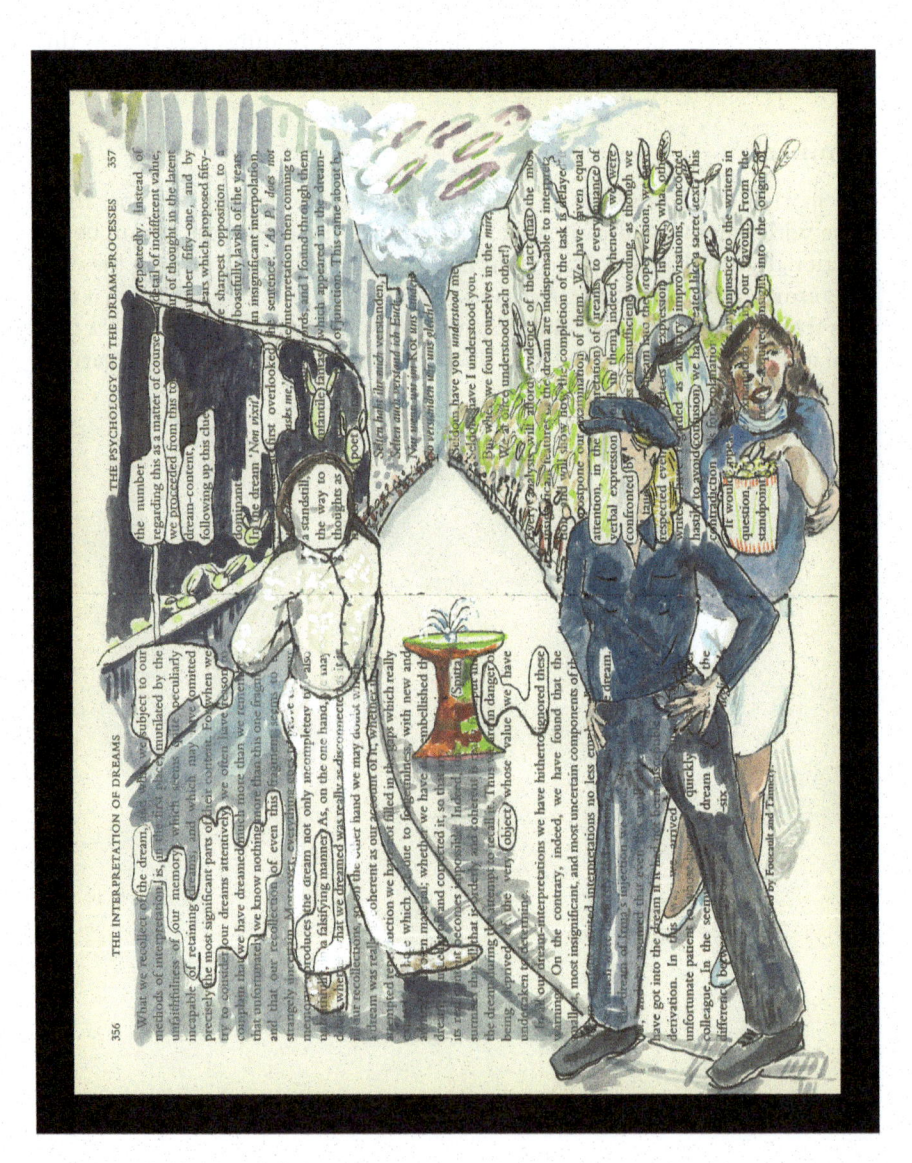

Figure 14.1 Dream of cop and apocalypse spores, 2021.

14 The DreamsID science and art collaboration

Surrealism and the socialising of dreams

This dream was told during our event at Surrealisms 2021, a conference of the International Society for the Study of Surrealism.

DREAM NARRATIVE: *I'm in a busy wide street in New York City. A woman of colour is being arrested for eating popcorn because she has no mask. I am also eating popcorn, outside a restaurant, and a cop who's next to me leans on the plate glass and says to me 'you know what's wrong with the world?' She continues, 'like why are we still using Xerox, so far into the pandemic?' I reply that maybe the problem with the world is a lack of personal responsibility. The cop has a hat with a visor and cannot arrest me because I am eating the popcorn out of a plastic mesh basket, which is within the regulations. The cop is angry and keeps talking to me but is also confiding in me. I look up and see lights in the sky, sparkling purple and green, in rings that are like aeroplanes or alien spaceships. There is also a water fountain which is orange and green. The fountain pops out a single alien spore that drifts and falls on a windowsill. The building collapses due to the spore and there is a botanical explosion with alien plants all over the building, coloured green and tan and beige, unlike the colours of plants on earth. More spores drift from the fountain: they are fist-size, with a round bottom that is pale off-white, and with two leaves sprouting from the top, like a helicopter spore. I know that the spores can destroy everything and I feel a heavy dread that all will soon be gone.*

DISCUSSION: In the discussion, the dream-sharer told of reading a lot on social media and online discussions about fears of the climate crisis and the collapse of civilization. We realised the possible relevance to the dream of a pun on 'cop', as the COP26 UN Climate Change Conference was happening at the time of the dream.

JULIA: (Painting shown as Figure 14.1) I first saw a triangle of white between the pages that I could use for the perspective in the street scene. The dreamer and police officer are shown in the foreground, on the pavement/sidewalk; the woman of colour, with popcorn, and the arresting officer, are on the right; the street stretches into the distance; and the spores are at the top with the collapsing building at the top right.

DOI: 10.4324/9781003037552-14

During the painting process, I found words of Freud that were appropriate to the dream. These *objets trouvés* include the following:

In the police officer's visor, the words:

attention, in the
verbal expression
confronted

And in the middle of the painting, and relevant to the apocalypse, the words:

in danger
we
ignored these

Regarding the realisation during the discussion of the relationship of the cop and apocalypse to the current COP26 conference, there is a found poem at the top of the right-hand page:

the number
regarding this as a matter of course
we proceeded from this to
dream-content,
following up this clue

The DreamsID science art collaboration

In the Summer of 2016, the British Science Association was due to hold its annual British Science Festival in Swansea. Following Mark's experiences and research in discussing dreams using the Ullman technique, he wanted to propose an evening session for the public coming to an open event in which he would discuss the dreams of anyone attending. This would use the Ullman method, as described in Chapter 10, but with a short time-frame of 15–20 minutes per person. The Festival planned to have an evening event, 'Creatures of the Night', in an educational, tourist attraction, rainforest-themed, nature centre, a striking glass-sided large pyramidal building, in Swansea. Mark talked this idea over with artist Julia Lockheart, who suggested that she could quickly paint each dream while the discussion of it occurred.

We agreed that each dreamer would be given the painting, to document their participation in the site-specific performance, and to enable them to use the painting to further consider the dream and the discussion at home with family and friends, and across time, after the event. On the evening, the event was magical, with dim light, trees everywhere and various arts-based science exhibits and performances. We sat at a table at the top of the

The DreamsID science and art collaboration: Surrealism 157

spiralling path, up through the rainforest-themed environment, and with a large screen behind us, on which was live-projected a film of each painting as it was being made.

As described in Chapter 10, the group dream discussion method (Ullman, 1996/2006) traces back the components of the dream to the dreamer's recent waking life experiences. In recognition of the discussion method being partly derived from the free association technique of Sigmund Freud, and to make the painting more memorable, Julia suggested that each painting could be made onto one or two pages taken from Freud's (1900/1997) book *The Interpretation of Dreams*. We obtained the kind permission of the publishers (Wordsworth Editions, Hertfordshire, UK) to do this, using the first English translation of the book. When the dream-sharer first tells their dream, Julia uses its narrative structure, for example, number of scenes, environmental features and presence of objects, to select pages from the book, by identifying visually relevant shapes in the paragraphs and text on the page, including shapes of any footnotes, bullet points or diagrams. This then structures the underlying composition of the painting. While the painting is being made, Julia incorporates relevant words from the page into the painting, as *objets trouvés*, found objects. As these words are not spotted when the pages are chosen, it is eerie how relevant these words can be, and it adds to the magic of the painting that words written by Freud (albeit originally in German) become part of the artwork, themselves like free associations.

We named our science art collaboration DreamsID (Dreams Illustrated and Discussed, or Dreams Interpreted and Drawn; with reference also to Freud's notion of the *id*). We started performing our dream salons at various places, such as conferences, art galleries, science festivals, the Freud Museum London (Figure 14.2 and Figure 14.3), University of California Los Angeles, Paris Institute for Advanced Study (Figure 14.4) and other places in mainland Europe and the US.

Our discussions of a dream are held in public, in venues or online, each lasting up to 90 minutes, with the painting produced in that time. The audience members can watch the painting process on a large screen, which is positioned directly behind Mark and the dream-sharer (see Figures 14.2–14.4). Though Mark can turn to see the painting process in order to collaboratively clarify visual and plot details of the dream, the dream-sharer is asked not to look at the emerging visual components of the painting so that it does not influence the dreamer's retelling. After the dream is told several times, Mark and the audience clarify visual and plot details of the dream, for example, colours, shapes, ages and sex of characters, and then discuss the dream, following Ullman's (1996/2006) method for this. It is a very captivating and engaging activity for the audience, and contributions and observations of the audience members have been a key component of all the performances. The performances are very much audio-visual, even immersive, in that audience members take part in the discussion while also watching the painting develop

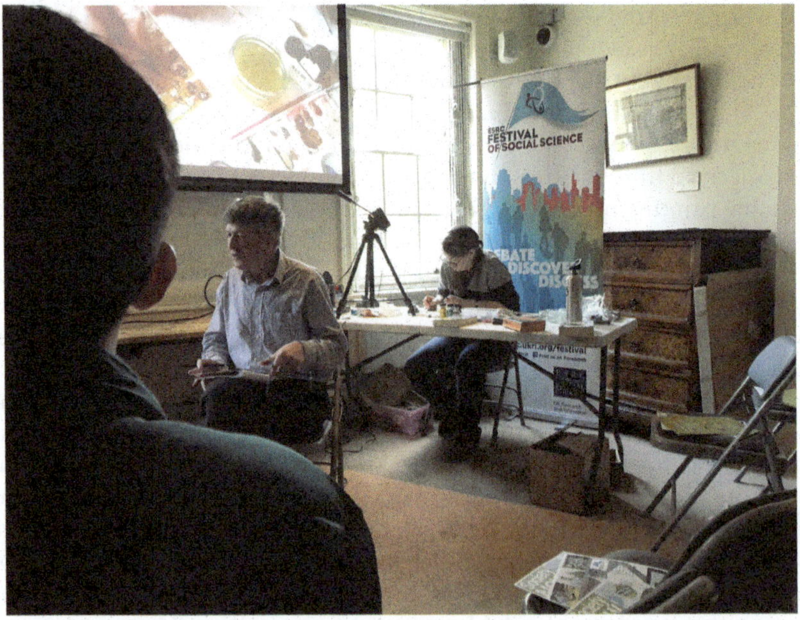

158 The DreamsID science and art collaboration: Surrealism

Figure 14.2 Julia Lockheart and Mark Blagrove at the Freud Museum London in 2018 (Courtesy of the Freud Museum London).

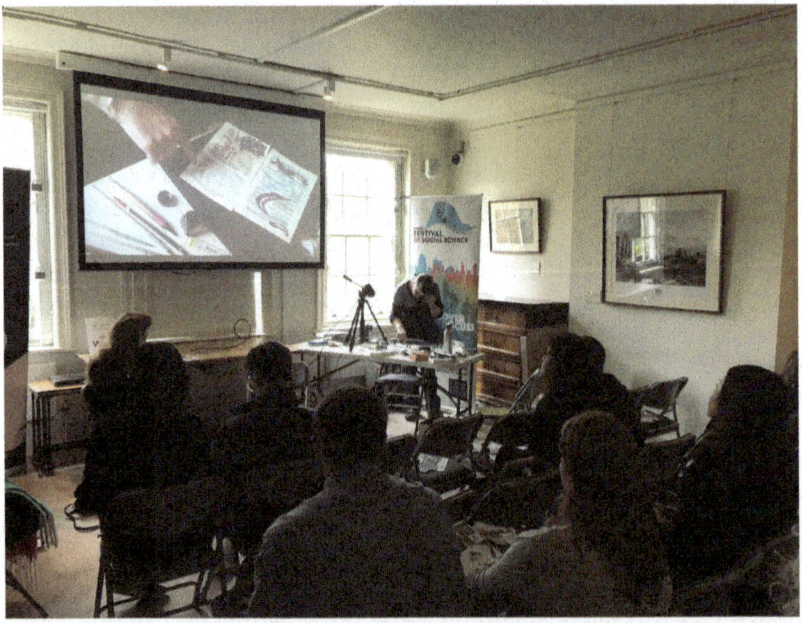

Figure 14.3 Julia Lockheart at the Freud Museum London in 2018 (Courtesy of the Freud Museum London).

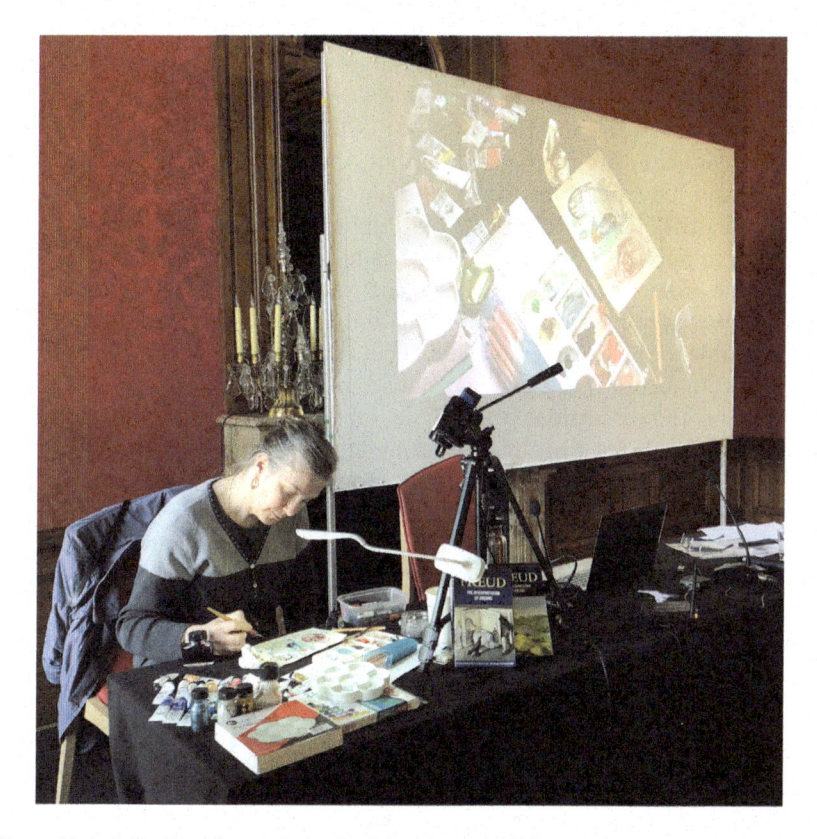

Figure 14.4 Julia Lockheart at the Paris Institute of Advanced Study in 2019.

on-screen. The audience and dream-sharer see and comment on the final painting at the end of the event.

After the event, the painting is scanned and an enlarged giclée print is made of it, which is combined with the printed text of the dream, underneath the image, as the final artwork. An art-quality print is used because we found that the original book pages that we gave to dreamers at the beginning of the project began to yellow due to sunlight and were noticeably affected by humidity and temperature fluctuations. Giclée prints give the work a longevity and allow us to use conservation-grade, acid-free paper; also, the use of conservation grade inks mean colours do not change with time. A further purpose of using an enlarged print is that the details of the artwork can be better seen from a distance, including any of Freud's words on the pages that are highlighted in the artwork. The carefully produced and enlarged gicleé print is the final artwork and is the only one made. This is given to the dream-sharer, with signed and dated documentation to show their participation in the situated DreamsID performance, and for display at home, so that they can discuss it and the dream with others, as part of a socialisation of the dream.

Outcomes of DreamsID events

Paintings from the DreamsID collaboration can be seen throughout this book, on the Gallery page of the website DreamsID.com, and in Lockheart (2022b) and Lockheart and Blagrove (2019, 2020). Paintings from the collaboration have been displayed at exhibitions, including at the Freud Museum London, and have been described in documentaries on the BBC, Australian Broadcasting Corporation and US Public Service Broadcasts, as well as appearing in publications such as New Scientist.

After the project had developed over two years, our original aim was being fulfilled. We were providing discussions and artworks that were meaningful and enjoyable to the dreamer and audiences and which provided some insight for the dream-sharer into their life. But we then started to notice the effects these dreams and discussions were having on us, and on some audience members, and realised that this dream-sharing and emergent image-making was evoking empathy from us and the audience towards the dream-sharer. The first dream where this clearly happened was described at the start of Chapter 13, with the painting of the dream also presented there. In this, and other dreams afterwards, we came to realise how the dream-sharer was speedily disclosing aspects of their life, and that we and the audience were partly seeing the world from their perspective, and having some understanding of their emotions and life experiences. We decided to investigate the effects of dream-sharing on empathy in experiments at the School of Psychology, Swansea University. This resulted in our paper on the effects of dream-sharing on empathy, published in June 2019 in the journal *Frontiers in Psychology* (Blagrove et al., 2019b), and a subsequent replication experiment (Blagrove et al., 2021), which we describe in Chapter 13. The experiments addressed only the discussion part of dream-sharing and not our additional creation of an artwork, which will be investigated experimentally in the future as it involves longer timespans than for the immediate effects of the discussions.

Art and the socialisation of dreams

The purpose of painting dreams at DreamsID events is to aid the socialisation of the dream, through the use of the painting as a cue to meaningful new discussions about the dream, and a cue to revisiting the original event and discussion. The aim is to increase self-understanding and the understanding of others towards the life circumstances of the dreamer, and to generate empathy towards the dreamer. This method is especially useful for people who might not engage with the dream in its written or spoken form, or who would also value a visual depiction of the dream. Whereas in our work for this the dream is painted by Julia, an artist, another approach is for the dreamer to draw their dream, so as to discuss the drawing and the dream with a group, for example, Berry's (2021) Drawn into the Dream method, and Mersky and Sievers' (2018) Social Dream Drawing. Mersky and Sievers make an interesting comparison of such drawings to transitional objects, a term used by psychoanalyst Donald Winnicott to describe an object or possession where inner desires and external reality are brought together and explored (Caldwell, 2022; Winnicott, 1953), and for which he gave examples of children's special blankets and stuffed animals.

Dreams can be used as inspiration in the production of art (Barcaro & Paoli, 2015; Barrett, 2001), including the Romantics with Fuseli and Blake (Brown, 2001, pp.316–320), and, as will be seen later in this chapter and chapter 16, the Surrealists. But art is included in the DreamsID events not just for its beauty but also for its social and epistemic importance. That is, for its communicative nature, eliciting socio-epistemic skills such as self- and other-understanding, and as 'a source of moral understanding and self-development' (Sherman & Morrissey, 2017). The latter authors present evidence that there can be emotional sharing between the artist and current and future viewers of the art, with the enhancement of mutual-understanding and affective and cognitive empathy. This is described well by King (2002), who holds that whereas physics, and science more generally, narrow down the sensorium to measurable quantities, art practice is an enquiry that opens up the sensorium, and to also include emotions. In science, knowledge is tested against sense-data, the sense-data being sought out. In contrast, sense-data are produced in art, and rather than validate theories or hypotheses, they validate the experiences to which the art refers. So, for our events, the artwork aims to honour the original dream, to show that the dream is valued, rather than dismissed as, say, a delirium, or as having no connection with the dreamer's waking life, or as not a worthy subject for the time of others. The art is also playful and contingent on the circumstances of the event, such as which pages of Freud's book are chosen on which to paint, and which later provide words that can be incorporated into the artwork. This use of found objects is akin to the uses of automatic writing, frottage, collage and chance described by King (2002) as occurring in Dadaist and surrealist works, and this valuing and socialising of dreams is part of Surrealism, to which we now turn.

DreamsID, Dadaism and Surrealism

During the painting process at our DreamsID events, found words are incorporated into the artwork, forming a palimpsest. Such *objets trouvés* (Oneto, 2017) and found poems are a waking life counterpart of the automatistic and playful incorporation and mergings of memories into dreams. The events combine dream and reality, a maxim of the *Manifesto of Surrealism* (Breton, 1924/1972, p.14), and the use of everyday dreams aims to fulfil Lautréamont's exhortation that 'Poetry must be made by all. Not by one' (quoted by Rosemont, in Breton 1924/1978, p.26). It also fulfils Czech avant-garde artist Karel Teige's exhortation that 'The dream expressed in a poem or in a picture becomes a force tending to materialise and to identify itself with life' (quoted by Rosemont, in Breton 1924/1978, p.547).

The DreamsID paintings and performances fit within Dadaism and Surrealism in six ways:

- The process demonstrates a valuing of the dream, such valuing being a key component of Surrealism.
- The dream is what in Surrealism is termed an 'automatism', something produced without conscious control.
- The paintings are made rapidly, in contrast to slow deliberation (Grant, 2005, p.115).
- The performances are one-time events, with audience participation. Experiential group events were prized by Dadaists and Surrealists and would more recently be called *happenings,* a word coined by performance artist Allan Kaprow (1993).
- The painting process and artworks incorporate *objets trouvés*, that is, objects that are found by chance on the page being painted on. In some places, these constitute *found poems*, which reflect a Dadaist influence.
- The associative reaction of each dream to the social and personal circumstances of the dream-sharer follows the 'disinterested play of thought' (Breton, 1924/1972, p.26; cf. Bulkeley, 2019), as do the reactions of dreamers and audiences to the finished artworks.

We thus now move to a description of the history, theory and art of Surrealism, and its relationship to dreaming.

Surrealism and the valuing of dreams

Surrealism grew out of Dadaism in the early 1920s (Hopkins, 2004; Legge, 2016). Dadaism had started in 1916 when German poet Hugo Ball founded the Cabaret Voltaire in Zurich, with offshoots starting in Paris, Berlin, New York and other cities. Dadaism was very internationalist and was partly a response to the horrors of the First World War. It was highly performative, with costumes and masks, music, dances, talks about artworks, such as by Hans Arp on his collages and the reciting of sound poetry. It partly allied itself with Futurism and Cubism (Lewer, 2016).

One of the early members of the Dada group was André Breton, who trained as a psychiatrist, and thus knew the work of Freud, including Freud's work on dreams and on the unconscious. In treating the injured at the front in the First World War, he 'realized the poetic quality of the free association writing sessions he prescribed to his patients' (Susik, 2016). Susik relates that unlike the Dadaist chance meeting of banal objects, such as paper and string, Breton emphasised psychological and linguistic associations. This led to the use of automatic writing and to waking dream séances and to automatic drawing and found objects. Surrealism arose due to André Breton's revolt against the chaos of some Dadaist activities. In 'After Dada' (Breton,

1924/1996), Breton writes that, regarding events organized by Dada, 'I have no wish to be amused. It seems to me that sanctioning a series of utterly futile "Dada" acts means seriously compromising one of the attempts at liberation to which I remain the most strongly attached.' For Breton, the professed leader of the new movement, Surrealism was to be more coherent and theoretically based than Dadaism.

As a political, cultural and artistic movement Surrealism greatly valued dreaming (Jiménez, 2013). From 1919 onwards, its proponents described its main aim as to bring together the waking and dreaming realms. Indeed, the need to find artistic analogues of dreams, as non-linear responses to human and world situations, was elucidated in 'The Mediums Enter' (Breton, 1924/1996) and the *Manifesto of Surrealism* (Breton, 1924/1972).

In 'The Mediums Enter' (1924/1996), Breton writes that in 1919 his attention was drawn to how, when falling asleep, phrases or sentences 'became perceptible to my mind'. With others he tried to recreate this state, using abbreviations so as to rapidly transcribe these trance-like images onto paper. In October 1924, the Surrealists founded the Bureau de Recherches Surréalistes in Paris. Dream performances were held there as part of the Surrealists' experiments into unconscious and semi-unconscious states (Groth & Lusty, 2013, chapter 6). The series of hypnotic or waking dream séances involved the questioning by the attendees of the automatist adepts such as Robert Desnos and René Crevel, and is shown in a well-known photograph *Waking Dream Séance* (1924), by Man Ray. However, Breton decided that there were 'incursions of conscious elements' into these gatherings, and this intrusion of waking human thoughts or literary form led him to instead devote his attention to actual dream narratives.

The Surrealists were publishing their own dream narratives. Georges Sebbag (2013) describes how in March 1922 the Surrealist magazine *Littérature* published three dream narratives by Breton, subsequent issues had dreams of other members of the group, and the first issue of *La Révolution surréaliste* in December 1924 had a dream of Georgio de Chirico, three dreams of Breton, and the dreams of other members of the movement. One of Breton's dreams was of a moveable urinal at a railway station, followed by a flying urinal which the dreamer thought was dangerous, an obvious reference here to Marcel Duchamp's use of a urinal in his readymade *Fountain* (1917). Spector (1989) describes these published dreams of Breton and suggests their waking life correspondences, including how they refer to many of the leading Surrealists, such as Pablo Picasso, and the poet and play-write Guillaume Apollinaire, who had died in 1918 and had coined the word Surrealism in 1917. In another dream reported by Spector, Breton is in a funeral procession which, to his surprise, is going in the opposite direction to the cemetery. He finds himself abreast of the hearse:

> On the coffin sits an older man, extremely pale, in deep mourning and wearing a top hat, who can be none other than the dead man who,

turning alternately left and right, returns the greetings of the passers-by. The procession enters into a match factory.

Spector's (1989) fascinating paper outlines the importance of dreams to Surrealism, and relates André Breton's dreams to what was occurring in the Surrealist movement and to its members at the time.

More dream texts were included in later issues of *La Révolution surréaliste*, and the final issue had 16 photo booth portraits of the main Surrealists, all with eyes closed, as if asleep. The development of thinking about dreaming by the Surrealists is described by Sebbag (2013), including an account of Max Ernst's painting *Two Children are Threatened by a Nightingale* (1924). This shows two small children in a much larger landscape of a house and surroundings, with a small physical gate fixed to the frame, and a very small nightingale, and was inspired by a vision Ernst had during a fever as a child.

It is of note that the valuing of dreams was extended to an extent by the Surrealists to the general public. The Bureau de Recherches Surréalistes was open to the public every day for two hours, staffed by two Surrealists on a rota, during which time visitors would be welcomed and encouraged to tell their dreams (Ades, 2013). Also, an archive of dreams was collected from 1937 to 1948 as part of the UK government's Mass Observation project, aimed to assess subjective psychic life as a counterpart to the wider observation of behaviours and attitudes assessed by the project. This subjective component of the much larger Mass Observation project was partly inspired by the ideas and individuals involved in 'surrealist ethnography' (Groth & Lusty, 2013, chapter 7).

Surrealist theory and dreams

To underline the importance of dreaming to Surrealism, in the *Manifesto of Surrealism* (Breton, 1924/1972), Breton states that, aside from Freud, dreaming has been 'grossly neglected', and that he would like to sleep 'in order to stop imposing, in this [waking] realm, the conscious rhythm of my thought.' Breton continues that he gives thanks to Freud that 'a part of our mental world which we pretended not to be concerned with any longer – and, in my opinion, by far the most important part – has been brought back to light.' As a result of this, Breton continues, 'The imagination is perhaps on the point of reasserting itself, of reclaiming its rights.' Central to this is dreaming and he states:

> Surrealism is based on the belief in the superior reality of certain forms of previously neglected associations, in the omnipotence of dream, in the disinterested play of thought. It tends to ruin once and for all all other psychic mechanisms and to substitute itself for them in solving all the principal problems of life.
>
> (*Manifesto of Surrealism*, Breton, 1924/1972, p.26.)

Surrealism aimed for 'the future resolution of these two states, dream and reality, which are seemingly so contradictory, into a kind of absolute reality, a *surreality*' (*Manifesto of Surrealism*, Breton, 1924/1972, p.14).

Surrealists saw this merging of dreams and reality as a path to freedom, and as countering 'the *hate of the marvelous* which rages in certain men' (*Manifesto of Surrealism*, Breton, 1924/1972, p.14). Along these lines, José Jiménez (2013), writing in the catalogue of a major surrealist exhibition, quotes René Magritte from 1938, 'Surrealism demands for waking life a freedom similar to the freedom we have when dreaming'. For Jiménez (p.50), reflecting on the purposes of Surrealism, invoking dreams is

> the manifestation of a revolt against the 'realistic' acceptance of an illmade' world, against an attitude of resigned acceptance of pain and suffering. The Surrealist invocation of the dream transmits a utopia of total liberation of the mind, the dream of a freedom without limits.

Yet, importantly, Surrealism is a very social worldview. For its first decades, the Surrealists lived and loved as a community, albeit a disputatious community (Chadwick, 2021a). Indeed, the first line of Breton's (1928/1999) semi-autobiographical novel *Nadja*, about his tumultuous love affair with the eponymous young women, reads: 'Who am I? If this once I were to rely on a proverb, then perhaps everything would amount to knowing who I "haunt."' The social nature of the movement is also seen in their use of surveys, with questions such as whether they have secret desires, and the role of will and conscience:

> Surveys were a popular tool of the surrealist movement, in part because they stimulated debate and in part because the responses illuminated the question of the extent to which a person's opinions were individual or shaped by the views of the collective.
>
> (Mundy, 2001)

The surveys and group events aimed to explore a shift away from rational orthodox thinking, for example, asking each other regarding paintings, 'where would you hide in this painting?' or 'where would you make love?' (In architectural environment-based works, such as de Chirico's *The Enigma of a Day* (1914), these questions are very thought-provoking.) It is the social nature of Surrealism and its emphasis on desire (Mundy, 2001) and the representation and recognition of desire, that again draws a parallel with dreaming, and the social and emotional content of dreams.

Surrealist methods and their relationships to dreams

Sinclair's (2021) chapter 'Psychoanalysis and Dada' describes the Dadaist performances that started at the Cabaret Voltaire in Zurich, during and as a response to the First World War, and describes the cut-up method of Tristan Tzara's manifesto 'To Make a Dadaist Poem,' originally published in 1920 (Tzara, 2013, p.39), in which words are cut-out from a newspaper article and randomly put together. The movement's use of automatic writing had similarities to Freud's method of free association, in that it aimed to bypass inhibition and censorship, unveiling latent associations and interconnections, such as in photomontage. The creation of art thus moved away from skill, intention and reason, and towards spontaneity and the production of novel associations. This led to methods such as collage, which would result in unplanned juxtapositions of printed or made materials, and Cadavre Exquis, or Exquisite Corpse, in which a long sheet of paper is folded so that consecutive drawings can be made by different people, each of whom does not see what has been drawn or written by previous contributors.

In May 1921, Max Ernst was exhibiting collaged photographs and collaged readymade images from scientific catalogues. Breton (1924/1996), in his essay 'Max Ernst,' wrote of Ernst's work in terms of poetry, on 'the marvellous ability to reach out, without leaving the field of our experience, to two distinct realities and bring them together to create a spark' and concluded 'we do not hesitate to see Max Ernst as the man of these infinite possibilities.' Such a creative bringing together of distinct realities is seen also in May Ray's photograph *Glass Tears* (1932), in which a model's eyes, looking up, have glass tears running from them, giving to the viewer a feeling of the physicalness and permanence of the tears, and of the distress causing them.

Another surrealist artform is the often-intriguing surrealist or symbolic object. Hopkins (2004, p.87) relates that Breton in 1924 had a dream of encountering an enigmatic book:

> The back of the book was formed of a wooden gnome whose white beard, clipped in the Assyrian manner, reached to his feet. The statue was of ordinary thickness, but did not prevent me from turning the pages which were of heavy black cloth.

Hopkins writes of Breton's conviction from the dream of the need for the production and circulation of such surrealist 'symbolically functioning objects'. Examples of these include Salvador Dali's *Lobster Telephone* (1936), and Meret Oppenheim's *My Nurse* (1936) and *Object* (1936, titled *Lunch in Fur* by Breton, a bowl and spoon that are lined with fur). These were to become some of the best-known works of Surrealism.

Interestingly, as Surrealism was becoming defined, and after the creation of surreal ballet, sculpture and poetry, there were arguments from the first issue of *La Révolution surréaliste* in 1924 about whether there could be surrealist painting. Some held painting to not be automatist enough, that it required too much deliberation and thought. The many arguments and personalities involved are described by Grant (2005, pp.89–115). Finally, in July 1925, André Breton wrote an article in the fourth issue of the magazine

La Révolution surréaliste in which he gave approval for surrealist painting, followed by his lengthy appraisal and cataloguing of Surrealist paintings in *Surrealism and Painting* (Breton, 1928/2002). The fourth issue of *La Révolution surréaliste* praised imagination in the visual arts and this followed the welcome already given over some years to the paintings of Picasso. However, there was concern about the commercial aspect of visual art, which was especially true for how they saw Picasso. On this, Grant reports (p.105) a dream of Breton in which Picasso 'draws distractedly in a notebook' and then sells these quick automatist lines for an enormous price, a dream which is thus referring to these fears of commercialisation.

Surrealist art, paintings and photography

Despite this initial suspicion regarding painting, and although Surrealism started as a literary movement, it is nowadays mainly renowned for painting. Examples of the wild combinations in surrealist artworks include Rene Magritte's *The Empire of Light* (1954), showing a dark street, house and park scene but with the bright blue sky in full daylight, and Duchamp's *L.H.O.O.Q.* (1919), a cheap reproduction postcard of the Mona Lisa onto which he drew a moustache and beard, and added the eponymous initials which function as a homophonic pun. (An engaging description of Duchamp's artworks and readymades and their place in his life, imagination and intellect can be read in Rabinovitch, 2020.) These works show the playfulness of Surrealism. Surrealist paintings, however, in general were not based on particular dreams, despite their oneiric qualities and also the valuing of dreams by the Surrealists. For Ades (2013), such images might spring from 'dream-work' processes and experiences that have escaped everyday logic and rationality, but 'not necessarily literally from a dream'. Examples of such processes of condensation and representation in the work of Ernst are described by Hopkins (2004, pp.100–101) and by psychologist and surrealist painter Grace Pailthorpe in her short essay 'The Scientific Aspect of Surrealism' (1938/39). A later example of oneiric processes in artworks can be seen with Dorothea Tanning. In *Birthday* (1942), she depicts doors intriguingly left ajar, and in many works, there are bright magical scenes showing environments that are partly real but partly fantastic. She also described her dreams as fantastical: 'bristling with objects which relate to nothing in the dictionary. On waking, they lose their clarity. Dreams one reads in books are composed as known symbols [but] it is the strangeness of dreams that distinguishes them' (Chadwick, 2021b, p.177, [but] in original).

Although there are few examples of surrealist artworks for which a specific dream is the inspiration, an exception is the depiction, socialisation and politicisation of dreams seen in the work of German-born photographer Grete Stern, whose main work was produced in Argentina. From 1948 to 1951 Stern produced 140 photocollages for a self-help column ('Psicoanalisis le ayudara' [Psychology will help you]) in a weekly women's magazine *Idilio*

[*Idyll*] (Marcoci & Meister, 2015; Montgomery, 2021). The photomontages were surreal depictions of dreams that women readers sent to the column and to its psychologist. Although based on the women readers' dreams, the photomontages commentated on and protested the social conditions of the readers. For example, one depicted a worried-looking woman on the telephone as if trying to speak, but with no mouth, in another, a woman is shocked and recoils from a man in a suit whose head is a camera, and, in another, a man, presumably a deceased husband, reaches out to the woman from a photograph. Marcoci and Meister (2015) describe how the magazine asked readers to categorise the dreams they submitted, such as of 'dreams of obstacles', 'dreams of discontent', 'mask dreams', 'dreams of dolls', 'anxiety dreams' and others.

There are only 46 preserved original negatives, now in a series termed Sueños [Dreams]. They include: *Dream No. 28: Love Without Illusion*, 1951, a cowering woman being held by a man in a suit, but who has the head of a lizard; *Dream No.15: Untitled*, 1949, a woman walking up a stony hill pulling a rope with a large boulder at the end of it; *Dream No. 7: Who Will She Be?*, 1949, a woman looking at multiples of her shocked reflection in a mirror; *Dream No. 18: Café Concert*, 1948, a woman on a concert stage playing a piano that has a typewriter keyboard; *Dream No. 43: Untitled*, 1949, a woman looking out of a window at a tree that is floating, with its roots hanging down; *Dream No. 22: Last Kiss* 1949, a woman kissing an inert man's head which is lying amongst graves; *Dream No. 45: Untitled*, 1949, a smartly dressed woman sitting in a chair in a birdcage; *Dream No. 24: Surprise*, 1949, a woman hiding her face in shock from a large baby doll which is approaching her. The techniques used for creating the photomontages are described by Stern in Marcoci and Meister (2015), where she states that 'numerous possibilities for the composition arise, among them the juxtaposition of implausible elements.' (p.241.) It is this artistic choice between possibilities for composition that characterises the work as surrealist, rather than as the *trompe-l'œil* still-life depiction of a dream cautioned against by Breton (1941/2002, p.70).

Contemporary legacy of Surrealism

The large-scale Dorothea Tanning exhibition at the Tate Modern gallery in London in 2019, in collaboration with the Museo Nacional Centro de Arts Reina Sofia in Madrid, showed Tanning's ability to rewrite the language of Surrealism. Her *Eine Kleine Nachtmusik* (1943) includes a girl standing but apparently asleep, and another girl with flying hair standing next to a giant sunflower, and was described by her as 'a confrontation between the forces of grown-up logic and the bottomless psyche of a child' (Mahon, 2018, p.7). However, it is Tanning's anamorphic mannequins and soft sculptural body parts, such as are seen in *Nue Couchée* (1969–70), that have been referenced by contemporary artist Sarah Lucas. Hopkins (2004, xvi–xvii) states that Lucas' painting and sculptural work 'relies on the achievements of Dadaists and Surrealists such as Marcel Duchamp, May Ray, and René Magritte' as do other so-called Young British Artists (YBAs) who used ready-mades or found objects and anti-art to embrace such surrealist and Dadaist approaches. For Cornelia Parker, who utilises a very wide variety of found objects in her artworks, or indeed as her artworks, these found objects have their own past, but can 'inhale some fresh meanings and values' through their new use, and can be a proxy for neglected emotions (Iversen, 2022).

There is thus a contemporary re-examination of the themes and theories of Surrealism. Indeed, the title of the 2022 Venice Biennale, *The Milk of Dreams* is named after Leonora Carrington's surreal, macabre, children's book *The Milk of Dreams* (2013). Occurring at the same time as the Biennale was the *Surrealisms Beyond Borders* exhibition, at the Tate Modern gallery with work which toured from The Metropolitan Museum of Art in New York (D'Alessandro & Gale, 2021). The show aimed to rewrite the Paris-centred narrative of the movement, framed and controlled by self-proclaimed gatekeeper Breton, by displaying the work of artists from around the world, exploring the revolutionary approaches to Surrealism, many of which had not previously been exhibited as part of a global surrealist movement. Prior to this, in *Phantoms of Surrealism*, the Whitechapel Gallery, London, in 2021, explored the British surrealist movement and the pivotal role women played in it.

In the 2022 exhibition *The Woven Child,* the Hayward Gallery, London, exhibited Louise Bourgeois' first major retrospective (Rugoff, 2022). Bourgeois, although not directly referencing particular dreams or dreaming, combines metaphorical references to waking life in physical pieces and environments. For example, *Untitled* (2005) has hanging, sagging cheesecloth sacks, bringing to mind the flaccidity of ageing skin and body. Many works also have a narrative, either within the piece or by referencing narratives from her life, such as of relationships with her parents. A narrative experience occurs for the viewer in *The Reticent Child* (2003), which is a melancholic diorama in a long display case. It shows the heavily pregnant Bourgeois on the left side, next is her giving birth in a labour ward, then her lying in a bed, and finally her young son, standing, covering his face. The narrative feel of this piece is boosted by a concave mirror at the back of the diorama, in which distorted, animated reflections and shapes of the viewer and other viewers are seen. The piece explores the origins of the reticence and withdrawal of her youngest son. The bringing together of disparate and uncomfortable memories, and their depiction with physical, soft or hard objects, sometimes with discomforting environments, is truly oneiric and captivatingly macabre. This, and many other exhibitions, and encyclopaedic works such as D'Alessandro & Gale (2021), Hopkins (2016) and Strom (2023) show the contemporary relevance of Surrealism.

Summary

Surrealism is one of the theoretical, social, cultural and artistic peaks of human creativity, whose artistic and theoretical role is currently being re-evaluated in relation to contemporary culture. Surrealism values the most innovative forms of human creativity and of novel combinations, including what occurs in dreams. The DreamsID collaboration likewise values dreams and uses public events and artworks which reflect a Dadaist and surrealist influence to socialise dreams and explore them publicly with the dreamer. Until the start of 2020 our dream salons took place in live venues. With the start of the pandemic, we moved our performances online, to discuss the dreams of key workers. The next chapter describes those online dream salons, the effect of the pandemic on sleep and dreams, and the paintings made of those dreams.

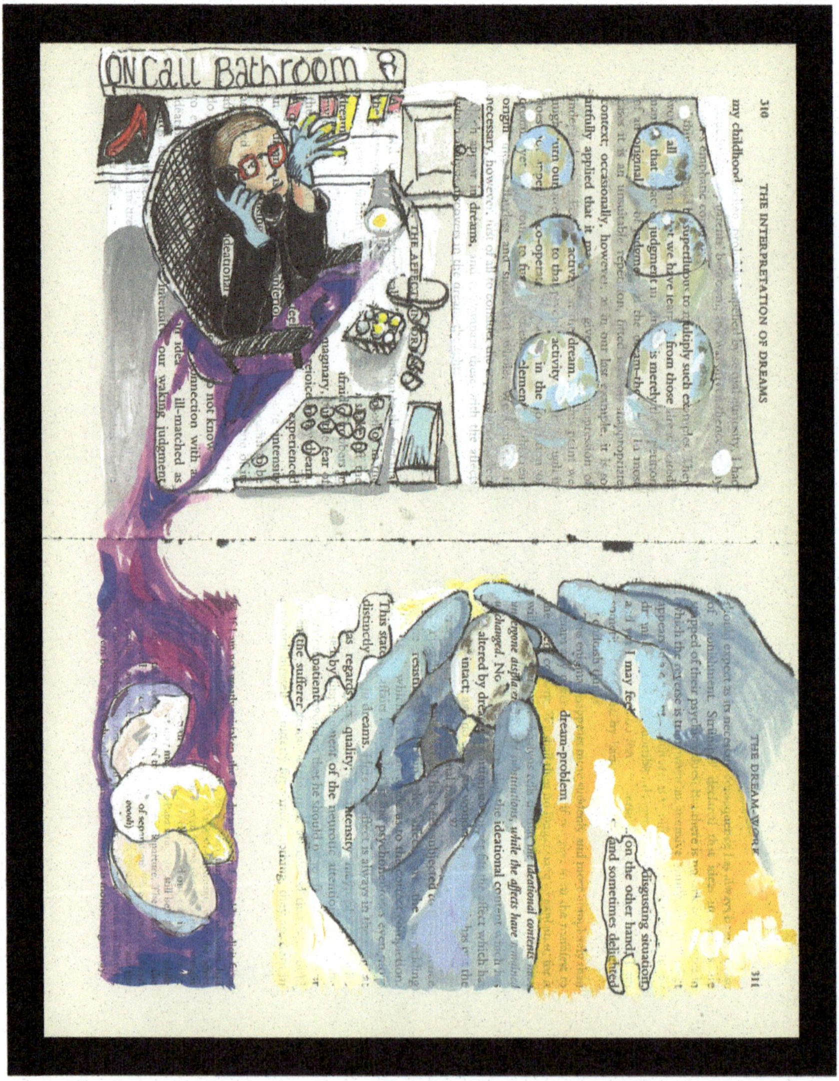

Figure 15.1 Dream of peeling quails' eggs for cure for Covid-19, 2020.

15 Sleep and dreaming during the Covid-19 pandemic

Exploring and painting Covid-19 and Lockdown dreams

The following dream, of Elaine, a National Health Service clinical lab doctor, was told to us online in April 2020 soon after the first Lockdown had started.

DREAM NARRATIVE: *I am sitting at my desk in the hospital at work with blue, latex medical gloves on, and a purple, woollen, furry blanket on my lap. I have quails' eggs in an egg box and am trying to peel them but cannot grip the cracks in them so as to pull off the shell. They are to be used to treat Covid-19 patients. The phone rings and I am being asked lots of questions about the eggs, but I am not sure they will work as a treatment. More eggs are being heated in a white medical bath, but they are soft, and egg yolk spills when I try to crack them open. I look around as I know I need to get the next batch of eggs on, but I can't see any, and there's no time to get more. Then the phone starts ringing and I can't answer it as I'm covered in yolk and bits of shell. I sit there crying, trying to peel the rest, and pushing my red glasses up with my wrist so I don't get yolk on my lenses.*

DISCUSSION: Elaine said that the purple blanket in the dream is actually at her home, and that she had recently bought chocolate quails' eggs as a gift for her husband. We discussed the developing blurred relationship between work and home during Lockdown. Elaine also discussed the pressure on her and other National Health Service (NHS) workers regarding treating Covid-19.

JULIA: (Painting shown as Figure 15.1) There are four paragraphs on the pages of the book that I used to paint this dream. These hold: the quails' eggs in their box, the dreamer at her desk, her hands with blue medical gloves shelling the eggs, and the eggs splitting open. The following interwoven phrases in Freud's text are fitting to the dream:

I may feel
disgusting situation
on the other hand
and sometimes delighted
dream-problem

DOI: 10.4324/9781003037552-15

Studies on dreams during the Covid-19 pandemic

Soon after the Covid-19 Lockdown started, there were many media reports of increases in dream recall and changes in dream content. However, as Covid-19 was unexpected, studying the changes in dreaming in the ways outlined in Chapter 1 would have been difficult. This is because of the need to find baseline dream data with which to compare the pandemic data. A similar problem occurred when researchers aimed to study how dreams changed due to the events of 9/11, as with the study by Ruth Propper and colleagues (2007) reviewed in Chapter 1.

One method used for studying pandemic dreams was to ask participants whether their dreams had changed during the pandemic, compared to previously. A representative sample in the US was contacted by YouGov in March and May 2020, with responses from a sample of 3,031 US adults, which were analysed by Schredl and Bulkeley (2020b). In their study, 29% of the participants reported that their dream recall had increased, whereas only 7.5% reported a decrease. Dreams were also reported to have become emotionally more negative. The study found that those people most strongly affected by the pandemic also reported the strongest effects on their dreams (heightened dream recall, more negatively toned dreams, and pandemic-related dreams). However, only 8% of respondents reported that they had had a dream with content related to Covid-19. Using a similar design, again with a very large sample of 15,292, Holzinger and colleagues (2022) found that the percentage of people experiencing one or more nightmares per week during the pandemic was 22.35%, whereas 13.24% stated that they were having one or more nightmares per week before the pandemic. Factors associated with this difference included self-reported posttraumatic stress, other mental disorders and various sleep disorders or problems. Gorgoni and colleagues (2021) found for their 1,091 participants that dream frequency, report length, and dream negative emotions, vividness and bizarreness were higher during the first Lockdown, compared to participants' recall of the characteristics of their dreams before the Lockdown period. The increase in negative emotions in dreams was greater for women, younger participants, and individuals with poor sleep or poor mental health.

The above studies had a limitation that they used retrospective recall of what dream characteristics were before the pandemic, and such recall might not be accuracte or might be subject to biases. Thus, a second method was to collect reports of dreams and to compare them to normative data collected from before the pandemic.

Dream reports were collected by Mota and colleagues before (September and November 2019) and during (March and April 2020) the Brazilian Lockdown (Mota et al., 2020). The two groups of participants were well-matched for education level, age and sex distribution. The study assessed all dreams recalled by the participants during each period, and used Linguistic Inquiry and Word Count (LIWC), a computerised text analysis method that identifies emotions and other content categories. The machine learning was supported by a database of Portuguese dictionary-derived synonyms. In their paper on this, Mota and colleagues reported:

- Pandemic-period dream reports were longer, when measured in words, than pre-pandemic reports.
- Pandemic dreams had more anger and sadness related-content than did pre-pandemic dreams. This effect was found even when the length of the dream reports was taken into account.
- The level of anger and sadness in dreams was related to how much the individual had mental suffering related to social isolation. The researchers stated that this is consistent with the Emotional Regulation Theory of dreaming.
- Pandemic dreams also had more references to contamination and cleanness. The authors link this to the Threat Simulation Theory, which holds that we practice overcoming threats in the virtual reality of the dream.

At the end of the study participants rated how much they observed their dreams or told them to others during the study. These behaviours occurred more if the person was happy (versus sad), energetic (versus tired), peaceful (versus aggressive), altruistic (versus selfish) and creative (versus confused). Mota and colleagues concluded that paying attention to and telling our dreams is a 'relatively safe way for self-observation and mental health management that can be recommended during this period of uncertainty'.

Whereas the Mota study investigated all dreams that occurred to participants during the pandemic, the online survey posted by Harvard Medical School researcher Deirdre Barrett, from March to July 2020, requested the submission of 'any dreams you have had related to the COVID-19 coronavirus'. Dreams from 2,888 individuals were processed by LIWC. In her (2020a) paper on this, Barrett reports that women showed significantly lower positive emotions in their dreams and higher rates of negative emotions, anxiety, sadness, anger, body content, references to biological processes, poor health, and death, whereas for male respondents only the poor health variable was as affected as it was for women. This she relates to the inequalities and stresses more prevalent to women during the pandemic.

The above studies addressed how the pandemic affected dreams, usually early in the pandemic. Scarpelli and colleagues (2021) extended those results in a longitudinal study that addressed how the dream variables changed from the first to the second wave of Covid-19. Their 611 participants completed a web survey in Spring 2020 and also December 2020 to January 2021. These participants were found to have lower dream-recall frequency, nightmare frequency, lucid dream frequency, emotional intensity and nightmare distress during the second than the first wave of the pandemic. (The finding of decreased lucid dream frequency in the second Lockdown compared to the first accords with Kelly et al.'s (2022) finding of an increased occurrence of lucid dreams during the first Lockdown compared to pre-Lockdown.)

Sleep and dreaming during the Covid-19 pandemic

The findings of these studies on dreams were explained by factors such as that many people were sleeping for longer during the pandemic, and waking without alarm clocks or an immediate work schedule (Nielsen, 2020). Also, some people were having more stressful lives, which, as we discussed in Chapters 1 and 3, can also alter dreaming. Examples of many such dreams and explanations of the science behind them were published in Deirdre Barrett's (2020b) book *Pandemic Dreams*. Although some people in Lockdown may have been having boring and uneventful days, the enforced family or social aspect of Lockdown may have resulted in more emotional experiences, which are then incorporated into dreams. As discussed in Chapter 2, these more vivid dreams may themselves be more memorable. In addition, dreams are usually forgotten quickly, and especially if one is distracted or busy upon waking. During Lockdown, more people had time to pay attention to and recollect and memorise the dreams that they woke up with. There would also have been for some people more unstructured time after waking, which would give greater opportunities to share dreams with significant others. This might result in more positive attitudes towards dreams and towards dream-sharing, and of greater empathy between people, because more time was available for the consideration, appreciation, sharing and discussion of dreams. It was these changes in sleep and dreaming that led us to begin our Lockdown project.

DreamsID Covid-19 Lockdown dreams project, April to July 2020

Due to the reports of people dreaming more vividly during Lockdown and due to a dream that Mark had at the start of Lockdown, which is reported next, we decided to start holding our now-established *dream salons* online, with dreamers participating by Skype. Also, so as to encourage a global audience to see, hear and engage with the process, we broadcast the events on Facebook Live. We were particularly interested in supporting those on the front line of the pandemic, and so we advertised via a range of social media platforms for people working in health, caring or other key professions. Apart from Mark's dream below, the dreams were told to us in online events, each with participation from a worldwide audience, from April to July 2020. Each event lasted approximately 90 minutes and the painting of each dream was completed by Julia in that time, and seen on the live broadcast simultaneously with the discussion. As well as wishing to support keyworkers by listening to and discussing their dreams, and gifting an artwork to them, we were also interested in how the waking life changed circumstances may have been depicted in a dream. Julia also had an interest in this aspect, as when she moved from practising her art full time to teaching, writing and text-based work, her dreams, which had been colourful and had been the inspiration for her paintings, as well as a regular talking point with friends and relatives, ceased abruptly. The effects of changed circumstances on dreams were thus of interest to Julia.

The following four dreams were discussed and painted as part of our pandemic dreams project. The other dreams of the project can be seen at the start of this chapter, and at the start of Chapters 3, 5 and 8. After the project, we also discussed and painted author and poet Michael Rosen's dream of 'pulling through' from Covid-19, which is at the start of Chapter 11.

Dream of Mark from the start of the Covid-19 Lockdown in March 2020, as a result of which, and the painting of it, we began our Lockdown dreams project.

DREAM NARRATIVE: *I leave a room by revolving so as to get past a strap on the doorway. I go down a corridor to see my wife. She is in the next room and has a present for me on the table, a box about 30x60cm, and about 5cm thick with a clear plastic top. It has various novelties and small activities in it. In the middle is a table tennis set with green bats. On one side of the box, there is an old black mobile phone, with a few other small components, and the words 'Funeral Preparation Kit'. The kit is partly a joke rather than being serious.*

DISCUSSION: On the day before the dream Mark had heard of a distant acquaintance who had died from Covid-19. As Mark only vaguely knew the person, the death was only a little unsettling, but it showed that Covid-19 was real and deadly.

JULIA: (Painting shown as Figure 15.2) I structured the narrative and painting into five paragraphs from two of Freud's pages: Mark revolving on the threshold (Black); the box left on the classroom table (White); the wife (Dark clothes and white background); the present, split into two (Green, silver, black and white). Words that jumped out of Freud's text related to the *present,* which has two meanings – the gift that was given and the current Covid-19 timeframe during which the dream took place.

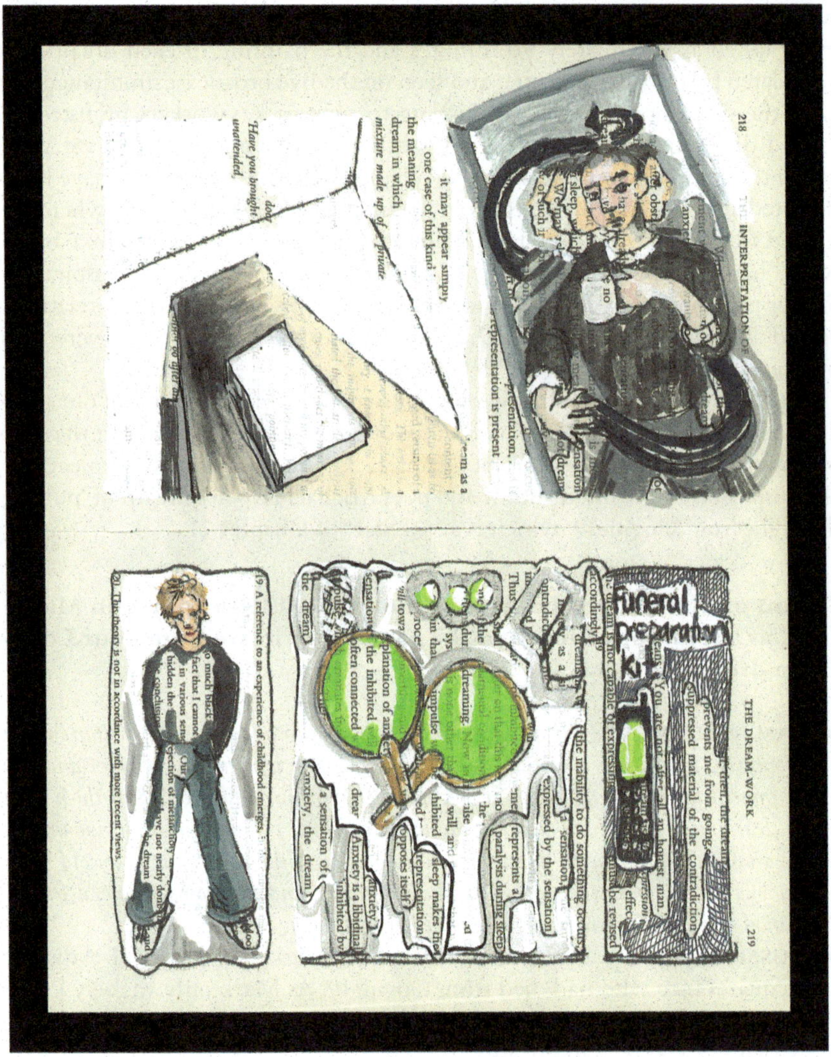

178 *Sleep and dreaming during the Covid-19 pandemic*

Figure 15.2 Dream of gift including death preparation kit, 2020.

Dream of Mason, a US delivery driver keyworker, who had recently stopped his delivery job so as to relocate across the country to start work elsewhere.

DREAM NARRATIVE: *I am trying to drive up the incline from a suburban house garage. I can't get the car into gear and so I can't move into the busy road to join the traffic there. I release the clutch but find the car is not in gear and it moves backward and stops. I get out to check that it did not hit the white garage door and am surprised to see that it has damaged the door badly. I get back in the car and see*

Sleep and dreaming during the Covid-19 pandemic 179

a man and a woman in an old white van looking at me almost with disgust. I feel embarrassed as I was not being able to drive the car, even though I should be able to do so and as it is my job to drive. The car was a brown Mazda Miata, which is not a car I drive in waking life and is a color that I would not choose.

DISCUSSION: We discussed that the dream, with the UPS-style brown colour, was linked to the dreamer's delivery work and to a lack of control in what would normally be a familiar task, that of driving.

JULIA: (Painting shown as Figure 15.3) I chose two pages with four distinct paragraphs to encapsulate this dream. The composition has a sense of a

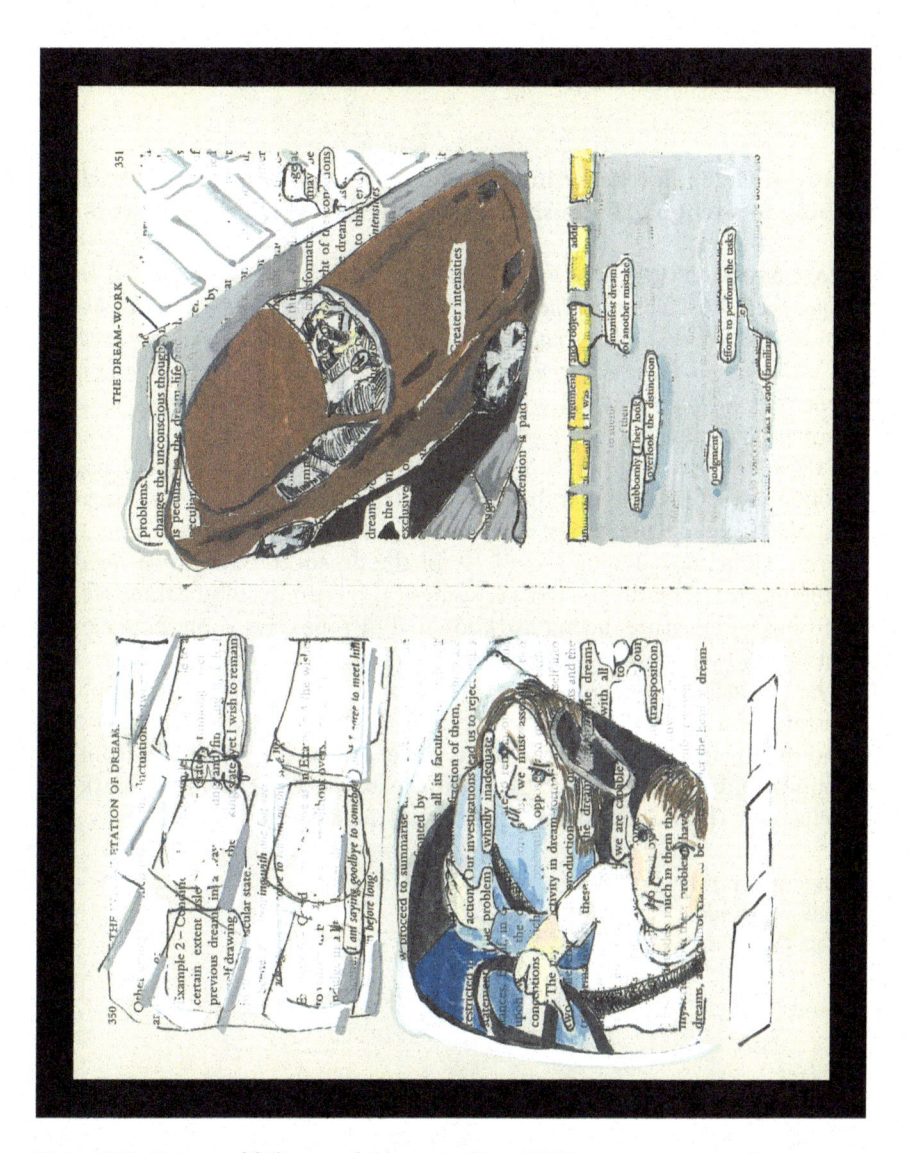

Figure 15.3 Dream of failing to drive up incline, 2020.

woven set of motifs: the warp contains the brown car trying to move up the hill, and weft, the white garage doors that it smashes into and the busy road which crosses in front of the driveway. The two judgemental onlookers watch from their white van. Eerily appropriate words come together in the road as a found poem:

manifest dream
of another mistake
stubbornly. They look
overlook the distinction
judgement
efforts to perform the tasks
familiar

Dream of Chloe, a teacher in Scotland who was waiting to go back to teaching in a school. Her husband and daughter were both key workers.

DREAM NARRATIVE: *I am inside a body, possibly my own. It feels small, and is blood-red. I feel confined. The lungs and heart can be seen as the skin lets through some light. I see a robin scratching and picking with its beak and feet at black, tar-like Covid-19, which is all around the lungs. The robin is working to move the black substance to a pile, so as to remove it. The robin is also looking for small worms to feed itself.*

DISCUSSION: We discussed how in Lockdown, on walks or in gardens, we often see robins, and that they are very friendly to humans. The dreamer spoke of these being a sign that life and the natural world continues, and even flourishes, despite Covid-19. In the dream, the robin was healing the person. The dream is a very physical picture of the healing we get from seeing nature during Lockdown. The robin was also taking care of itself, by looking for worms to eat. This was a very life-affirming dream.

JULIA: (Painting shown as Figure 15.4) I chose bullet-pointed paragraphs to form the ribs or chamber surrounding the lungs. There were two sides to the dream: one where the robin clears the tar-like Covid-19 from the lungs, and the other where the dreamer sits watching, inside the dark red chamber. The following words of Freud are incorporated:

under treatment
what difficulties
continuing the treatment

and

plant
flowers
friends of mine

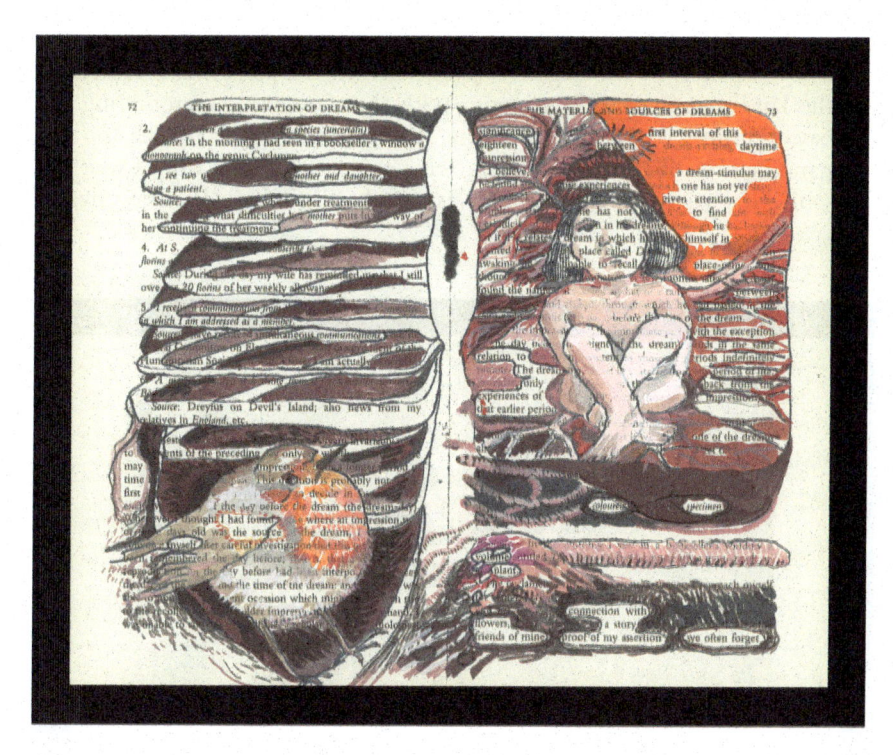

Sleep and dreaming during the Covid-19 pandemic 181

Figure 15.4 Dream of robin pecking Covid-19 from lungs, 2020.

Dream of Mai, a health-care worker at a hospital in Melbourne, Australia, whose work was not directly related to Covid-19.

DREAM NARRATIVE: *I am in darkness, it is cold and I hear a deep natural rumbling sound. I can hear water trickling behind me. I can only move my left arm, and feel a smooth surface behind me. This is all gently rocking me, like a lullaby. I see an opening in front of me, with natural light coming through. Now I can move my head and my neck and I look to my left. I see blue and green shiny colours, with the opening getting bigger. I realise that I am in a paua shell, a blue and green abalone shell. It looks amazing and I wish I could take a photo to show people, and I want all this to last longer. I then look out of the side of the shell and see the ocean and some land in the distance. I can then move more and see a playful, loving, brown seal pup with beautiful eyes. The dream was beautiful, I was in nature and loved the whole dream.*

DISCUSSION: The dreamer told how she is originally from New Zealand. Her dream reminded her of her idyllic childhood there, and of how she should go back there after the pandemic. It was a very positive and joyful dream.

182 *Sleep and dreaming during the Covid-19 pandemic*

JULIA: (Painting shown as Figure 15.5) I chose two pages and turned them on their side to give depth to the composition. The composition is divided into six panels by the negative space between the paragraphs. However, the landscape appears continuous with the mountains surrounding the bay, running across the top of the image. Demarcated by the top left paragraph is a beach with the exterior of the paua shell full of writing, while the paragraph below depicts the dark, concealed, silky interior

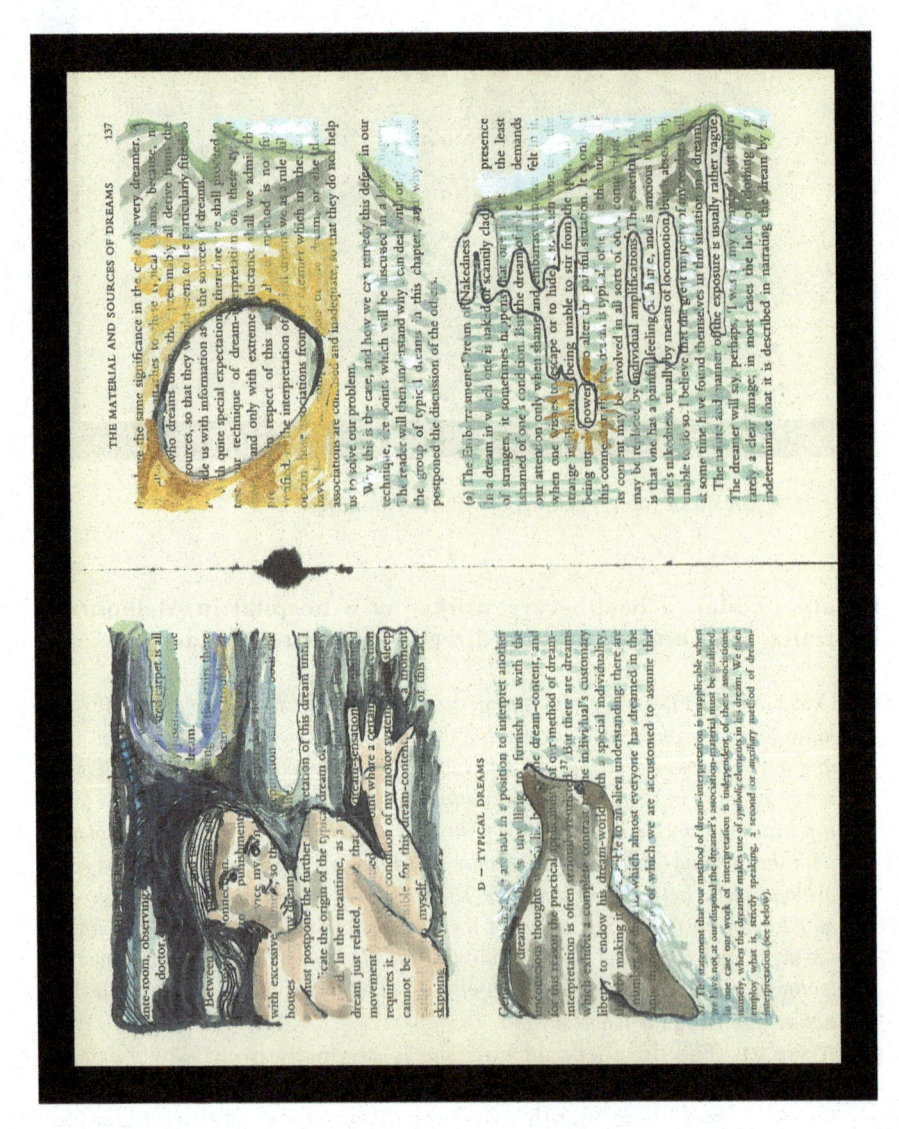

Figure 15.5 Dream of emerging from shell and seeing seal pup in the ocean, 2020.

containing the dreamer. Her hand, which she used to touch and feel around the interior of the paua shell, is made up of the words:

dream-sensation
where a certain
condition of my motor system
for this dream-content

On the other side of the page, the bottom right depicts the frolicking seal pup, while the top right paragraph contains the following found poem:

Nakedness
or scantily clad
the dream
and
escape or to hide
being unable to stir from
power

I circled the homophone *power* with strips of gold paint to make it stand out. I also highlighted a sentence fragment:

the exposure is rather vague

This was in response to the dreamer's stated visual adjustment from the dark paua shell to the bright sunlit landscape, the colours and light in the painting are subtle and there is little contrast; this is noted in this highlighted phrase.

The videos of the above paintings being created, and of the online discussions, can be seen on the DreamsID YouTube channel. Four of these paintings (Dream of new life by a beach (Figure 5.1); Dream of walking alone and then dancing with friends (Figure 8.1); Dream of peeling quails' eggs for cure for Covid-19 (Figure 15.1); and Dream of robin pecking Covid-19 from lungs (Figure 15.4) were chosen to be part of the exhibition *1920/2020: Freud and Pandemic* held at the Freud Museum London in 2021. The paintings and texts of some of the dreams can also be seen in Barrett (2020b) and Lockheart and Blagrove (2020).

We are grateful to everyone for sharing these dreams publicly. The events and discussions showed that the experiences of their waking lives were influencing and becoming part of their dreams. We were glad that the project enabled them to express not only their dreams but themselves and their work and home lives, with a wide audience. As a result of our pandemic dreams project, we became part of a longer collaboration with the National Health Service regarding the continuing impact of the Covid-19 pandemic and other stresses on the health of staff, and the role of conversations and art about dreams in ameliorating this stress. This is the NHS *Finding Hope* project for all staff, including porters, cleaning staff, doctors and nurses.

Summary

Many scientific papers have shown the impact of the Covid-19 pandemic on people's mental health, sleep and dreams. Keyworkers from around the world shared their dreams with us online during the early months of the Covid-19 pandemic. These dreams were discussed by a worldwide audience who also saw each dream being painted live. The dreams depicted in a metaphorical way, the very much altered waking life circumstances of the dreamers.

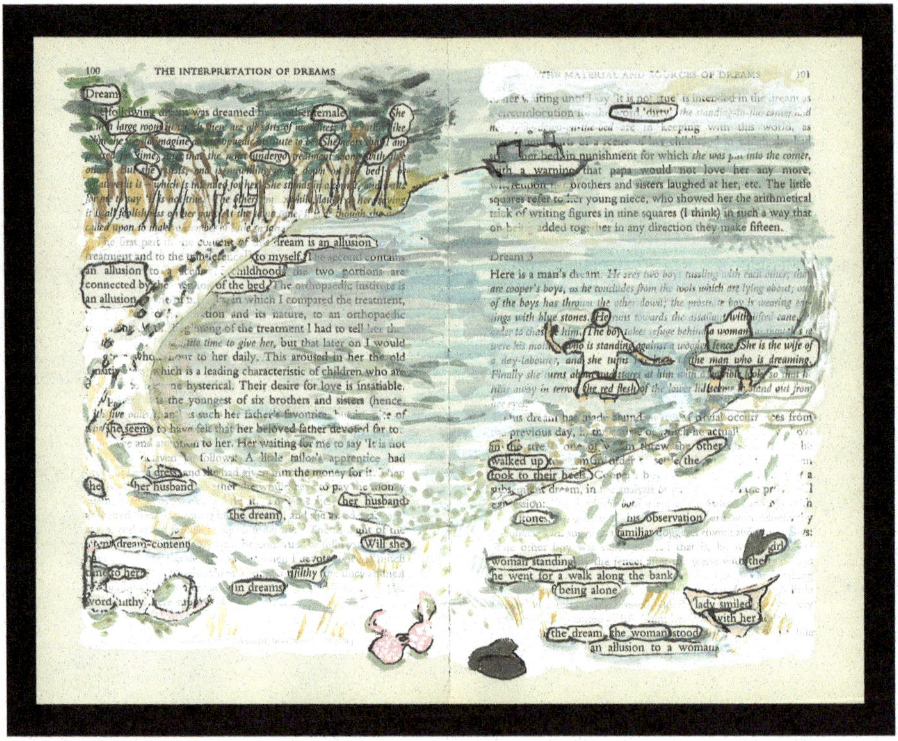

Figure 16.1 Dream of snowy beach, underclothes and ferry, 2022.

16 Dreaming, films and Surrealism

This dream was told to us at an online event organised by the International Society for the Study of Surrealism in February 2022.

DREAM NARRATIVE: *I walk out of woods and onto a bay with a snow-covered marsh that leads to the sea. The sea has stones under it. Along the paths, there are some footsteps but no one is around. My wife is present but unseen. The snow is knee high, I am wearing shorts or swimming trunks, as if it was Summer. I then see clothing and underclothes strewn on the ground, there are frilly brassieres and Ugg boots, as if some young people had discarded them to go into the water. I am fleetingly bemused by this, thinking that they must be cold in this weather. But I also wonder that when I go into the water maybe it will not be as cold as the marshy surroundings. As I step into the water I wake up. However, at this point or earlier, I was on my way to a ferry and my wife and I had to stay overnight in a hotel so as to catch the ferry the next day. I was hoping that we had reserved a room, but my wife and I agreed that we could always sleep in the hotel or ferry lounge if not.*

DISCUSSION: The dream-sharer, Jonathan, said that the dream was related to ageing, and also to nostalgia as he had known ferry areas next to the sea like this when younger.

JULIA: (Painting shown as Figure 16.1) I composed the painting using an area in italics at the right to depict part of the sea. This paragraph, where the dreamer and his wife are represented in the sea, begins:

Here is a man's dream

And on the outlined figure of the dreamer's wife, to the right of the man, are the words:

with
a woman
She is the wife of
the man who is dreaming.

DOI: 10.4324/9781003037552-16

Above the two figures, near the horizon of the sea, is the word *fifteen*, the age of the dreamer's child, which was briefly mentioned in the discussion. It is compositionally linked to the ferry boat on the horizon at the top of the right page, which includes two lines:

her bed
with a warning

These were highlighted because, in the discussion, the dreamer couldn't remember if he and his wife had booked a room at the hotel and thought they might have to sleep in the hotel or ferry lounge.

To make the footprints I combined pairs of words, like the heel and toe of a footprint, across the bottom of the composition:

The dream
Her husband
Will she
In dreams

And in the same section, I also highlighted:

An allusion to a woman

This was because the dreamer suggested his wife was present in his thoughts in the dream but he did not physically see her. This is mirrored in the way I depicted the wife as an outlined figure made of words.

Dreams and film

This book has so far addressed the science and art of dreams, with dreams as an object to be studied or used as a stimulus for personal growth or for art. Part of the artistic use of dreams, however, concerns their depiction in films, and this depiction has occurred from the early days of cinema. This chapter does not aim to be a comprehensive account of the use of dreams in films, but instead to give examples of the use of dreams in linear narrative films, sometimes as plot devices, and then to compare this with films that are oneiric, that is, films that have sequences, often disjointed, that are inspired by common understandings of what dreams are like. Such oneiric films might not overtly include any dreams, and might even deny a link to dreaming, but aim to give the viewer an experience akin to dreaming. The chapter concludes that the insights of surrealist filmmakers are very relevant to the phenomenology of dreams.

The use of dreams in linear films

Many dreams in films are part of a linear plot and often aim to show the psychological state of the protagonist. For example, in Ingmar Bergman's (1957)

Wild Strawberries. The plot of the film concerns retired professor Isak Borg, who drives from his home in Stockholm to Lund to receive an honorary degree from his former university. He is an angry, old, solitary, disputatious character, and travels to Lund with his daughter-in-law, who does not like him, and who tells him along the way that his son hates him. On the journey he is reminded of his younger life, including his cousin Sara, with whom he was in love, but who chose to marry his more lively and fun brother rather than him. The film addresses the course of his life, with flashbacks to when he was younger.

At the start of the film, Isak is seen asleep, having a dream, or rather nightmare, as he describes it as 'very unpleasant'. The dream is of being in a deserted town or city street. He looks up at a clock over an optician's shop and sees that the clock has no hands. He looks down to check his pocket watch, which on opening he sees also has no hands. The viewer of the film, seeing Isak's age, would understand the metaphor of time has ended, and would connect this to the end of life. Similar to a ticking clock, his heartbeat is heard as he looks again, confused, at the clockface. Walking slowly along the street he sees a man from behind, who turns around and has no face and who collapses into a pool of blood; the repetitive rhythm of a church bell starts to toll. A hearse drawn by two horses appears, and, due to an accident, the coffin falls to the ground, opens, and a hand grabs Isak, who then sees his own dead body in the coffin. The dream is a captivating depiction of life drawing to a close and nearing its end.

For part of the journey to the honorary degree ceremony, the car is driven by Isak's daughter-in-law. Isak falls asleep, and has what he calls a humiliating dream. In the dream, he is his current self, an old man. He meets Sara, as she was when a young woman, and she asks him to look into a mirror, and not to look away, and says that he is an old man who will soon be dead. She says she is going to marry his brother and that they 'love one another as if it were a game', and she says that Isak 'is a professor emeritus who knows so much but doesn't really know anything'. She leaves to look after a baby, and Isak follows and sees her in their childhood country house, with his brother, playing music lovingly and having a meal with wine. He then goes to an examination, the components of which he fails, and is told that he is incompetent, that his wife thinks him callous, selfish and ruthless, and that his punishment will be loneliness. He wakes and says 'It is as if I am telling myself something I don't want to hear when I am awake'. For the viewer the dream is captivating, showing the historical and internal world of Isak, and his (literal) awakening, insight and growth of self-awareness.

A further example of a linear narrative, realist film, that similarly involves a dream depicting the psychological life of a protagonist, is Stanley Kubrick's *Eyes Wide Shut* (1999). This was based on Arthur Schnitzler's atmospheric short story *Traumnovelle*, published in 1926 in German, and titled *Dream Story* in English (Schnitzler, 1999). In the film, Dr. Bill Harford (played by Tom Cruise) and his wife, Alice Harford (played by Nicole Kidman), live in New York City and are a successful and beautiful couple. She tells him that on a holiday with him she had encountered a naval officer and fantasized about him enough that she considered leaving Bill and their daughter. Bill is distraught at this revelation and goes out alone, where he has some lengthy but unconsummated sexual meetings. Later in the film, Alice tells him she has had a dream in which she was having sex with the naval officer and other men, and laughing at the idea of Bill witnessing the scene. Eventually, he tells her of his near-infidelities of the past two days and apologises to Alice. At the end of the film, in response to Bill reminding her of her dream, she says:

> Maybe I think we should be grateful. Grateful that we've managed to survive through all of our adventures, whether they were real, or only a dream.

He says: '*And no dream is ever just a dream*'.
To which she replies: '*The important thing is we're awake now and hopefully for a long time to come*'.
She and Bill thus now have their eyes wide open to the need to resist infidelity, and of knowing not to act on the contents of the dream.

The science fiction film *Vanilla Sky* (2001, director Cameron Crowe), in contrast, has a dream more clearly related to a waking life wish. David Aames, played by Tom Cruise, is a rich playboy who is having a casual sexual relationship with Julie, played by Cameron Diaz. He has a birthday party and his best friend David introduces him to Sofia, who is David's girlfriend. David and Sofia spend the night together at Sofia's apartment and fall in love. There follow many scenes with David developing a loving relationship with Sofia, but having strange experiences, including of killing Julie. After many plot complications, he realises that almost all of the relationship with Sofia after they met has been a dream, and, in places, a nightmare. The film poignantly depicts dreaming of a very meaningful wish, a long loving relationship with Sofia, and at the end, the film characters discuss how the dream was produced, including the incorporation of memories into dreams, and how a non-lucid dream can become a nightmare, but with instances of recognising puzzles and incongruities in the dream. The use of dreams in films can thus sometimes involve the film also being about dreaming.

Another example of a film depicting dreams but also about dreaming is *A Nightmare on Elm Street* (1984, director Wes Craven). Here, teenagers dream of a man, Freddy Krueger (played by Robert Englund), whose face is disfigured by fire and who has knife extensions to the fingers of his gloves, and who attempts to murder the children in their dreams. Freddy partially enters their waking reality and the teenagers start to avoid sleep, but then realise they need to confront him in their dreams by becoming lucid. The film draws on the science of dreams, including a scene in a sleep clinic, and was followed by several sequels. The final film in the series, *Wes Craven's New Nightmare* (1994), or Nightmare on Elm Street 7, is wonderfully meta and self-referential. Wes Craven and the actors play themselves, even Robert Englund, and the plot has Freddy now reappearing to some of the original cast.

Other films with dreams integral to the plot and with a generally linear narrative draw upon Surrealism. Jan Švankmajer's (2010) *Surviving Life* is about a middle-aged man who is very unhappy in his marriage and begins a wonderful relationship with a woman in his dreams. His wife finds out about the infidelity and he has to choose between his emotionally and materially impoverished waking life and his exciting and warm life in his dreams. Although *Surviving Life* is Švankmajer's only film directly referring to dreams, it and his other films use wild and creative juxtapositions to give surreal and oneiric effects, and he was included in the *Surrealism Beyond Borders* exhibition at Tate Modern in 2022, discussed in Chapter 14. One of these, *The flat* [*Byt*], is described below. Švankmajer started making films in the 1960s, using stop-motion filming, animation, puppets, claymation, cut-outs and live-action with actors. For O'Pray (1986), Švankmajer's Surrealism has a psychoanalytical framework, because of its brutal bodily concerns, mixtures of media, free associations, and depictions of aggression and love.

Surreal imagery and juxtapositions occur also in *The Science of Sleep* (2006, director Michel Gondry) which tells the story of Stéphane (played by Gael García Bernal), who wishes to work creatively but instead has a menial job making calendars, and who develops a close friendship with his apartment neighbour, Stéphanie (played by Charlotte Gainsbourg). Stéphane's dreams start to intrude into and merge with reality. This results in astounding images of a spider typewriting, a one-second time machine, cardboard cars and houses, and of Stéphane as a homunculus creating his own dreams.

Also full of strange images is arguably the most famous dream scene in film, in Hitchcock's (1945) *Spellbound*. The dream is of the protagonist, played by Gregory Peck, playing cards with an older man in a gambling house, and then in the next scene seeing the older man die; this is related in the film to a repressed memory. Although Dalí was chosen by Hitchcock to write and create the dream scene, Hitchcock said that this was not because of Dalí's fame, nor his ability to create surreal images, many of which were in fact cut after filming. It was due to his artwork being 'very solid and very sharp', producing a very real 'hard image', in contrast to the usual clichéd blurred images of dreams in films at the time (quotations of Hitchcock in King, 2007, p.79).

The tangential incorporation of dreams into films

Some films are more tangential in their use of dreams, with dreams only being hinted at. David Lynch's (2001) *Mulholland Drive* appears at the start to be about a murder and about a young female actor arriving in Hollywood, and about the rivalries that result. Its developing complexity and lack of linear time, however, make this film surreal and oneiric, with elements of the film being perplexing or indeed incomprehensible when they occur, and even in retrospect. The film combines strong emotions, conflicting characters, deception, dreams, reality and imagination. It is the complex clash between imagination and reality that makes the film surreal.

The distinction between fantasy and reality is similarly blurred in Buñuel's *Belle de Jour* (1967). For Matthews (1971), that film illustrates the surrealist thesis of dream and reality being bound together, and with Séverine/Belle de Jour (played by Catherine Deneuve) unable to 'keep apart the dream where her sexual fantasies are acted out and the world where she lives in frustration at her husband's side.' (p.174.) Matthews concludes that whether we are watching something true or false is less important than whether it seems real or unreal to the heroine.

A similar sense of not knowing whether a film depicts reality or a dream of one of its characters occurs with *Last Year at Marienbad* (1961, director Alain Resnais). The film tells of a man living with many others in a palatial chateau and telling a woman how she had met him the year before in Marienbad. She does not believe him, but the film's use of flashbacks results in ambiguity about whether that meeting had occurred, and has led some to propose that either he is lying to her, or that she has forgotten the meeting, or that one of them is dreaming. The unreal atmosphere, with ponderous organ music in the background, stylised unemotional characters and non-linear timeline, makes this one of the most captivating oneiric films.

History of realist and non-realist dream films

Sharot (2015) distinguishes dreams used as part of a realist film, in which they might be a plot device, such as for warning about the future or disclosing a memory or depicting the inner life of a character, and the 'dream film', which appropriates the dream state, and which is referred to as oneiric. Sharot details the history of film, with the earliest films using dreams for comic effect or to enable special effects, to dreams being then developed as portraying a subjective state. He finds that from 1915, as feature-length films became standard, the number of films with dream sequences declined substantially, as earlier dream scenes were seen as unsophisticatedly comic or moralistic. He shows that there were few feature films that included dreams in the 1920s and early 1930s, and that it was the public knowledge of psychoanalysis from the late 1930s that led to dreams in films becoming more frequent, and often showing insights into a protagonist's waking life. In many of these films, from early in cinema to later, a dream was signified by visual and aural effects. These effects reinforced the viewer being a spectator rather than an experiencer, and it was this distinction between a protagonist's dream and the waking life of the protagonist in the film and the waking life of the viewer that the Surrealists sought to dissolve, using wild associations and the juxtapositioning of images. To achieve this effect they thus favoured films with a discontinuous narrative.

Surrealist oneiric films

Thus in contrast to popular films where a dream was inserted within a realist or linear or magical realist frame, Surrealists favoured dream-like and bizarre experiences, which could thus omit any mention of dreaming itself. The expectations and hopes of the Surrealists for the new medium, with examples of their films, are reviewed by Short (2008a). A precursor to surrealist films was the Dadaist film *Entr'acte* (1924), a 21-minute film, directed by René Clair. The film starts with a cannon being fired by artist Francis Picabia over Paris, and then has various humorous scenes, such as Man Ray and Marcel Duchamp playing chess and being hosed down by Picabia, and the chess board being sent flying above Paris. There is a spinning ballerina seen from below who is later seen to be a bearded lady, which O'Donoghue (2004) suggests was inspired by Duchamp's artwork *L.H.O.O.Q.* (1919), in which Duchamp painted a moustache onto a postcard of the Mona Lisa. A final long sequence has a hearse pulled by a camel, with slow-motion mourners running and prancing behind. They run faster and faster, this being intercut with film of a roller-coaster, and then see the hearse crash. The coffin opens, a magician comes out who makes each mourner in turn disappear, and he then disappears himself. As a Dadaist film, there is no conventional narrative and the fast-paced scenes make it impossible to identify with the characters.

The juxtapositions in this film are a hallmark of Dada and later Surrealism. Kuenzli (1996) quotes Picabia, who wrote much of the screenplay, that '*Entr'acte* does not believe in very much, in the pleasure of life perhaps; it believes in the pleasure of inventing, it respects nothing except the desire to *burst out laughing*'. Kuenzli (1996) describes the development from early non-narrative Dadaist films, some of them depicting only moving geometrical shapes, or using optical techniques such as slow motion and montage, to the longer, more complex surrealist films, with discontinuous narrative, and cites Breton's hopes for the use of film in Surrealism. He describes Breton's practice of dropping in on cinema films at any point in the show, and leaving so as to do the same with another film, and without even knowing the titles of the films.

La Coquille et le Clergyman/The Seashell and the Clergyman (director Germaine Dulac) was released in 1928 and was subsequently described by its co-screenwriter Antonin Artaud as the precursor to all surrealist films. The clergyman is first seen filling numerous shell-like glasses with liquid, following which there are many scenes of his lust for the wife of a general, who appears with an extremely long sword and often as photomontage. Dulac uses fades, superimpositions, split screens and many other visual devices. However, Surrealists objected at its inaugural screening because the director labelled the film a 'dream' in her press release before its screening. Another press release was titled *A dream on the screen*, stating that 'someone else's dream (if we were able to see it) would be capable of moving us as effectively as any other spectacle' (reproduced in Flitterman-Lewis, 1996). Artaud objected to this, warning 'I will not seek to find excuse for its apparent incoherence through the facile loophole of the dream' (Matthews, 1971, p.79). Indeed, according to Flitterman-Lewis (1996), Artaud emphasised that it was a film of self-sufficient pure images, with no hidden psychological significance, and each viewer was to derive their own meaning for it. Artaud stated that 'This scenario is not the reproduction of a dream', even though it had been inspired by the dream of a close friend, and could be 'related to *the mechanism of a dream* without actually being a dream itself' (Flitterman-Lewis, 1996). For Flitterman-Lewis, it has the unconscious logic of a dream, its action operating almost intuitively on the brain, without claiming to be a representation of a dream, and evoking 'the marvelous' through unexpected and incongruous images.

Flitterman-Lewis concludes that Artaud wanted to recreate the experience of the dream for the spectator, as something deeply felt, rather than just giving an impression of incoherence. She quotes Artaud in his *Cinema and Abstraction* as writing: '*The Seashell and the Clergyman* does not tell a story, but develops a series of states of mind, just as one thought derives from another, without needing to reproduce a logical sequence of events.' This occurs through 'the clash of objects and gestures' and through new associations of colliding images. This fits within Artaud's wider film theory, which for us relates to the tension between the interpretation and experience of dreams that we will address later in this chapter. That film theory 'formulates a confrontation with representation, with the aim of tearing the image away from representation, to transplant it directly into the film spectator's ocular nerves and sensation' (Barber, 2008, pp.46–47).

The next surrealist film was the 21-minute *L'Etoile de mer/The starfish* (1928, directed by Man Ray, scenario by Robet Desnos). It has the perturbing early scene of a man and woman going upstairs to her apartment and bedroom, where the woman carefully undresses, the man remaining seated on the bed. She lies on the bed and he gets up, they shake hands and he leaves. The word 'Adieu' appears. A filter is used to blur this scene. The viewer may be expecting eroticism but none is present. At the end of the film, she reappears with the intertitle 'vous ne révez [sic] pas' [you are not dreaming].

Such a sequence of disconnected scenes occurs also in the most famous early surrealist film, *Un Chain andalou/An Andalusian dog* (1929, directed by Luis Buñuel and Salvador Dalí). In his chapter 'Surrealism (1929–1933)' in his (1994) autobiography *My Last Breath*, Buñuel writes that he told Dalí a dream 'in which a long, tapering cloud sliced the moon in half, like a razor blade slicing through an eye'. Dalí then told Buñuel his dream of the previous night, of a hand crawling with ants. In less than a week they wrote the script for *Un Chien andalou*, using these dreams. The film's prologue is followed by a scene that takes place eight years later. For Matthews (1971), the absence of a consecutive plot makes this prologue offensively gratuitous, it being followed by many scenes with a 'pantomime of passion and stylized gesture' and an 'unrelated succession of incidents and responses'. It includes grotesque juxtapositions, such as of the white teeth of a rotting donkey and the white keys of a piano. Matthews concludes that the pattern of the film is of the generation of dramatic interest, which piques the wish to psychoanalyse, but which is dissipated each time by humorous surprise. For Finkelstein (1996), whereas in

The Seashell and the Clergyman there are cinematic devices that cause transformations, in *Un Chien andalou* the narrative dislocations are naturalistic, with humour and absurdities. There are oneiric scenes, such as of the passive heroine arguing with a male protagonist, and opening a door of their apartment which we, the audience, surprisingly see leads to a beach.

Buñuel mainly relied on juxtaposition in *Un Chien andalou*. As with Artaud, Buñuel insisted that he and Dalí had not attempted to reconstruct a dream but to profit from a 'mechanism analogous to that of dreams' (Matthews, 1971, p.90). The films were not to be interpreted, but experienced. As Flitterman-Lewis (1996, p.117) says of Artaud, 'to recreate the impact of the dream *as it is being dreamed*' (italics in original). To achieve this, Dalí and Buñuel rejected sequences in the film that would be dictated by rational associations. Automatic writing was used to generate the plot, and the use of intertitles that give various time sequences makes the sequence of events even less logical (Liebman, 1996, p.145; Matthews, 1971, pp.84–90). This thus mixes reality and fancy, and the instinctive and the irrational, without the need for unusual angles or complex shots.

There is more of a narrative in *L'Age d'Or/The age of gold* (1930, directed by Luis Buñuel, screenplay by Buñuel and Salvador Dalí) than in *Un Chien andalou*, with a series of incidents in which would-be lovers are continually interrupted; there are also fewer cinematic techniques than in the earlier film. In Buñuel's later films the dreams are of particular characters, and can be narratively interpreted by the viewer, such as in *The Discreet Charm of the Bourgeoise* (1972). But surreality remains, with a disturbing dream sequence in *Los Olvidados (1950)*, the beggars dining at a large table in *Viridiana* (1961), their pose evoking da Vinci's *The Last Supper*, and a bizarre juxtaposition of Brahms' romantic music in *Las Hurdes/Land Without Bread (1933)*, a documentary about rural communities with severe poverty. Matthews (1971, p.107) makes the point that this jarring juxtaposition of music also occurs at the end of *L'Age d'Or*, where de Sadean horror is placed together with a fast military march.

Buñuel's *The Phantom of Liberty* (1974) uses a sequence of short scenes, some tangentially connected. There are bizarre often comic themes, such as a child reported as disappeared by parents and school while the child is still present and protesting unheeded that she has not disappeared, or guests eating dinner alone, but defecating together.

Yet even when the film time is linear, a film can be surreal and oneiric. Matthews (1971, p.161) writes of Buñuel's *El Angel exterminador/The exterminating Angel* (1962) that Buñuel thought it an 'absolutely irrational' subject. In the film, upper-class guests arrive for dinner at a large house but are unable to leave at the end of the evening. There is no explanation for this, even though at the start of the film the servants themselves did urgently and mysteriously leave. A crowd gathers outside to watch the house while the guests degenerate in their actions towards each other. There is a hint at the start of the film of its surreal character, the guests are filmed twice arriving at the house. (This being so strange that one DVD version of the film erroneously includes only one of the arrival scenes.) At the end of the film three sheep wander into the house, and the dinner guests now leave and go to a church, where they are again imprisoned. Matthews (1971, p.161) reproduces Buñuel's screening note for the film:

> If the film you are going to see seems to you enigmatic or incongruous, life is that way also. It is as repetitive as life, and similarly subject to many interpretations. The author declares he has not wished to play upon symbols, at least consciously. Perhaps the best explanation of *El Angel exterminador* is that, reasonably, it does not have one.

Matthews then describes and discounts various symbolic interpretations of the film, including relationships with the Old and New Testaments. The film has also been seen as symbolic of the stasis during the Francoist dictatorship in Spain at the time. But if we take Buñuel's claim of no conscious symbolism, we are left with seeing the film as an experience. Maybe the audience experiencing such mental and physical stuckness is the aim of the film, its bizarre surface is all there is. This unexplained immobilisation can be contrasted with the fast-moving theme of *The Discreet Charm of the Bourgeoisie* (1972), in which a group of friends who wish to have dinner together is continually thwarted, such as by the death of a restaurant owner, or mistaking the date of the dinner, or a dinner changing to be on a stage, with an audience, which is then a dream. It becomes more a comedy, or farce, and comedies were appreciated by the Surrealists, but *The exterminating Angel* in contrast provides no explanations for the disconcerting incongruity of the immobility of the guests.

Turning to films of other directors, a similar lack of explanation for a predicament occurs in Švankmajer's (1968) film *The flat* [Byt], which shows a man locked in a room, and being thwarted in many everyday activities. He tries to look at himself in a mirror that only shows the back of his head, and despite his attempts in turning around he cannot see his face. He finds his piece of bread is hollow and that his soup spoon has holes in it. A glass of beer becomes smaller as he drinks it, he cannot break open an egg, which breaks his plate, and when turning on a tap, a stone falls out of it. He lies down on his bed, but the bed turns into sawdust which engulfs him, his clothes then become nailed to the wall and table. Throughout, the music is incongruous with a beautiful choir during one macabre scene. He finally tries to escape using an axe but finds on a wall the names of previous inhabitants of the flat, and he uses a pencil that is hanging down to write his own name. There is no dramatic arc, no escape, just endless thwarting and failures, with stuck oneiric dismay. This film contrasts with the exuberant, zany, sensuous adventures of two young women in Věra Chytilová's surreal (1966) film Daisies [Sedmikrásky], also made in Czechoslovakia at that time (Bittencourt, 2022). More recent surrealist films by Roy Andersson, such as *You, the Living* (2007) and *Songs from the Second Floor (2000)* have short vignettes, with little connection except as themes. In the latter film, one protagonist has burnt down his furniture store so as to seek insurance money, and is railing at his son in a psychiatric hospital for becoming insane due to writing poetry. The scenes are often disconnected, but are all bleak. Buñuel's influence of surreal disconnected films has thus continued (Short, 2008b). We now turn to his inspiration and love, his dreams.

Buñuel – a love for dreams

Luis Buñuel demonstrated his love for dreaming in his chapter 'Dreams and Reveries,' in his (1994) autobiography *My Last Breath*, as follows:

> 'IF SOMEONE were to tell me I had 20 years left, and asked me how I'd like to spend them, I'd reply: "Give me two hours a day of activity, and I'll take the other twenty-two in dreams … provided I can remember them."' He goes on: 'I love dreams, even when they're nightmares, which is usually the case. My dreams are always full of the same familiar obstacles, but it doesn't matter. My *amour fou* - for the dreams themselves as well as the pleasure of dreaming - is the single most important thing I shared with the surrealists. *Un Chien andalou* was born of the encounter between my dreams and Dalí's. Later, I brought dreams directly into my films, trying as hard as I could to avoid any analysis. "Don't worry if the movie's too short," I once told a Mexican producer. "I'll just put in a dream." (He was not impressed.)'
>
> (p.92)

Buñuel then writes of common dream themes he has, such as of taking his final exams all over again, being back in uniform doing military service, eating dinner with his deceased father while knowing not to tell him he is dead, and of needing to go on stage in just a few minutes to play a role he has not learned. He describes how he included the latter in *The Discreet Charm of the Bourgeoisie* (1972), and also how he reproduced in that film a dream he had at 70 years old of meeting his deceased cousin Rafael in an empty street: '"What are you doing here?" I ask him, surprised. "Oh, I come here every day," he replies sadly'. Buñuel later calls for his mother in the dream, and asks her 'What are you doing wandering about among all these ghosts?' (Buñuel, 1994, p.94.)

Cocteau – the film is a dream

In contrast to Buñuel, Cocteau is a master auteur of oneiric films that do not explicitly mention dreams. *Le Sang d'un Poète/The Blood of a Poet* (1930) tells of a statue that comes to life, with the protagonist going through a mirror to a surreal world of hotel rooms that can be viewed through keyholes. The film is dreamlike without the presence of any dreams, but in the sequencing and juxtaposition of images, and in the use of a mirror that is gone through to reach the other world, the film refers to the mechanisms of dreams and also the distinction between the dream and waking world. This film has the quotation 'Mirrors should reflect a bit more before sending back images' (Cocteau, 1930, 27:14; 1985, p.36.), which might also be said of dreams. Cocteau (1985, p.4) said of the film:

> *The Blood of a Poet* draws nothing from either dreams or symbols. As far as the former are concerned, it initiates their mechanism, and by letting the mind relax, as in sleep, it lets memories entwine, move and express themselves freely. As for the latter, it rejects them, and substitutes acts, or allegories of these acts, that the spectator can make symbols of if he wishes.

Orphée/Orpheus (1950) tells of a contemporary French poet who, watched over and loved by an angel, visits the underworld through a mirror so as to retrieve his deceased wife. Props from the film, with many other memories from Cocteau's films and life, appear in *Le Testament d'Orphée/The Testament of Orpheus* (1960), which has many bizarre occurrences, including time travel and disappearing characters. Of this film, he said: 'In Le Testament, events follow one another as they do in sleep, when our habits no longer control the forces within us or the logic of the unconscious, foreign to reason' (Tolton, 1999).

In the (1994) collection of his writings, Cocteau makes the wider point that:

> A film is not the telling of a dream, but a dream in which we all participate together through a kind of hypnosis, and the slightest breakdown in the mechanics of the dream wakens the dreamer, who loses interest in a sleep that is no longer his own.
>
> By dream, I mean a succession of real events that follow on from one another with the magnificent absurdity of dreams, since the spectators would not have linked them together in the same way or have imagined them for themselves, but experienced them in their seats as they might experience, in their beds, strange adventures for which they are not responsible…
>
> (p.40)

Fellini – from neorealist to oneiric films

Cocteau's creation of oneiric films from the start of his film-making contrasts with how the films of Federico Fellini developed. Having produced neorealist films in his early career, Fellini began keeping a dream diary in 1960, which he extensively and lavishly illustrated, and which has been published as his immense work *The Book of Dreams* (Fellini, 2020). Kezich (2020) details how the dreams, on the nearly 400 pages of the original diary, and which were collated across 22 years, relate so colourfully to the events and people in Fellini's professional and personal life. Kezich (2007, pp.221–227) describes how Fellini started the illustrated dream diary between his films *La dolce vita* and *8½*, and that from *8½* (which starts with a nightmare of a traffic jam), his films became 'primarily oneiric'.

Contrasting realist and oneiric films

The distinction between oneiric films and realist films (which can include magical realism, such as Kurosawa's, 1990, *Dreams*, and science fiction, such as Kon's, 2006, *Paprika*) is examined by Earle (1987/2017). He writes that 'Movies took two directions right at the start' with films such as of the arrival of a train at a railway station, in contrast to films depicting what the audience had never or could never see. There was thus a tendency towards the documentary or realist, and, on the other hand, towards the imaginary or surrealistic. The realist sensibility, Earle says, includes 'narrative plot, continuity and integration within the film, a conceptualizable gist or moral for the whole affair, social commentary, psychoanalytic depth-meanings'. Obviously, as explored in Chapter 1, dreams can include these realist characteristics, some of which are identified by Domhoff and Foulkes, but they also have the wild associations characterised by Stickgold, Hobson and Hartmann. It's the latter characterisation that has its analogue in surrealist movies, where, as summarised by Earle (1987/2017), the story told is incoherent, actions without motivation, and the absence of locale, which produce 'a disquieting experience which might appeal to each spectator's dreaming psyche, but which had no summarizable meaning' (p.58). *Meshes of the Afternoon* (1943, directed by Maya Deren and Alexander Hammid), shows such disquieting incoherence, with repetitive time loops and a woman dreaming, who watches the dream as if real, and whose sleeping body is watched by herself.

Earle (1987/2017, pp.20–21) gives the example of a filmmaker, having made a conventionally ordered film, gathering together all the outtakes, the scraps lying on the cutting room floor, and putting them together without order in whatever position they happen to be lying and then projecting the whole chaotic mess on the screen. Earle says that this 'chance composition' will exhibit poetry that is unforeseen by any voluntary will, but with a good deal of 'meaningless rubbish' as well. He says the chance composition 'has a suggestive power never present in any willed composition'. This results, he says, in the conflict between the carefree world of Dada and the surrealist marvelous on the one hand, which can appear frivolous, and people's serious preoccupations in life on the other.

To summarise this chapter so far, for Surrealism, art and films can be oneiric but need not explicitly refer to dreams. The aim is for an oneiric experience. Indeed, in Hans Richter's (1947) *Dreams That Money Can Buy*, the third vignette or case, written by Man Ray, and titled *Ruth, Roses and Revolvers*, depicts people in a cinema standing and copying the poses and gestures of a man on the screen. With this emphasis on experience, it is thus understandable that Max Ernst and René Magritte did not want their paintings to be seen as just copying a dream onto canvas, because important waking life freedom would be lost in producing such mimetic art (Jiménez, 2013). Surrealism thus emphasises experience and freedom in art, and, as above, in oneiric films, all with the aim of encouraging experience and freedom in life. The counterpart in dreams to this emphasis on experience and freedom is the phenomenological tradition, to which we now turn.

Phenomenology and dreams

Following Medard Boss, Gendlin (1977) asks of a dream: what is the bearing of the dreamer in the dream and what are the possibilities shown in the dream? This phenomenological approach aims not to interpret the dream, to translate it, but to consider the experience of being in the dream. Dreaming and waking experiences then come together, aided by questions such as what in your life is like that, or feels like that, or what does it feel like to be each of the characters in the dream? The dream is thus a space for discovering or rehearsing possibilities, leading to the freer more meaningful existence that was the hallmark of existentialism, and which is oriented more to the future than to the past.

Boss (1957, pp.77–90) illustrates his phenomenological approach to dreams with the dream of a 32-year-old woman, 'A Strange Dream of an Urn'. In this dream the woman is sitting at the dinner table with her husband and children, she feels safe and peaceful in an environment so dear to her. She could see and smell the roast dinner, and feel her mouth water for the 'delicious juiciness of the lettuce'. She asks her husband whether he remembers that they had the same menu on their honeymoon, he confirmed this with a smile adding 'It was exactly a year ago'. She is not disturbed by this assertion even though they have been married for ten years. She feels gratitude, happiness and fondness for her family. She feels very near to all of them, especially her eldest son, who is suddenly transported from the opposite end of the table to right next to her. This changing places without any movement did not appear strange to her. She then sees colourful bridges like bright rainbows extending across the table between her and her family, with a large golden urn hovering on the bridges. The dream continues with her worries about the country being invaded, but she dispels these dark images. On waking she was confused to find herself in bed because the lunch had been so real and vivid. 'At first I could not decide which of the two was real: the luncheon which I had just dreamt of, or my bed.'

Boss relates that although the woman had been hungry before going to bed, and that this might therefore be seen as a wish fulfilment dream, at a phenomenological level there was no wish in the dream. 'Our dreamer is supplied with food from the very start of her dream, and therefore does not need to wish it but only to eat it.' Boss notes absurdities in the dream, such as the contention of the husband that they had been on honeymoon only a year before, and that her favourite son is suddenly seated at her right side, and the hovering golden urn, which cannot be explained from any external point of view. He also sees the bridges and urn not as symbols but as objects in themselves. People and objects in dreams thus do not symbolise something in waking life, nor do they symbolise parts of the dreamer, but are as much real in the dream as in waking life.

Boss then gives details of a deeply depressed middle-aged engineer, with few emotional relationships in life, who dreamt of dead, grey mathematical machinery (pp.113–115). During psychoanalytic treatment, the man's dreams slowly changed to include plants and animals. It is difficult for us to see how these dream contents and changes are not symbolic of the man's waking life, but Boss' emphasis on the felt dream and its phenomenology remain useful. He also emphasises the complexity of dreams, that we live in them rather than experience them as hallucinations, and can have volition, reflective behaviour, mistakes, lies, artistic appreciation and moral evaluation in dreams. He concludes that alternative ways of being can reveal themselves and be evaluated in our dreams, and that the only difference between the dream and waking worlds is that we always find ourselves in the same world each time we wake up, but that in dreams we are transported each time into a different world.

Implications of the phenomenological approach to dreams

Although earlier parts of this book addressed wake-life memory sources and metaphorical characteristics and interpretations of dreams, Boss' approach is striking for emphasising the dream in itself. This can be useful for where the dreamer has a very impactful and vivid dream (Kuiken et al., 2006), and the second stage of the Ullman technique, described in Chapter 10, encourages approaching a dream in this way, in terms of how being in the dream would feel. One type of dream that would benefit from a phenomenological approach is where no believable or plausible wake-life source can be found for the dream. For example, at the 2014 annual conference of the International Association for the Study of Dreams, psychotherapist and researcher Professor Clara Hill described her cognitive-experiential model for working with dreams, which facilitates exploration of the dream and its relationship to waking life memories, insight about the dream and consequent action (Hill, 2004). But, she asked, what of dreams for which no waking life counterpart can be found? What if someone who is very happily married dreams of the partner being unfaithful? She suggested that such a puzzling dream could be considered solely as an experience in itself, unrelated to any reality of waking life, with the only conclusion for the dreamer that, well, if this happened, this is what it would feel like. The following dream of Buñuel might also fall into this category of a dream that depicts very unlikely waking life circumstances.

He describes in his autobiography (Buñuel, 1994, p.97) the very bad relationship he had with Dalí's wife Gala, including their mutual dislike and how he physically attacked and choked her during an argument, and relates a dream of her that he had 50 years later:

> She was sitting in a box at the theatre with her back to me. I called her softly, she turned around, stood up, and kissed me lovingly on the lips. I can still smell her perfume and feel the incredible softness of her skin.

He says that he was more surprised by this dream than by any other he had had.

We come back to the funeral scene in *Entr'acte*, and the immobilisation theme in *The exterminating Angel*; if we cannot relate these absurdities to waking life maybe just experiencing the absurdity feeds our playfulness, our wish to explore, and the sense of wonder that the Surrealists so valued. And it is this playfulness, with its links to dreaming and to oneiric art and Surrealism, that takes us to the next chapter, on human social evolution.

Summary

Since the birth of cinema, films have depicted dreams. Sometimes this has been as a plot device, so as to reveal the inner life of a protagonist, or for comic effect. From early in the surrealist movement, oneiric films were produced, using the processes that form dreams even if a dream was not overtly depicted. This emphasis on oneiric experience supports the exploration of human freedom and playfulness, and is in accord with the phenomenological approach to dreams. Although it can be argued that an interpretative approach to dreams can still sit with a phenomenological approach, the latter does have the merit of emphasising the felt reality of dreams. It is that feeling of reality that often intrigues us and urges us to tell the dream. In the next chapter, we explore the social and even social evolutionary consequences of the sharing of dreams.

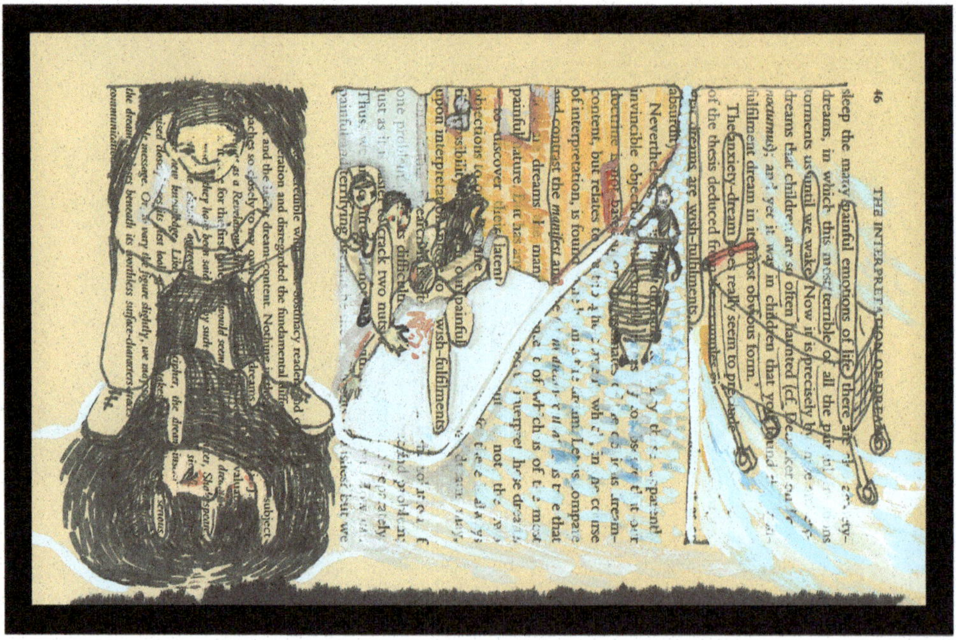

Figure 17.1 Dream of unfair blame, 2017.

17 Dream-sharing, evolution and human self-domestication

An important aspect of human self-domestication (HSD) is empathy. This dream incorporates in a complex way an instance of empathy that had been felt in waking life.

DREAM NARRATIVE: *I push a shopping trolley and release it down a steep hill and it almost causes an accident. Three angry men beat up a man who they think pushed the trolley. I hide in a house and can see the attack through a window. The attackers leave and I go outside and see the man lying on the ground, he is almost dead. He is in a dip in the road. I do not want to admit my involvement as they would then attack me. They have covered him in black oil and his face is half-submerged in the oil. I wonder how to help him without letting my involvement in the near-accident be known.*

DISCUSSION: The dreamer had heard of a young relative who had been unfairly blamed by a friend for what could be a criminal action. Despite the unfairness of the relative being blamed, the dreamer had empathised with the other young person who, out of fear, had attempted to shift the blame onto the young relative. In the dream, the dreamer is himself trying to avoid blame for an action and sees the effect of this on the person who is unfairly blamed.

JULIA: (Painting shown as Figure 17.1) This painting was made on a single page which was divided into three sections. The section on the right has the trolley going down the hill.

The central section shows a fight and a person watching it from a window. Arms flail about and this section contains the found poem:

painful
latent
painful
wish-fulfilments
crack two nuts
terrifying

DOI: 10.4324/9781003037552-17

The words demonstrate the confusion of the dream's street fight.

The section with the dreamer looking at the man's face in the oil used a large, footnoted section in smaller font.

At the top of the page, this scenario and its waking life causes are summarised with the poignant words:

painful emotions of life

Dream-sharing and empathy

This book has so far reviewed the many theories of the function of dreams, such as memory consolidation (Chapter 5), emotion processing (Chapter 12), threat simulation (Chapter 3) and social simulation (Chapter 12). Although differing in what they propose as the adaptive role for dreams, these theories all hold that the proposed function occurs for unremembered dreams as well as for remembered dreams. In contrast to these theories of within-sleep functions of dreaming, Chapter 13 described how dreams have an adaptive function at the point of being told to others, in that they enhance empathy between the dream-sharer and those with whom the dream is told and discussed.

We extended these findings and possible function in Blagrove et al. (2019b) by proposing the *empathy theory of dreaming*. This suggests that across human evolution there has been a selection for fictional and story-like aspects of dream content that support this function, and also a selection for the highly social and emotional characteristics of dream content. These functional and evolutionarily adaptive consequences of dream content would occur after sleep, as a result of the sharing of dreams, such sharing taking advantage of the long Rapid Eye Movement (REM) periods that occur for biological reasons near the end of the night. Dreaming might have originated from memory consolidation or threat rehearsal or other functions, in early humans and other animals, or indeed might be no more than a spandrel (the definition and derivation of spandrel are given in Chapter 12), an epiphenomenon of sleep (Flanagan, 2000): the theory proposed here is that when dream-sharing started, new selective pressures began for the components of dream content. As described by Barrett (2007), if spandrels become useful they can then become subject to evolutionary selection.

Dream content that supports empathy and bonding when the dream is shared may thus have been selected for during early human evolution. This would have occurred after complex speech had developed, on a timescale similar to that for the evolution of human language and story-telling as part of group cohesion and cooperation in humans (Smith et al., 2017), and parallel with the evolution of the social brain (Dunbar, 2009).

These dream content characteristics that support empathy would also have been subject to sexual selection, where an inherited feature leads to the individual being more attractive to the opposite sex for mating (Verweij et al.,

2014), as occurs for artistic virtuosity (Miller, 2000, 2001), and story-telling. The creativity of male story-tellers contributes to their attractiveness beyond physical appearance (Watkins, 2017), and they are seen as more appealing when completing verbal and physical tasks (Prokosch et al., 2009). Individuals skilled at story-telling are also preferred social partners for cooperation, extending the benefits outside the domain of sexual reproduction (Smith et al., 2017). Creative individuals may thus benefit from creative signals both directly, in that it increases attractiveness, and indirectly, in that increased cooperation from others leads to wider social networks.

McNamara et al. (2007) also proposed that there are social evolutionary benefits of dream-sharing and of REM sleep. Such social effects have been a frequent topic in anthropology (Tedlock, 1987), but the empathy theory prioritises the emphasis on fiction and narrative that has to be explored by the dreamer and recipients, and with a self-disclosure function. The proposal for a post-sleep empathic and group bonding function to dreaming has the advantage over within-sleep function theories in that measurement of hypothesised behaviour changes, such as interactions and feelings of intimacy with a partner (Selterman et al., 2014), and measurement of empathy, are easily undertaken.

This chapter now addresses a possible wider theoretical context for this proposal of adaptive effects of dreams and dream-sharing, which places dream-sharing as part of human self-domestication (HSD), which is a major theory of human social evolution, and specifically as part of the more recent language-based mechanisms for HSD.

The human self-domestication hypothesis of human social evolution

The HSD hypothesis proposes that in human evolution there has been a selection for humans having reduced emotional reactivity, and, in particular, reduced aggression within their social group (Hare, 2017; Hare & Woods, 2020; Price, 2019). This selection has resulted in humans exhibiting prosociality, self-control, tolerance, co-operation, and the ability to mentalise, that is, to recognise what others perceive, feel, intend and know.

Wrangham (2019) provides a history of the idea of humans being self-domesticated. He writes that the term domestication had been applied to humans by the ancient Greeks and so predates theories of evolution, and that although Darwin considered the possibility of humans being domesticated, he rejected it as it was not clear how the selection would have occurred. It was only later that the mechanism for domestication was identified. As a fascinating example of how domestication evolves, Wrangham (2019) reviews the work of Dmitri Belyaev in the Soviet Union in the 1950s on the domestication of foxes, which was based on selection for docility. This followed the model that the domestication of dogs resulted from wolves that were less aggressive approaching human settlements and starting to coexist with humans. According to Wrangham, Belyaev found that after three generations of selective breeding some foxes would no longer show aggression or fearful responses to humans, and that, by the thirtieth to thirty-fifth generation of breeding, 70%–80% of foxes were domesticated, which included approaching the experimenters to sniff and lick them. The foxes would also wag their tails and follow human gestures. In this domestication of foxes, a less reactive temperament may have replaced being naturally fearful of humans, resulting in an attraction to humans. Wrangham also addresses that such selection by humans for reduced emotional reactivity changes not only temperament but also results in unrelated phenotypic traits, such as floppy ears and altered face shape, and, for dogs, social skills.

Wrangham (2019) states that selection against reactive aggression has occurred for humans across the last 300,000 years, and that this also caused a reduction in face size, which is a characteristic of domesticated species. He states that, with language starting to develop from 100,000 to 60,000 years ago, individuals were then able to form coalitions so as to counter the most aggressive members. Wrangham (2019) reviews Hare's (2017) work on how reduced reactive aggression decreases fear responses to other humans, which gives more time for individuals to read other humans' signals, including gaze direction, aided by attention to the white of the eye (sclera), leading to increased co-operation. Wrangham concludes that the differences between Homo sapiens and Neanderthals 'may have been due more to emotion than to intellect' (p.197), and that our prosociality is underpinned by embarrassment and guilt, and the pain, and danger, of being ostracised. So as to illustrate prosociality, he contrasts bonobos with chimpanzees, the former being non-aggressive, trusting and very playful towards each other, and very accepting and welcoming of stranger bonobos joining the group. Bonobos have far lower aggression than other apes and no tendency to kill members of the same species. According to Hare (2017), bonobos evolved to be less aggressive because females were able to express a mating preference for less aggressive males; this was thus that species' mechanism for self-domestication.

Human levels of co-operative communication are, for Hare, a result of an increase in social tolerance generated by a decrease in emotional reactivity. According to this hypothesis, an increase in tolerance in humans allowed inherited cognitive skills to be expressed in new social situations. For example, Hare notes that infants with the least aggressive and most socially reserved temperaments show the earliest expression of the false belief understanding that supports co-operative forms of communication. The HSD theory states that increases in self-control and reductions in reactivity, as a result of an increase in brain size, steadily drove the evolution of tolerance and social cognitive skills, including empathy, and mentalising (the attribution of mental states to others), mediated by the white sclera of the eyes, prefrontal mechanisms and oxytocin. Hare (2017) details how the widening of developmental windows in the young, which is a common consequence of domestication, resulted in an extended juvenile period, which facilitates participation in cultural forms of learning, including the explosion of cultural artefacts that began around 80,000 years ago.

Cultural and language extensions of HSD

The above stance on HSD is highly biological, including, for Wrangham, the use of legal and extra-legal executions so as to rid the group of over-aggressive and anti-social individuals, and hence of their genes. A more psychological and cultural extension of HSD is explored at length by Shilton et al. (2020), who ask whether the above evidence could better be described as selection for co-operation and emotional control, as is observed in many other highly social mammals, rather than as self-domestication. They propose the first stage of human social evolution involving mimetic communication, with mimetic speech developing half a million years ago, and the beginnings of musical engagement. Engagement with music is proposed to bond the group together through emotional and embodied unity.

The second stage involves an increased sophistication of language (see also Dor, 2015), which goes beyond the immediate communication event, and allows the communication of experiences, norms, skills and worldviews beyond what was possible through mimesis. With language, individuals begin to take into account things they themselves have never experienced, things they have only heard about, as well as sharing conceptual thinking, complaining and making complex plans. Here, Shilton et al. (2020) emphasise the importance of communication by stories. We propose that this culturally evolved communication system could have involved the sharing of dreams upon waking, allied to the evolution of story-telling.

Story-telling, fiction, dreaming and human evolution

According to Boyd (2018), early in human evolution, narratives would be limited to what had already happened or was happening, they would be mimetic, but when this became combined with play, fiction arose. Boyd continues that there would be a craving for understanding our world not only in terms of our own direct experience, but through the experience of others, whether those others were real or, as occurs in fiction, imagined. Boyd (2018) details the personal, social and cultural benefits of fictional and non-fictional narratives, and of their sharing, including understanding causality and the perspectives of others. Fiction would thus have arisen as one characteristic of play, and would be a learning, bonding and corrective mechanism. Language, narrative, play and sociality would all then synergise each other.

To summarise, humans have evolved to have reduced emotionality and increased prosociality, mentalising and empathy, and this selection has been described as HSD (Hare, 2017; Wrangham, 2019) or as prosocial motivation and self-control (Shilton et al., 2020). These processes may be aided by mimetic and, more recently, fictional narratives (Boyd, 2018; Dunbar, 2009), which may have developed around campfires (Dunbar, 2014). However, fictional narratives are not only produced during wakefulness, but also during sleep, as dreams. We will now introduce dreaming into this line of argument about social evolution, with a quotation from Boyd (2018, p. 9):

> And every night, too, the actor–scene network was already active. Dreaming appears to occur in many species. It too combines memories into new configurations. We experience dreams as immediately present to the inner eye and as engaging both attention and emotion. To that extent dreams resemble and probably anticipated fictional narrative, and would have had more raw material to play with the more frequently and more elaborately factual narrative had begun to circulate. But dreams recombine elements of memory in apparently stochastic and therefore arbitrary and usually poorly retrieved ways, even if they can be triggered by current preoccupations or moods. They mostly provide meager direct hints either for waking life or for fiction. I suggest that the main function of dreams may be to keep the retrieval and recombinatorial mechanisms of the default or actor-scene network in good running order for daytime retrieval and planning—with the consequence that the network was also already available for idle daydreaming and could easily be coopted for purposeful fictional invention.

Though Boyd's inclusion of dreaming into human social evolution is intriguing, his characterisation of dreams as providing 'meager direct hints either for waking life or for fiction' suggests a cognitive deficiency view of dream cognition that much work in the field has countered. For example, Domhoff (1996) shows extensive continuities between wake-life conceptualisations and dream content; Edwards et al. (2015) and Blagrove et al. (2019a) show personal insight gains from group consideration of dreams; and high levels of complexity in terms of self-representation and interactions of characters are found even in children's dreams, by Sándor et al. (2015, 2016).

Regarding narrative complexity, Pace-Schott's (2013) paper 'Dreaming as Story-telling' shows similarities between the basis of story production in the brain and dream production. There may indeed be common processes between dreaming and story-telling, in that both are narrative representations (or simulations) of waking life, and story grammar methods show that there is a greater length and complexity of reports collected from the fourth compared to the second REM period of the night, and greater for a 10-minute compared to a 5-minute REM duration (Cipolli et al., 2015). The advantage of morning dream-recall referred to earlier as a result of longer REM periods is thus augmented by the greater complexity of the narrative. We therefore consider that Boyd was correct to link the processes of dreaming to the processes of waking life fiction production, but may have underestimated the possible direct personal and social effects of recalling and telling dreams. (A fascinating exploration of the complex and disturbing narratives and stories that can result from dreams and from the experience of sleep disorders is provided by Vernon, 2022.)

We suggest that the timescale for dreams becoming functional in humans, through sharing, is the same timescale for story-telling having emerged, which is estimated by Pagel (2017) as occurring from 40,000 years BCE, with cave art depicting series of events, and the creation of other art and cultural artefacts, in parallel with the development of complex grammatical language. Although the use of dreams in human pre-history cannot be shown or studied, there is considerable evidence for their use currently and recently in hunter-gatherer societies (e.g., Gregor, 1981; Pandya, 2004; Peluso, 2004; Wax, 2004), and so dreams in pre-history may have been treated as worthy narratives in themselves, and may also have provided some of the first fiction that humans could tell. Many of these hunter-gatherer dreams are socially important, and some may be passed down in folklore, and have been termed 'big dreams', which may even have had a part to play in religion (Bulkeley, 2016; Jung, 1948/2002b, p.78). But with the valuing of these 'big dreams' comes the possibility that the telling of ordinary dreams may have occurred, and bonding and self-revelation could have resulted from this, given that the method of interpretation of dreams by relating them to waking life is evidenced by historical materials from ancient cultures (Hughes, 2000).

HSD and within-sleep and post-sleep functions of dreaming

The HSD theory emphasises the importance of play, and of domesticated species having extensive periods of the lifespan in which play can occur. As reviewed above, one of the facets of play is the production of fiction. Play has also been related to dreaming by Bulkeley (2019), who states that dreaming is imaginative play in sleep, play being incompletely functional, spontaneous, initiated in the absence of stress, and often part of an animals juvenile period. The sharing of the night-time fictions produced by this imaginative play would be expected to show many of the interpersonal and social benefits proposed by the HSD theory.

Following the reasoning in this chapter, and in Chapters 12 and 13 of this book, we suggest that the function of dreams resides in their waking use, and that remembering them is essential to this function. We can contrast this suggested post-sleep function of dreams with the emotion regulation theory of dreaming, which holds that emotions are processed during our dreams (Cartwright, 2010; Scarpelli et al., 2019). We can ask, what if dreams have a role in emotion processing not during sleep, but when awake, as a result of telling and considering the dream? Such processing of emotions with others, as a result of the group or social consideration of the dream, is part of the hypothesised role of dream-sharing within HSD, as to explore dreams as a group activity enhances levels of mentalising and emotional understanding between people. Rimé (2009) similarly contrasts the individualistic view of emotion regulation to a social sharing view of emotion regulation at interpersonal and collective levels.

To illustrate how data that may support claims for within-sleep effects or even functions for dreams can also be interpreted in favour of a post-sleep dream-sharing effect or function, we address here first the interesting findings of Bergman et al. (2020). These authors report a content analysis of 632 dreams of 150 Polish Auschwitz survivors, collected in the 1970s, and comprising retrospectively recalled dreams from before the Second World War, during imprisonment, and after the war. They found that war-related and threat dreams were more common after the war than during imprisonment, and dreams involving family and freedom-related themes were more common during imprisonment than they were before or after the war.

Bergman et al. (2020) discuss which theories of dream function and of post-trauma nightmares can account for this pattern of results, and give reasons why the data do not accord with some theories. The authors focus on the emotional processing that a dream may be performing for the individual, and the relationship of dream content to waking life experiences occurring at the time of the dream. In contrast, the empathy theory of dreaming, and the proposal for the inclusion of dream-sharing within HSD, would lead to consideration of the effects of sharing these dreams. Although dream-sharing was not addressed in the Bergman et al. (2020) paper, we can use their dream content data to suggest possible effects of sharing dreams that have such content. In this regard, sharing during imprisonment a dream of one's prior life, worth and identity would aid the encouragement of social bonding and empathy during the terrible circumstances of the concentration camp. However, after the war, sharing dreams of the concentration camp encourages social bonding and empathy towards the dreamer for what they have experienced, this sharing sometimes occurring in the face of social, political and cultural downplaying, ignoring or even denial of those experiences. The sharing of dreams with these contents would thus be adaptive and of benefit to the group, in that self-disclosure and group bonding are promoted, even if from the standpoint of the individual the post-war dreams bring back painful memories.

To further demonstrate this distinction between within-sleep and post-sleep functions of dreams, we can return to the NEXTUP theory of dreaming (Zadra & Stickgold, 2021), which was considered in Chapter 12, and which holds that in REM dreams the brain combines memories 'into a dream narrative that explores associations the brain would never normally consider' (p.109). Zadra and Stickgold illustrate the theory with a dream that Stickgold had in his first faculty position when helping to lead a lab class in which anaesthetised dogs would be operated on by medical students, a class that he says he was 'too squeamish' for. He reports a dream from that time in which, as a dog's chest was being cut open, he 'suddenly realized that it wasn't a dog; it was my five-year-old daughter, Jessie' (p.113). On waking, Bob told the dream to his wife and discussed it with her. Zadra and Stickgold conclude that

> This association, Jessie and the dog lab, was a valuable one. Something was uncovered about the fragility or sacredness of life that was important, something worth marking and strengthening and keeping available for the future. Once these connections were strengthened, the brain's job was done. Whether Bob remembered the dream when he woke up or not didn't really matter.
>
> (p.113)

In our view, the dream's novel association between a vulnerable dog and Bob's daughter may well have been produced during sleep. However, the strengthened connection that results might be initially between dream-sharer and listener, when the dream is told and discussed, rather than between neurons during sleep, although, obviously, the dream recall and discussion also make permanent the newfound very poignant link the dream created between vulnerable dog and daughter.

Costs and benefits of dream-sharing

Any theory of benefits of dream-sharing needs to take into account balancing these benefits with possible costs. Regarding benefits, it is not necessary to hypothesise that dream-sharing contributes more to group cohesion than does fiction-sharing, as they may have similar levels of effect. Instead, the suggestion by us is that dreams are an additional source of instances of fiction, they increase the amount of fiction that is shared, but with some characteristics that make them different from fiction that is produced in waking life, such as being created spontaneously and without intention or plan. And people are motivated to share dreams. In Graf et al. (2021), the highest-ranked motives for participants' most recent instance of sharing a dream were, with highest first, 'Because I was interested what the other person would think about the dream', 'To emotionally relieve me', and 'Because I wanted to better understand the dream'. Lower scores were given for 'For entertaining reasons', and 'Because the other person occurred within the dream'. A benefit of dream-sharing is thus that it fulfils these motivations, and we would note that even telling a dream for entertainment or humour can be bonding.

There are, however, costs in that some dreams might be confusing or simply bizarre and with no recognisable benefit to dreamer or listener. Some dreams might also be embarrassing to the dreamer or disclose personal information that disadvantages the dreamer. There is thus the intriguing similarity between dream telling and blushing, in that both signal the emotional state of the person to others. Because the blush is involuntary, it is a believable signal about regret, embarrassment and shame. It can be distressing and embarrassing to the person blushing, but provides a benefit to the group by signalling emotional states to others (Crozier & de Jong, 2013). Dreams may similarly be distressing to the individual, but act as a useful means for forcing self-disclosure between people.

Dream recall also has to be balanced with the need for forgetting the dream experiences, so that they are not mixed with waking life real events, as with the source memory deficits for dreams in narcoleptic patients which result in the detrimental mixing of real with dreamt memories (Wamsley et al., 2014). Having a source memory deficit may be detrimental to the social standing of individuals in the group. Related to this, Bardina (2021) explores how, as with eye-witness reports, the dream-sharer must show that they are a reliable source for recounting what happened in the dream. Although the sharer recounts what may be strange or even impossible, they must show that they are a normal and reliable agent for the reporting.

The cost-benefit analysis is further complicated by the occurrence of nightmares and troubling dreams that might be difficult to forget and which might be adverse to mental health or happiness in waking life. Nevertheless, there may often be benefits to sharing negatively toned dreams, just as there are benefits to the revelation and expression of negative thoughts and memories (Ruini & Mortara, 2022). Sliwinski (2017) gives examples of the nightmares of people in very distressing political circumstances: Nelson Mandela dreaming in prison of being released and of finding his home empty, with no one there, and the nightmares of people subject to colonial violence in Algeria. For certain nightmares, Sliwinski suggests that a function of dreams within sleep might be impaired under conditions of severe stress. In contrast, we would suggest that extremely adverse waking-life circumstances and nightmares will be highly distressing to the individual, but that seen in the light of HSD the nightmare, and even a Post-Traumatic Stress Disorder (PTSD) nightmare, is still expressive of those waking-life circumstances that caused the nightmare, and hence sharing the nightmare after waking might still be beneficial. The proposed post-sleep function of dreams would thus still be maintained, even though proposed within-sleep functions would be expected to be disrupted. Importantly, the content of dreams does not itself have to be domesticated, in the sense of being emotionally unreactive and affiliative, to have a domesticating effect when shared. Dreams may have aggression and other anti-social activities, but the same is true for films, be they horror, drama or thrillers. It may be that the sharing of such negativity and drama brings people together through experiencing troubling narratives together, much as the experience of tragedy in drama for adults, or Halloween for children can do.

Future research

Although the majority of the human population may be characterised by HSD there may also be alternative evolutionary strategies for a small proportion of the population, and that proportion might not have had the same dream content or dream-sharing characteristics as is hypothesised here for the majority of the population. For example, Lyons et al. (2019) found that the frequency of aggressive dreams is predicted by the traits Machiavellianism and psychopathy. Future research on the characteristics of dreams that result in post-sleep prosocial effects for the majority of the population should take into account such individual difference factors.

Future research should also address empathy for positive experiences. In a study in everyday circumstances rather than in a laboratory, Depow et al. (2021) found that empathy for positive experiences is as common as for negative experiences, and that empathy more often occurs for those to whom we are close than to strangers. They conclude that laboratory studies have led to a priority for emphasising empathy for the negative situations of strangers. Depow and colleague's findings are very relevant to the proposal for dream-sharing being important for empathy and for HSD, as dreams are as likely to be emotionally positive as negative (Schredl & Doll, 1998), and sharing of them usually occurs between people who have a close relationship (Graf et al., 2021). Finally, it is also important to address tentative sharing, where the sharer is unsure of whether to tell a dream due to what it unwittingly reveals (Rycroft, 1981), or, alternatively, where the sharer is using the dream as a way to broach a subject with the listener.

Of course, it is unknown what dreams occurred to individuals in pre-history hunter-gatherer societies, and any effects of sharing those dreams. The closest we can get now to studying dreams from pre-history is to investigate whether current hunter-gatherer groups engage in dream-sharing, which we know they do: The extensive importance of dreams and dream-sharing across many cultures and times is reviewed by Sheriff (2021), and within this, the distinction between sensory or physical, personal, and cultural metaphors in dreams is explored by Mageo (2021). But, we do not know whether the sharing of such dreams has an effect of self-disclosure for the individuals, and this needs to be investigated.

Implications for a function of consciousness

We can extend the arguments about dreaming in this chapter to consciousness more generally. Oatley's (2016) paper 'Fiction: Simulation of social worlds,' ' states that people who read fiction improve their understanding of others, because fiction has complex characters and circumstances that we might not encounter in daily life. He concludes:

> While some everyday consciousness can remain inside the individual mind and be externalized in small pieces during conversations, fictional stories can be thought of as larger pieces of consciousness that can be externalized by authors in forms that can be passed to others so that these others can internalize them as wholes, and make them their own.

This chapter is proposing that dreams can, like fictional stories, be passed to others who internalise them as wholes, they are pieces of consciousness. But what is being said of dreaming consciousness could also be said of the scenarios and narratives present in waking consciousness. A function of human consciousness could thus be that its content and narratives can be passed to and engaged with by others, rather than just experienced by the individual in the first person for access to their emotional and cognitive processes.

Summary

Dream-sharing might have occurred in human history and pre-history and caused empathy between people, and increased social bonding. We propose that this may have resulted in an evolutionary pressure for dream content that refers to social and emotional relations between people. Dream-sharing would thus contribute to HSD. A key component of HSD is play, which can be seen in children and adults, can result in the different varieties of fiction and art, and extends into sleep as the production of dreams. The sharing of dreams may sometimes be uncomfortable for the dreamer, but the benefit to the group may have ensured the development across evolutionary time of this method of self-disclosure. Evidence that dreams are involved in the processing of emotions and memories during sleep can be interpreted alternatively as the dream-content eliciting this processing socially when the dream is shared after waking.

Acknowledgement: Part of this chapter was published by Blagrove and Lockheart (2022) in the *International Journal of Dream Research*. We thank the journal for the helpful reviewer and editor comments.

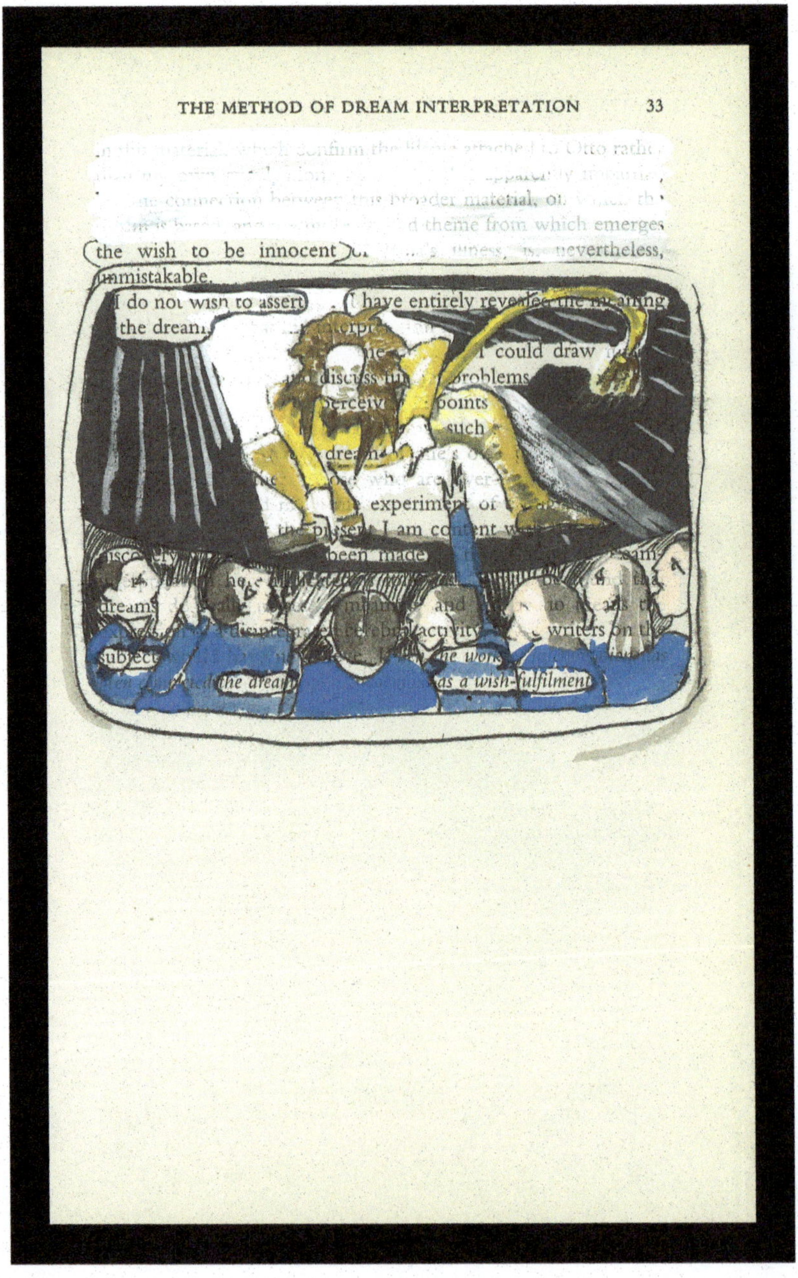

Figure 18.1 Dream of boss on stage at festival, 2019.

18 Conclusions and summary

For the concluding chapter, we include here a dream told to us at a science festival, and which was painted on the final page of one of the chapters from *The Interpretation of Dreams*.

DREAM NARRATIVE: *I am watching the Glastonbury festival, and am surprised to see on the main stage my boss, who, despite her age, is dancing and doing acrobatics while singing. She is wearing a lion suit, which covers all of her body except for her face, which I can see. My work colleagues are at the front of the audience, all wearing their blue uniforms, and they greatly enjoy the performance; they were expecting to see her. For me it is like watching it on a television, I am not there and can see shots of it from different directions.*

DISCUSSION: We discussed with the dreamer, Laura, how the dream refers to relationships with her colleagues and the boss at work.

JULIA: (Painting shown as Figure 18.1) I chose the single paragraph at the end of a chapter as it was well suited to depict the idea of a main stage. It was also particularly suited to show the screen through which the isolated dreamer experienced the image, as the dreamer was apart from the work colleagues in the audience, but all were watching the boss live.

People differ in how seriously they take dreams, ranging from deep interest to indifference, and even hostility. The scientific community similarly varies: ranging from intrigue at the relationship of dreams to neuroscience and to the science of consciousness, to dismissal of dreams as a delirium, a waste of time at best, or, at worst, a source of losing touch with the real world.

We aimed with this book to show readers the breadth of research on dreaming, spanning many decades, as well as how that research shows that there is good reason for people to consider and discuss their own dreams.

We reviewed how dreams are far from an amorphous delirium. Indeed, despite the novelty of each dream, they have meaningful relationships with waking life, principally incorporating waking-life emotional rather than mundane or unemotional experiences. Furthermore, we now know more about the relationship of the brain to the recall and production of dreams, although personality factors of interest in and positive attitude towards dreams may also be involved.

Given that sleep has been found to consolidate memories, and that dreams prioritise the incorporation of emotional waking-life experiences and concerns, there has been a longstanding view that dreams play a role in these processes during sleep. As a common understanding across many theories, it may be possible to agree that dreams might start with the memories that the brain is processing during the night, whether or not dreams contribute anything to that processing. There is also a common understanding across many theories that dreams depict waking-life concerns and concepts in a tangential or metaphorical manner, and it is here that there may be a meeting place with Freud, and with the cognitive science of metaphor. We hope we have shown that meeting place with our re-readings and paintings of the dreams of Freud's heroic patient Dora. The Dora dreams illustrate how metaphorical relationships between dream content and waking life can be identified, given time and dedication to exploring the dream and exploring free associations to it.

We hope that readers will use the gentle but searching Ullman method we have outlined for exploring their own dreams, and in light of our review of the research into that method. It was our wish to undertake this fascinating dream exploration method with members of the public at open events that led to our science art collaboration. Each individual event has brought together so many different people, online or at venues, but they have all, during each event, honoured and concentrated on a single dream of one person, and helped that person to explore the relationship of their dream to their waking life. These events aim to socialise each dream, with the art returning the dream to its visual form, and also enabling the dream and the discussion of the dream to be revisited later with others.

It is because of this collaboration that the next stage of our research began, with the realisation that dreams may have their greatest effect socially rather than in the mind or brain of the dreamer while asleep. At the risk of being grandiose, we have placed those social effects within the theory of human self-domestication, held by many researchers to be the primary driver of the evolution of human prosociality, empathy, tolerance and reduced emotional reactivity.

We have therefore linked our findings to social evolution. And we also place the artworks produced by Julia within another field of inquiry, that of art, and have drawn on two art and cultural movements in this, Dadaism and Surrealism. Dadaism valued public performances, what would later be called *happenings*. Surrealism greatly valued dreams, dream-like processes, and the community that these can engender. Surrealism continues to be one of the high-points of human creativity and playfulness; playfulness also being a characteristic of human social and cognitive evolution, and of human self-domestication, and of dreaming. Julia has also contemporised these approaches by drawing her own links to the emergent synergistic and collaborative field of metadesign (Lockheart, 2022a, 2022b; Wood, 2022).

Conclusions and summary 221

We are glad and honoured to have brought all these areas of science and art together in one book. Our intention is for this to lead to greater scientific, artistic, personal, and community engagement with dreaming. And, for humanity, that the use of dream discussions and visualisations can be a source of creative, meaningful conversations and mutual understanding.

We conclude with a quotation from the end of Act 4 scene 1 (lines 208-209) of *A Midsummer Night's Dream* (Shakespeare, 1600/2016). As Hermia, Lysander, Helena and Demetrius wake, they are asked to follow the Duke back from the oneiric world of the wood to the formal world of the palace, and say:

> Why, then, we are awake. Let's follow him,
> And by the way let us recount our dreams.

We hope that this book inspires readers to know more about dreaming, to recall and consider their own dreams, and to recount and share their dreams with others.

References

Ades, D. (2013). Dreams in surrealist discourse and the unusual case of Miró's photo: This is the color of my dreams. In J. Jiménez (Ed.), *Surrealism and the dream* (pp. 75–95). Madrid: Museo Thyssen-Bornemisza.
Adler, K. (2018). *Ida*. Hamburg: Rowohlt Verlag.
Andersson, R. (2000). *Songs from the Second Floor* [Film]. Roy Andersson Filmproduktion. Sweden.
Andersson, R. (2007). *You, the Living* [Film]. Roy Andersson Filmproduktion. Sweden.
Andrews-Hanna, J. R. (2012). The brain's default network and its adaptive role in internal mentation. *Neuroscientist, 18*, 251–270.
Antrobus, J. S. (1977). The dream as metaphor: An information-processing and learning model. *Journal of Mental Imagery, 2*, 327–338.
Antrobus, J. (1983). REM and NREM sleep reports: Comparison of word frequencies by cognitive classes. *Psychophysiology, 20*, 562–568.
Aron, E. N., & Aron, A. (1997). Sensory-processing sensitivity and its relation to introversion and emotionality. *Journal of Personality and Social Psychology, 73*, 345–368.
Aserinsky, E., & Kleitman, N. (1953). Regularly occurring periods of eye motility, and concomitant phenomena, during sleep. *Science, 118*, 273–274.
Ashton, J. E., Staresina, B. P., & Cairney, S. A. (2022) Sleep bolsters schematically incongruent memories. *PLoS ONE, 17*(6): e0269439.
Askitopoulou, H. (2015). Sleep and dreams: From myth to medicine in Ancient Greece. *Journal of Anesthesia History, 1*, 70–75.
Aviram, L., & Soffer-Dudek, N. (2018). Lucid dreaming: Intensity, but not frequency, is inversely related to psychopathology. *Frontiers in Psychology, 9*, 384.
Baird, B., Aparicio, M. K., Alauddin, T., Riedner, B., Boly, M., & Tononi, G. (2022a). Episodic thought distinguishes spontaneous cognition in waking from REM and NREM sleep. *Consciousness and Cognition, 97*, 103247.
Baird, B., Castelnovo, A., Gosseries, O., & Tononi, G. (2018). Frequent lucid dreaming associated with increased functional connectivity between frontopolar cortex and temporoparietal association areas. *Scientific Reports, 8*, art. no. 17798.
Baird B., Tononi G., & LaBerge S. (2022b). Lucid dreaming occurs in activated rapid eye movement sleep, not a mixture of sleep and wakefulness. *Sleep, 45* (4), art. no. zsab294.
Barber, S. (2008). Extremities of the mind. In: R. Short (ed.), *The Age of Gold, Dalí, Buñuel, Artaud: Surrealist Cinema*, chapter 1, pp.33–49. Solar Books.
Barcaro, U., & Paoli, M. (2015). Dreaming and neuroesthetics. *Frontiers in Human Neuroscience, 9*, 348.

Bardina, S. (2022). 'That's what the dream says': The use of normalizing devices in dream reports. *Discourse Studies*, online first, doi:10.1177/14614456211001607

Baron-Cohen, S., Wheelwright, S., & Hill, J. (2001). The 'Reading the mind in the eyes' test revised version: A study with normal adults, and adults with Asperger Syndrome or High-Functioning autism. *Journal of Child Psychology and Psychiatry, 42*, 241–252.

Barrett, D. (1992). Just how lucid are lucid dreams? *Dreaming, 2*, 221–228.

Barrett, D. (2001). *The committee of sleep.* New York: Random House.

Barrett, D. (2007). An evolutionary theory of dreams and problem-solving In D. Barrett & P. McNamara (Eds.), *The new science of dreaming, Vol. 3. Cultural and theoretical perspectives* (pp. 133–153). Westport, CT: Praeger.

Barrett, D. (2020a). Dreams about COVID-19 versus normative dreams: Trends by gender. *Dreaming, 30*, 216–221.

Barrett, D. (2020b). *Pandemic dreams.* Oneiroi Press.

Baylor, G. W., & Cavallero, C. (2001). Memory sources associated with REM and NREM dream reports throughout the night: A new look at the data. *Sleep: Journal of Sleep and Sleep Disorders Research, 24*, 165–170.

Beaulieu-Prévost, D., & Zadra, A. (2005). How dream recall frequency shapes people's beliefs about the content of their dreams. *North American Journal of Psychology, 7*, 253–264.

Beaulieu-Prévost, D., & Zadra, A. (2007). Absorption, psychological boundaries and attitude towards dreams as correlates of dream recall: Two decades of research seen through a meta-analysis. *Journal of Sleep Research, 16*, 51–59.

Belicki, K. (1992). The relationship of nightmare frequency to nightmare suffering with implications for treatment and research. *Dreaming, 2*, 143–148.

Bergman, I. (1957). *Wild Strawberries / Smultronstället* [Film]. Svensk Filmindustri. Sweden.

Bergman, M., MacGregor, O., Olkoniemi, H., Owczarski, W., Revonsuo, A., & Valli, K. (2020). The Holocaust as a lifelong nightmare: Posttraumatic symptoms and dream content in Polish Auschwitz survivors 30 years after World War II. *The American Journal of Psychology, 133*, 143–166.

Bernheimer, C., & Kahane, C. (Eds.) (1990). *In Dora's Case: Freud – hysteria – feminism.* Columbia University Press.

Berry, W. (2021). *Drawn into the Dream: How Drawing Your Dreams can take you to the Land of Awes.* Los Angeles, CA: Precocity Press.

Bittencourt, E. (2022). Surrealist cinema's drive towards freedom. *Frieze*, issue 228, 5th July 2022.

Black, J., Belicki, K., & Emberley-Ralph, J. (2019). Who dreams of the deceased? The roles of dream recall, grief intensity, attachment, and openness to experience. *Dreaming, 29*, 57–78.

Blagrove, M. (1992). Dreams as the reflection of our waking concerns and abilities: A critique of the problem-solving paradigm in dream research. *Dreaming, 2*, 205–220.

Blagrove, M. (2009). Dreaming – motivated or meaningless? *The Psychologist, 22* (number 8; August), 680–683.

Blagrove, M. (2011). Distinguishing continuity/discontinuity, function and insight when investigating dream content. *International Journal of Dream Research, 4*, 45–47.

Blagrove, M., Bell, E., & Wilkinson, A. (2010). Association of lucid dreaming frequency with Stroop task performance. *Dreaming, 20*, 280–287.

Blagrove, M., Edwards, C., van Rijn, E., Reid, A., Malinowski, J., Bennett, P., Carr, M., Eichenlaub, J-B., McGee, S., Evans, K., & Ruby, P. (2019a). Insight from the consideration of REM dreams, non-REM dreams and daydreams. *Psychology of Consciousness, 6*, 138–162.

Blagrove, M., Farmer, L., & Williams, E. (2004). The relationship of nightmare frequency and nightmare distress to well-being. *Journal of Sleep Research, 13*, 129–136.

Blagrove, M., Fouquet, N., Henley-Einion, J., Pace-Schott, E., Davies, A., Neuschaffer, J., & Turnbull, O. (2011a). Assessing the dream-lag effect for REM and NREM stage 2 dreams. *PLoS ONE, 6*, e26708.

Blagrove, M., French, C. C., & Jones, G. (2006). Probabilistic reasoning, affirmative bias and belief in precognitive dreams. *Applied Cognitive Psychology, 20*, 65–83.

Blagrove, M., Hale, S., Lockheart, J., Carr, M., Jones, A., & Valli, K. (2019b). Testing the empathy theory of dreaming: The relationships between dream sharing and trait and state empathy. *Frontiers in Psychology, 10*, 1351.

Blagrove, M., & Hartnell, S. J. (2000). Lucid dreaming: Associations with internal locus of control, need for cognition and creativity. *Personality and Individual Differences, 28*, 41–47.

Blagrove, M., Henley-Einion, J., Barnett, A., Edwards, D., & Seage, C. (2011b). A replication of the 5–7 day dream-lag effect with comparison of dreams to future events as control for baseline matching. *Consciousness and Cognition, 20*, 384–391.

Blagrove, M., Lockheart, J., Carr, M., Basra, S., Graham, H., Lewis, H., Murphy, E., Sakalauskaite, A., Trotman, C., & Valli, K. (2021). Dream sharing and the enhancement of empathy: Theoretical and applied implications. *Dreaming, 31*, 128–139.

Blagrove, M., Neuschaffer, J., & Henley-Einion, J. (2010). Assessing dream impactfulness, session depth and dream understanding in a dream group. Paper presented at the 27th Annual Conference of the International Association for the Study of Dreams, June 27th – July 1st 2010, Ashville, NC. Abstract available at: *International Journal of Dream Research, 3*, Supplement 1, S1.

Blagrove, M., & Pace-Schott, E. F. (2010). Trait and neurobiological correlates of individual differences in dream recall and dream content. *International Review of Neurobiology, 92*, 155–180.

Blechner, M. J. (2001). *The dream frontier.* Hillsdale, NJ: The Analytic Press.

Boag, S. (2017). On dreams and motivation: Comparison of Freud's and Hobson's views. *Frontiers in Psychology, 7*, 2001.

Boss, M. (1957). *The analysis of dreams.* (Translated by A. J. Pomerans.) London: Rider.

Boyd, B. (2018). The evolution of stories: From mimesis to language, from fact to fiction. *Cognitive Science, 9*, e1444.

Breton, A. (1924/1972). *Manifestoes of surrealism.* Translation by R. Seaver & H. R. Lane. Ann Arbor Paperbacks, University of Michigan Press.

Breton, A. (1924/1978). *What is surrealism? Selected writings.* (Edited and introduced by F. Rosemont). Pathfinder.

Breton, A. (1924/1996). After Dada. In *The lost steps* (pp. 74–76). Translation by M. Polizzotti. University of Nebraska Press.

Breton, A. (1924/1996). Max Ernst. In *The lost steps* (pp. 60–61). Translation by M. Polizzotti. University of Nebraska Press.

Breton, A. (1924/1996). The mediums enter. In *The lost steps* (pp. 89–95). Translation by M. Polizzotti. University of Nebraska Press.

Breton, A. (1928/1999). *Nadja.* Penguin Modern Classics.

Breton, A. (1928/2002). Surrealism and painting. Part I in *Surrealism and painting* (Translated by S. W. Taylor). Boston Museum of Fine Arts: Artworks.

Breton, A. (1941/2002). Artistic genesis and perspective of surrealism. Part II in *Surrealism and painting* (Translated by S. W. Taylor). Boston Museum of Fine Arts: Artworks.

Brown, D. B. (2001). *Romanticism*. London: Phaidon Press.

Bryant, R. A., Wyzenbeek, M., & Weinstein, J. (2011). Dream rebound of suppressed emotional thoughts: The influence of cognitive load. *Consciousness and Cognition, 20*, 515–522.

Bulkeley, K. (2016). *Big dreams: The science of dreaming and the origins of religion*. Oxford: Oxford University Press.

Bulkeley, K. (2019). Dreaming is imaginative play in sleep: A theory of the function of dreams. *Dreaming, 29*, 1–21.

Bulkeley, K., & Bulkley, P. (2005). *Dreaming beyond death: A guide to pre-death dreams and visions*. Boston, MA: Beacon Press.

Buñuel, L. (1930). *L'Age d'Or / The age of gold* [Film]. Corinth Films (1979 U.S. release). France.

Buñuel, L. (1933). *Land Without Bread / Las Hurdes* [Film]. Transflux (2013 DVD). Spain.

Buñuel, L. (1950). *The Forgotten Ones / Los Olvidados; known in the US as The Young and the Damned* [Film]. *Ultramar Films*. Mexico.

Buñuel, L. (1961). *Viridiana* [Film]. Kingsley-International Pictures. Spain.

Buñuel, L. (1962). *The exterminating Angel / El Angel exterminador* [Film]. Reel Media International [US], Facets, Hen's Tooth Video Inc. [US]. Mexico.

Buñuel, L. (1967). *Belle de Jour* [Film]. *Valoria, and Euro International Films*. France.

Buñuel, L. (1972). *Le Charme Discret de la Bourgeoisie / The Discreet Charm of the Bourgeoisie* [Film]. Greenwich Film Productions. France.

Buñuel, L. (1974). *Le Fantôme de la Liberté / The Phantom of Liberty* [Film]. Greenwich Film Productions. France/Italy.

Buñuel, L. & Dalí, S. (1929). *Un Chain andalou / An Andalusian dog* [Film]. Les Grands Films Classiques. France.

Buñuel, L. (1994). *My last breath*. New York: Vintage Books.

Caldwell, L. (2022), A discussion of three versions of Donald Winnicott's 'Transitional Objects and Transitional Phenomena', 1951–1971. *British Journal of Psychotherapy, 38*, 42–60.

Carr, M., Konkoly, K., Mallett, R., Edwards, C., Appel, K., & Blagrove, M. (2020). Combining presleep cognitive training and REM-sleep stimulation in a laboratory morning nap for lucid dream induction. *Psychology of Consciousness: Theory, Research, and Practice*. Advance online publication. https://doi.org/10.1037/cns0000227

Carr, M., Matthews, E., Williams, J., & Blagrove, M. (2021). Testing the theory of differential susceptibility to nightmares: The interaction of sensory processing sensitivity with the relationship of low mental wellbeing to nightmare frequency and nightmare distress. *Journal of Sleep Research, 30*, Article e13200.

Carr, M., & Nielsen, T. (2017). A novel differential susceptibility framework for the study of nightmares: Evidence for trait sensory processing sensitivity. *Clinical Psychology Review, 58*, 86–96.

Carr, M. Saint-Onge, K. Blanchette-Carrière, C. Paquette, T., & Nielsen, T. (2018). Elevated perseveration errors on a verbal fluency task in frequent nightmare recallers: A replication. *Journal of Sleep Research, 27*, e12644.

Carrington, L. (2013). *The milk of dreams*. New York: New York Review Children's Collection.
Cartwright, R. D. (1991). Dreams that work: The relation of dream incorporation to adaptation to stressful events. *Dreaming, 1*, 3–9.
Cartwright, R. D. (2010). *The twenty-four hour mind: The role of sleep and dreaming in our emotional lives*. Oxford: Oxford University Press.
Cernovsky, Z. Z. (1984). Dream recall and attitude toward dreams. *Perceptual and Motor Skills, 58*, 911–914.
Chadwick, W. (2021a). *The militant muse: Love, war and the women of surrealism*. London: Thames & Hudson.
Chadwick, W. (2021b). *Women artists and the surrealist movement*. London: Thames & Hudson.
Chopik, W. J., O'Brien, E., & Konrath, S. H. (2017). Differences in empathic concern and perspective taking across 63 countries. *Journal of Cross-Cultural Psychology, 48*, 23–38.
Cipolli, C., Guazzelli, M., Bellucci, C., Mazzetti, M., Palagini, L., Rosenlicht, N., & Feinberg, I. (2015). Time-of-night variations in the story-like organization of dream experience developed during rapid eye movement sleep. *Journal of Sleep Research, 24*, 234–240.
Cirelli, C., & Tononi, G. (2008). Is sleep essential? *PLOS Biology, 6*, e216.
Clair, R. (1924). *Entr'acte* [Film]. Société Nouvelle des Acacias. France.
Cocteau, J. (1930). *Le Sang d'un Poète / The Blood of a Poet* [Film]. Tamasa Distribution; The Criterion Collection. France.
Cocteau, J. (1950). *Orphée / Orpheus* [Film]. DisCina. France.
Cocteau, J. (1960). *Testament d'Orphée/The Testament of Orpheus* [Film]. Les Editions Cinégraphiques. France.
Cocteau, J. (1985). *Two screenplays: The blood of a poet and the testament of Orpheus*. (Originally published, 1968.) (Translated by C. Martin-Sperry.) London, New York: Marion Boyars Publishers.
Cocteau, J. (1994). *The art of cinema*. (Originally published, 1988). (Translated by R. Buss.) London: Marion Boyars Publishers.
Cohen, D. B. (1974). Presleep mood and dream recall. *Journal of Abnormal Psychology, 83*, 45–51.
Cohen, D. B., & Wolfe, G. (1973). Dream recall and repression: Evidence for an alternative hypothesis. *Journal of Consulting and Clinical Psychology, 41*, 349–355.
Colace, C. (2003). Dream bizarreness reconsidered. *Sleep and Hypnosis, 5*, 105–128.
Craven, W. (1984). *Nightmare on Elm Street* [Film]. New Line Cinema, Potsdam, NY.
Craven, W. (1994). *New Nightmare* [Film]. Craven/Maddalena Films.
Crowe, C. (2001). *Vanilla Sky* [Film]. Paramount Pictures.
Crozier, W. R., & de Jong, P. J. (Eds.). (2013). *The psychological significance of the blush*. Cambridge: Cambridge University Press.
Curci, A., & Rimé, B. (2008). Dreams, emotions, and social sharing of dreams. *Cognition and Emotion, 22*, 155–167.
D'Alessandro, S., & Gale, M. (2021). *Surrealism beyond borders*. New York: Metropolitan Museum of Art.
Davidson, J., & Lynch, S. (2012). Thematic, literal and associative dream imagery following a high-impact event. *Dreaming, 22*, 58–69.
Decker, H. S. (1991). *Dora and Vienna 1900*. New York: Macmillan.
De Koninck, J., Prévost, F., & Lortie-Lussier, M. (1996). Vertical inversion of the visual field and REM sleep mentation. *Journal of Sleep Research, 5*, 16–20.

De Koninck, J., Wong, C., & Hébert, G. (2012). Types of dream incorporations of language learning and learning efficiency. *Journal of Sleep Research, 21*(Suppl. S1), 190.

Dement, W. C., Kahn, E., & Roffwarg, H. P. (1965). The influence of the laboratory situation on the dreams of the experimental subject. *Journal of Nervous and Mental Disease, 140*, 119–131.

Dement, W., & Kleitman, N. (1957). The relation of eye movements during sleep to dream activity: An objective method for the study of dreaming. *Journal of Experimental Psychology, 53*, 339–346.

Dement, W., & Wolpert, E. A. (1958). The relation of eye movements, body motility, and external stimuli to dream content. *Journal of Experimental Psychology, 55*, 543–553.

Depow, G. J., Francis, Z., & Inzlicht, M. (2021). The experience of empathy in everyday life. *Psychological Science, 32*, 1198–1213.

Deren, M. & Hammid, A. (1943). *Meshes of the Afternoon* [Film]. Produced by Maya Deren, USA.

Deutsch, F. (1990). A footnote to Freud's "Fragment of an Analysis of a Case of Hysteria." In C. Bernheimer & C. Kahane (Eds.), *In Dora's Case: Freud – hysteria – feminism* (chapter 1, pp. 35–43). New York: Columbia University Press.

Diekelmann, S., & Born, J. (2010). The memory function of sleep. *Nature Reviews Neuroscience, 11*, 114–126.

Domhoff, G. W. (1996). *Finding meaning in dreams: A quantitative approach*. New York: Plenum.

Domhoff, G. W. (2001). A new neurocognitive theory of dreams. *Dreaming, 11*, 13–33.

Domhoff, G. W. (2003). *The scientific study of dreams: Neural networks, cognitive development, and content analysis*. Washington, DC: American Psychological Association.

Domhoff, G. W. (2007). Realistic simulation and bizarreness in dream content: Past findings and suggestions for future research. In D. Barrett & P. McNamara (Eds.), *The new science of dreaming: Content, recall, and personality characteristics* (Vol. 2, pp. 1–27). Westport, CT: Praeger Press.

Domhoff, G. W. (2011). Dreams are embodied simulations that dramatize conceptions and concerns: The continuity hypothesis in empirical, theoretical, and historical context. *International Journal of Dream Research, 4*, 50–62.

Domhoff, G. W. (2017). The invasion of the concept snatchers: The origins, distortions, and future of the continuity hypothesis. *Dreaming, 27*, 14–39.

Domhoff, G. W. (2018). *The emergence of dreaming: Mind-wandering, embodied simulation, and the default network*. Oxford: Oxford University Press.

Domhoff, G. W. (2019). The neurocognitive theory of dreams at age 20: An assessment and a comparison with four other theories of dreaming. *Dreaming, 29*, 265–302.

Domhoff, G. W., & Schneider, A. (1998). New rationales and methods for quantitative dream research outside the laboratory. *Sleep, 21*, 398–404.

Domhoff, G. W., & Schneider, A. (2018). Are dreams social simulations? Or are they enactments of conceptions and personal concerns. An empirical and theoretical comparison of two dream theories. *Dreaming, 28*, 1–23.

Dor, D. (2015). *The instruction of imagination: Language as a social communication technology*. Oxford: Oxford University Press.

Dorus, E., Dorus, W., & Rechtschaffen, A. (1971). The incidence of novelty in dreams. *Archives of General Psychiatry, 25*, 364–368.
Dresler, M., Koch, S. P., Wehrle, R., Spoormaker, V. I., Holsboer, F., Steiger, A., Sämann, P. G., Obrig, H., & Czisch, M. (2011). Dreamed movement elicits activation in the sensorimotor cortex. *Current Biology, 21*, 1833–1837.
Dresler, M., Wehrle, R., Spoormaker, V. I., Koch, S. P., Holsboer, F., Steiger, A., Obrig, H., Sämann, P. G., & Czisch, M. (2012). Neural correlates of dream lucidity obtained from contrasting lucid versus non-lucid REM sleep: A combined EEG/fMRI case study. *Sleep, 35*, 1017–1020.
Duffey, T. H., Wooten, H. R., Lumadue, C. A., & Comstock, D. C. (2004). The effects of dream sharing on marital intimacy and satisfaction. *Journal of Couple and Relationship Therapy, 3*, 53–68.
Dulac, G. (1928). *La Coquille et le Clergyman / The Seashell and the Clergyman* [Film]. France.
Dunbar, R. I. M. (2009). The social brain hypothesis and its implications for social evolution. *Annals of Human Biology, 36*, 562–572.
Dunbar, R. I. M. (2014). How conversations around campfires came to be. *Proceedings of the National Academy of Sciences of the United States of America, 30*, 14013–14014.
Earle, W. (1987/2017) *Surrealism in film: Beyond the realist sensibility*. Originally published 1987. Abingdon & New York: Routledge.
Edwards, C. L., Malinowski, J. E., McGee, S. L., Bennett, P. D., Ruby, P. M., & Blagrove, M. T. (2015). Comparing personal insight gains due to consideration of a recent dream and consideration of a recent event using the Ullman and Schredl dream group methods. *Frontiers in Psychology, 6*, 831.
Edwards, C. L., Ruby, P. M., Malinowski, J. E., Bennett, P. D., & Blagrove, M. T. (2013). Dreaming and insight. *Frontiers in Psychology, 4*, 979.
Eichenlaub, J.-B., Bertrand, O., Morlet, D., & Ruby, P. (2014). Brain reactivity differentiates subjects with high and low dream recall frequencies during both sleep and wakefulness. *Cerebral Cortex, 24*, 1206–1215.
Eichenlaub, J.-B., Nicolas, A., Daltrozzo, J., Redouté, J., Costes, N., & Ruby, P. (2014). Resting brain activity varies with dream recall frequency between subjects. *Neuropsychopharmacology, 39*, 1594–1602.
Eichenlaub, J.-B., van Rijn, E., Gaskell, M. G., Lewis, P. A., Maby, E., Malinowski, J. E., Walker, M. P., Boy, F., & Blagrove, M. (2018). Incorporation of recent waking-life experiences in dreams correlates with frontal theta activity in REM sleep. *Social Cognitive and Affective Neuroscience, 13*, 637–647.
Eichenlaub, J.-B., van Rijn, E., Phelan, M., Ryder, L., Gaskell, M., Lewis, P., Walker, M., & Blagrove, M. (2019). The nature of delayed dream incorporation ('dream-lag effect'): Personally significant events persist, but not major daily activities or concerns. *Journal of Sleep Research, 28*, e12697.
Ellis, A. W., Raitmayr, O., & Herbst, C. (2015). The Ks: The other couple in the case of Freud's "Dora". *Journal of Austrian Studies, 48*, 1–26.
Ellis, L. (2020). *A Clinician's Guide to Dream Therapy*. Abingdon & New York: Routledge.
Epel, N. (1993). *Writers Dreaming*. New York: Carol Southern Books.
Erlacher, D., & Stumbrys, T. (2020). Wake up, work on dreams, back to bed and lucid dream: A sleep laboratory study. *Frontiers in Psychology, 11*, art. no. 1383.
Fellini, F. (2020). *The Book of Dreams*. (S. Toffetti, editor; A. Maines & D. Stanton, translators. Originally published in 2007 in Italian.) New York & Milan: Rizzoli.

Fernandez, L. M. J., & Lüthi, A. (2020). Sleep spindles: Mechanisms and functions. *Physiological Reviews, 100*, 805–868.

Findlay, G., Tononi, G., & Cirelli, C. (2020). The evolving view of replay and its functions in wake and sleep. *SLEEP Advances, 1*, zpab002.

Finkelstein, H. (1996). Dalí and *Un Chien andalou*: The nature of a collaboration. In R. E. Kuenzl (Ed.), *Dada and surrealist film*, pp.128–142. Cambridge, MA: MIT Press.

Fisher, S., Wood, R. L., & Blagrove, M. (2004). The frequency of dreams and nightmares after brain injury. *Sleep, 27*, (Abstract supplement), A64.

Fitch, T., & Armitage, R. (1989). Variations in cognitive style among high and low frequency dream recallers. *Personality and Individual Differences, 10*, 869–875.

Flanagan, O. (2000). *Dreaming souls: Sleep, dreams and the evolution of the conscious mind*. Oxford: Oxford University Press.

Flitterman-Lewis, S. (1996). The image and the spark: Dulac and Artaud reviewed. In: R. E. Kuenzl (Ed.), *Dada and surrealist film*, pp.110-127. Cambridge, MA: MIT Press.

Forer, B. R. (1949). The fallacy of personal validation: A classroom demonstration of gullibility. *Journal of Abnormal and Social Psychology, 44*, 118–123.

Forget, D., Morin, C. M., & Bastien, C. H. (2011). The role of the spontaneous and evoked K-complex in good-sleeper controls and in individuals with insomnia. *Sleep, 34*, 1251–1260.

Fosse, M. J., Fosse, R., Hobson, J. A., & Stickgold, R. J. (2003). Dreaming and episodic memory: A functional dissociation? *Journal of Cognitive Neuroscience, 15*, 1–9.

Fosse, R., Stickgold, R., & Hobson, J. A. (2004). Thinking and hallucinating: reciprocal changes in sleep. *Psychophysiology, 41*, 298–305.

Foulkes, W. D. (1962). Dream reports from different stages of sleep. *Journal of Abnormal and Social Psychology, 65*, 14–25.

Foulkes, D. (1996). Misrepresentation of sleep-laboratory dream research with children. *Perceptual and Motor Skills, 83*, 205–206.

Foulkes, D. (1999). *Children's dreaming and the development of consciousness*. Cambridge, MA: Harvard University Press.

Foulkes, D., & Fleisher, S. (1975). Mental activity in relaxed wakefulness. *Journal of Abnormal Psychology, 84*, 66–75.

Fox, K. C., Nijeboer, S., Solomonova, E., Domhoff, G. W., & Christoff, K. (2013). Dreaming as mind wandering: Evidence from functional neuroimaging and first-person content reports. *Frontiers in Human Neuroscience, 7*, 412.

Freud, S. (1900/1997). *The interpretation of dreams*. Translation by A. A. Brill. Ware, Hertfordshire: Wordsworth Classics.

Freud, S. (1901/1966). *The psychopathology of everyday life*. Pelican Freud Library, volume 5. Translation by J. Strachey. London: Pelican.

Freud, S. (1905/1977). *Fragments of an analysis of a case of hysteria ('Dora')*. Pelican Freud Library, volume 8 Case Histories I. Translation by A. Strachey & J. Strachey. London: Pelican.

Freud, S. (1916–1917/1974). *Introductory lectures on psychoanalysis*. Pelican Freud Library, volume 1. Translation by J. Strachey. London: Pelican.

Gackenbach, J. (2006). Video game play and lucid dreams: Implications for the development of consciousness. *Dreaming, 16*, 96–110.

Gais, S., & Born, J. (2004). Declarative memory consolidation: Mechanisms acting during human sleep. *Learning & Memory, 11*, 679–685.

Gauchat, A., Zadra, A., Tremblay, R. E., Zelazo, P. D., & Séguin, J. R. (2009). Recurrent dreams and psychosocial adjustment in preteenaged children. *Dreaming, 19*, 75–84.

Gendlin, E. T. (1977). Phenomenological concept vs. Phenomenological method. A critique of medard boss on dreams. *Soundings: An Interdisciplinary Journal, 60*(3), 285–300.

Georgi, M., Schredl, M., Henley, J., & Blagrove, M. (2012). Gender differences in dreaming in childhood and adolescence: The UK Library study. *International Journal of Dream Research, 5*, 125–129.

Gieselmann, A., et al. (2019). Aetiology and treatment of nightmare disorder: State of the art and future perspectives. *Journal of Sleep Research, 28*, e12820.

Gillespie, A. K., Astudillo Maya, D. A., Denovellis, E. L., Liu, D. F., Kastner, D. B., Coulter, M. E., Roumis, D. K., Eden, U. T., & Frank, L. M. (2021). Hippocampal replay reflects specific past experiences rather than a plan for subsequent choice. *Neuron, 109*, 3149–3163.

Gondry, M. (2006). *The Science of Sleep* [Film]. France 3 Cinema, Canal+, and TPS Star. France.

Gorgoni, M., Scarpelli, S., Alfonsi, V., Annarumma, L., Cordone, S., Stravolo, S., & De Gennaro, L. (2021). Pandemic dreams: quantitative and qualitative features of the oneiric activity during the lockdown due to COVID-19 in Italy. *Sleep Medicine, 81*, 20–32.

Gott, J., Bovy, L., Peters, E., Tzioridou, S., Meo, S., Demirel, Ç., Esfahani, M. J., Oliveira, P. R., Houweling, T., Orticoni, A., Rademaker, A., Booltink, D., Varatheeswaran, R., van Hooijdonk, C., Chaabou, M., Mangiaruga, A., van den Berge, E., Weber, F. D., Ritter, S., & Dresler, M. (2021). Virtual reality training of lucid dreaming. *Philosophical Transactions of the Royal Society of London. Series B, Biological Sciences, 376*(1817), 20190697.

Graf, D., Schredl, M., & Göritz, A. S. (2021). Frequency and motives of sharing dreams: Personality correlates. *Personality and Individual Differences, 175*, 110699.

Grant, K. (2005). *Surrealism and the visual arts: Theory and reception*. Cambridge: Cambridge University Press.

Grant, P. C., Depner, R. M., Levy, K., Lafever, S. M., Tenzek, K. E., Wright, S. T., Kerr, C. W. (2020). Family caregiver perspectives on end-of-life dreams and visions during bereavement: A mixed methods approach. *Journal of Palliative Medicine, 23*, 48–53.

Gray, J. (2006). *Consciousness: Creeping up on the hard problem*. Oxford: Oxford University Press.

Gregor, T. (1981). "Far, far away my shadow wandered...": The dream symbolism and dream theories of the Mehinaku Indians of Brazil. *American Ethnologist, 8*, 709–720.

Gregoric, P., & Fink, J. L. (2022). Introduction sleeping and dreaming in Aristotle and the Aristotelian tradition. In C. T. Thörnqvist & J. Toivanen (Eds.), *Forms of representation in the Aristotelian Tradition. Volume Two: Dreaming.* (pp. 1–27.) Leiden: Koninklijke Brill NV.

Groth, H. & Lusty, N. (2013). *Dreams and Modernity: A Cultural History*. Abingdon & New York: Routledge.

Hall, C. S., & Nordby, V. J. (1972). *The individual and his dreams*. New York: New American Library.

Hall, C. S., & Van De Castle, R. L. (1966). *The content analysis of dreams*. Norfolk, CT: Appleton-Century-Crofts.

Hare, B. (2017). Survival of the friendliest: *Homo sapiens* evolved via selection for prosociality. *Annual Review of Psychology, 68,* 24.1–24.32.

Hare, B., & Woods, V. (2020). *Survival of the friendliest.* London: Oneworld Publications.

Hartmann, E. (1991). *Boundaries in the mind: A new psychology of personality.* New York: Basic Books.

Hartmann, E. (1995). Making connections in a safe place: Is dreaming psychotherapy? *Dreaming, 5,* 213–228.

Hartmann, E. (1996). Who develops PTSD nightmares and who doesn't? In D. Barrett (Ed.), *Trauma and dreams,* chapter 7, pp.100–113. Cambridge, MA: Harvard University Press.

Hartmann, E. (2000). We do not dream of the 3 R's: Implications for the nature of dreaming mentation. *Dreaming, 10,* 103–110.

Hartmann, E. (2011). *The nature and functions of dreaming.* Oxford: Oxford University Press.

Hartmann, E., Elkin, R., & Garg, M. (1991). Personality and dreaming: The dreams of people with very thick or very thin boundaries. *Dreaming, 1,* 311–324.

Heaton, K. J., Hill, C. E., Petersen, D. A., Rochlen, A. B., & Zack, J. S. (1998). A comparison of therapist-facilitated and self-guided dream interpretation sessions. *Journal of Counseling Psychology, 45,* 115–122.

Hill, C. E. (ed.) (2004). *Dream work in therapy: Facilitating exploration, insight, and action.* Washington, D.C.: American Psychological Association.

Hill, C. E., Diemer, R., Hess, S., Hilliger, A., & Seeman, R. (1993). Are the effects of dream interpretation on session quality due to the dream itself, to projection or the interpretation process? *Dreaming, 3,* 269–280.

Hitchcock, A. (1945). *Spellbound* [Film]. Culver City, CA: Selznick International Pictures.

Hobson, J. A., & McCarley, R. W. (1977). The brain as a dream-state generator: An activation-synthesis hypothesis of the dream process. *American Journal of Psychiatry, 134,* 1335–1348.

Hobson, J. A., & Schredl, M. (2011). The continuity and discontinuity between waking and dreaming: A dialogue between Michael Schredl and Allan Hobson concerning the adequacy and completeness of these notions. *International Journal of Dream Research, 4,* 4–7.

Hoel, E. (2021). The overfitted brain: Dreams evolved to assist generalization. *Patterns, 2,* 100244.

Holzinger, B., et al. (2022). Has the COVID-19 pandemic traumatized us collectively? The impact of the COVID-19 pandemic on mental health and sleep factors via traumatization: A multinational survey. *Nature and Science of Sleep, 14,* 1469–1483.

Holzinger, B., Klösch, G., & Saletu, B. (2015). Studies with lucid dreaming as add-on therapy to Gestalt therapy. *Acta Neurologica Scandinavica, 131,* 355–363.

Hopkins, D. (2004). *Dada and surrealism: A very short introduction.* Oxford: Oxford University Press.

Hopkins, D. (2016). *A Companion to Dada and Surrealism.* Chichester: Wiley Blackwell.

Horowitz, A.H., Cunningham, T. J., Maes, P., & Stickgold, R. (2020). Dormio: A targeted dream incubation device. *Consciousness and Cognition, 83,* 102938.

Hu, X., Cheng, L. Y., Chiu, M. H., & Paller, K. A. (2020). Promoting memory consolidation during sleep: A meta-analysis of targeted memory reactivation. *Psychological Bulletin, 146,* 218–244.

Hughes, J. D. (2000). Dream interpretation in ancient civilizations. *Dreaming, 10,* 7–18.

Iber, C., Ancoli-Israel, S., Chesson, A., Quan, S. F. for the American Academy of Sleep Medicine (2007). *The AASM manual for the scoring of sleep and associated events: Rules, terminology and technical specifications*. Westchester, IL: American Academy of Sleep Medicine.

Ijams, K., & Miller, L. D. (2000). Perceptions of dream-disclosure: An exploratory study. *Communication Studies, 51*, 135–148.

Iversen, M. (2022). On the positive value of destruction. In A. Schlieker (ed.) *Cornelia Parker* (pp.48–49). London: Tate Publishing.

Jenkins, J. G., & Dallenbach, K. M. (1924). Obliviscence during sleep and waking. *The American Journal of Psychology, 35*, 605–612.

Jiménez, J. (Ed.) (2013). *Surrealism and the dream*. Madrid: Museo Thyssen-Bornemisza.

Jung, C. G. (1931/2002). The practical use of dream analysis. In C. G. Jung (2002) *Dreams*, Part 3, Chapter 1, pp.87–108 (translator R. F. C. Hull). (First published as Die praktische Verwendbarkeit der Traumanalyse, 1931.) Abingdon & New York: Routledge Classics.

Jung, C. G. (1948/2002a). General aspects of dream psychology. In C. G. Jung (2002) *Dreams*, Part 2, Chapter 1, pp.25–68 (translator R. F. C. Hull). (First published as Allgemeine Gesichtspunkte zur Psychologie des Träumes, in über psychische Energetik und das Wesen der Träume, 1948.) Abingdon & New York: Routledge Classics.

Jung, C. G. (1948/2002b). On the nature of dreams. In C. G. Jung (2002) *Dreams*, Part 2, Chapter 2, pp.69–84 (translator R. F. C. Hull). (First published as Vom Wesen des Träumes, in über psychische Energetik und das Wesen der Träume, 1948.) Abingdon & New York: Routledge Classics.

Kahan, T. L., & LaBerge, S. (1996). Cognition and metacognition in dreaming and waking: Comparisons of first and third–person ratings. *Dreaming, 6*, 235–249.

Kaprow, A. (1993). *Essays on the blurring of art and life*. Oakland, CA: University of California Press.

Kelly, P., et al. (2022). Lucid dreaming increased during the COVID-19 pandemic: An online survey. *PLoS ONE, 17*(9), e0273281.

Kerr, C. W., Donnelly, J. P., Wright, S. T., Kuszczak, S. M., Banas, A., Grant, P. C., & Luczkiewicz, D. L. (2014). End-of-life dreams and visions: a longitudinal study of hospice patients' experiences. *Journal of Palliative Medicine, 17*, 296–303.

Kezich, T. (2007). *Federico Fellini: His Life and Work* (trans. M. Proctor.) London: I.B. Tauris.

Kezich, T. (2020). Somnii explanatio or in the realm where everything is possible. In Fellini, F. (2020). *The Book of Dreams*, pp.571–579. (S. Toffetti, editor; A. Maines & D. Stanton, translators. Originally published in 2007 in Italian.) New York & Milan: Rizzoli.

King, E. H. (2007). *Dalí, Surrealism and Cinema*. Harpenden: Kamera Books.

King, M. (2002). From Max Ernst to Ernst Mach: Epistemology in art and science. *Working Papers in Art and Design, volume 2*. https://www.herts.ac.uk/__data/assets/pdf_file/0013/12307/WPIAAD_vol2_king.pdf.

Kon, S. (2006). *Paprika* [film]. Kabushiki-gaisha Maddohausu / Madhouse. Japan.

Konkoly, K. R., Appel, K., Chabani, E., Mangiaruga, A., Gott, J., Mallett, R., Caughran, B., Witkowski, S., Whitmore, N. W., Mazurek, C. Y., Berent, J. B., Weber, F. D., Türker, B., Leu-Semenescu, S., Maranci, J. B., Pipa, G., Arnulf, I., Oudiette, D., Dresler, M., & Paller, K. A. (2021). Real-time dialogue between experimenters and dreamers during REM sleep. *Current Biology, 31*, 1417–1427.

Konrath, S. H., O'Brien, E. H., & Hsing, C. (2011). Changes in dispositional empathy in American college students over time: A meta-analysis. *Personality and Social Psychology Review, 15*, 180–198.

Koulack, D., & Goodenough, D. R. (1976). Dream recall and dream recall failure: An arousal-retrieval model. *Psychological Bulletin, 83*, 975–984.

Krakow, B., Melendrez, D., Warner, T. D., Dorin, R., Harper, R., & Hollifield, M. (2002). To breathe, perchance to sleep: sleep-disordered breathing and chronic insomnia among trauma survivors. *Sleep and Breathing, 6*, 189–202.

Kramer, M. (1994). Sigmund Freud's *The Interpretation of Dreams*: The initial response (1899–1908). *Dreaming, 4*, 47–52.

Krupic J. (2017). Wire together, fire apart. *Science, 357*(6355), 974–975.

Kubrick, S. (1999). *Eyes Wide Shut* [Film]. Warner Bros, USA.

Kuenzli, R. E. (1996). *Dada and surrealist film*. Cambridge, MA: MIT Press.

Kuiken, D., Lee, M-N., Eng, T., & Singh, T. (2006). The influence of impactful dreams on self-perceptual depth and spiritual transformation. *Dreaming, 16*, 258–279.

Kurosawa, A. (1990). *Dreams* [film]. Akira Kurosawa USA. Japan and US.

LaBerge, S. (1990). Lucid dreaming: Psychophysiological studies of consciousness during REM sleep. In R. R. Bootzen, J. F. Kihlstrom, & D. L. Schacter (Eds.), *Sleep and cognition* (pp. 109–126). Washington, D.C.: American Psychological Association.

LaBerge, S., LaMarca, K., & Baird, B. (2018). Pre-sleep treatment with galantamine stimulates lucid dreaming: A double-blind, placebo-controlled, crossover study. *PLoS ONE, 13*, art. no. e0201246.

LaBerge, S., & Levitan, L. (1995). Validity established of DreamLight cues for eliciting lucid dreaming. *Dreaming, 5*, 159–168.

LaBerge, S., Levitan, L., & Dement, W. (1986). Lucid dreaming: Physiological correlates of consciousness during REM sleep. *Journal of Mind and Behavior, 7*(2–3), 251–258.

Ladd, G. T. (1892). Contribution to the psychology of visual dreams. *Mind (New Series), 1*, 299–304.

Lakoff, G. (1993). How metaphor structures dreams: The theory of the conceptual metaphor applied to dream analysis. *Dreaming, 3*, 77–98.

Lakoff, G., & Johnson, M. (1980). *Metaphors we live by*. Chicago, IL: University of Chicago Press.

Legge, E. (2016). Nothing, ventured: Paris Dara into Surrealism. In D. Hopkins (Ed.), *A companion to Dada and Surrealism*, pp.89–109. Chichester: Wiley Blackwell.

Leonard, L., & Dawson, D. (2018). The marginalisation of dreams in clinical psychological practice. *Sleep Medicine Reviews, 42*, 10–18.

Levin, R., & Nielsen, T. A. (2007). Disturbed dreaming, posttraumatic stress disorder, and affect distress: A review and neurocognitive model. *Psychological Bulletin, 133*, 482–528.

Lewer, D. (2016). Dada's genesis: Zurich. In Hopkins, D. (Ed.), *A companion to Dada and Surrealism*, pp.21–37. Chichester: Wiley Blackwell.

Lewis, P. A., & Durrant, S. J. (2011). Overlapping memory replay during sleep builds cognitive schemata. *Trends in Cognitive Sciences, 15*, 343–351.

Lewis, P. A., Knoblich, G., & Poe, G. (2018). How memory replay in sleep boosts creative problem-solving. *Trends in Cognitive Sciences, 22*, 491–503.

Libet, B. (2005). *Mind time: The temporal factor in consciousness*. Cambridge, MA: Harvard University Press.

Liebman, S. (1996). *Un Chien andalou*: The talking cure. In: R. E. Kuenzl (Ed.), *Dada and surrealist film*, pp.143–158. Cambridge, MA: MIT Press.

Lipsky, J. (2008). *Dreaming Together: Exploring Your Dreams by Acting Them Out*. Burdett, NY: Larson Publications.

Lockheart, J. (2022a). Languaging design In: J. Wood (ed.) *Metadesigning Designing in the Anthropocene* (pp.46–54). London: Routledge

Lockheart, J. (2022b). Co-exploring the visual metaphors of the dream. In: J. Wood (ed.), *Metadesigning Designing in the Anthropocene* (pp.197–207). London: Routledge

Lockheart, J., & Blagrove, M. (2019). Dream sharing. *Sublime Magazine*, 2nd November 2019. https://sublimemagazine.com/dream-sharing

Lockheart, J., & Blagrove, M. (2020). Exploring lockdown dreams. *Sublime Magazine*, 17th July 2020. https://sublimemagazine.com/exploring-lockdown-dreams

Lockheart, J., Holzinger, B., Adler, K., Barrett, D., Nobus, D., Wessely, Z., & Blagrove, M. (2021). 120th anniversary event for 'Dora' telling her burning house dream to Freud. *International Journal of Dream Research, 14*, 202–208.

Louie, K., & Wilson, M. A. (2001). Temporally structured replay of awake hippocampal ensemble activity during rapid eye movement sleep. *Neuron, 29*, 145–156.

Lynch, D. (2001). *Mulholland Drive* [Film]. Universal Pictures. USA.

Lyons, M., Khan, S., Sandman, N., & Valli, K. (2019). Dark dreams are made of this: Aggressive and sexual dream content and the dark triad of personality. *Imagination, Cognition and Personality: Consciousness in Theory, Research, and Clinical Practice, 39*, 88–96.

Macêdo, T. C. F., Ferreira, G. H., Almondes, K. M., Kirov, R., & Mota-Rolim, S. A. (2019). My dream, my rules: Can lucid dreaming treat nightmares? *Frontiers in Psychology, 10*, 2618.

Mageo, J. (2021). Metaphors We Dream By: On the nature of Dream Cognition. In J. Mageo & R. E. Sheriff (eds.) *New Directions in the Anthropology of Dreaming* (chapter 3, pp.53-71). Abingdon, & New York: Routledge.

Mahon, A. (Ed.) (2018). *Dorothea Tanning*. London: Tate Enterprises Ltd.

Malinowski, J., Carr, M., Edwards, C., Ingarfill, A., & Pinto, A. (2019). The effects of dream rebound: Evidence for emotion-processing theories of dreaming. *Journal of Sleep Research, 28*, e12827.

Malinowski, J., & Horton, C. L. (2014). Evidence for the preferential incorporation of emotional waking-life experiences into dreams. *Dreaming, 24*, 18–31.

Malinowski, J. E., & Horton, C. L. (2015). Metaphor and hyperassociativity: The imagination mechanisms behind emotion assimilation in sleep and dreaming. *Frontiers in Psychology, 6*, 1132.

Maquet, P., Peters, J.-M., Aerts, J., Delfiore, G., Degueldre, C., Luxen, A., & Franck, G. (1996). Functional neuroanatomy of human rapid-eye-movement sleep and dreaming. *Nature, 383*, 163.

Mar, R. A., & Oatley, K. (2008). The function of fiction is the abstraction and simulation of social experience. *Perspectives on Psychological Science, 3*, 173–192.

Mar, R. A., Oatley, K., Hirsh, J., de la Paz, J., & Peterson, J. B. (2006). Bookworms versus nerds: Exposure to fiction versus non-fiction, divergent associations with social ability, and the simulation of fictional social worlds. *Journal of Research in Personality, 40*, 694–712.

Marcoci, R., & Meister, S. H. (2015). *From Bauhaus to Buenos Aires: Grete Stern and Horacio Coppola*. New York: Museum of Modern Art.

Matthews, J. H. (1971). *Surrealism and Film*. Ann Arbor, MI: University of Michigan.

Matthijs Bal, P., & Veltkamp, M. (2013). How does fiction reading influence empathy? An experimental investigation on the role of emotional transportation. *PLoS ONE, 8*, e55341.

McNamara, P. (1996). REM sleep: A social bonding mechanism. *New Ideas in Psychology, 14*, 35–46.

McNamara, P., Harris, E., & Kookoolis, A. (2007). Costly signalling theory of dream recall and dream sharing. In D. Barrett & P. McNamara (Eds.), Chapter 5 in *The new science of dreaming* (pp. 117–132). Westport, CT: Praeger.

Mersky, R. R., & Sievers, B. (2019) Social photo-matrix and social dream-drawing. In: Stamenova, K. & Hinshelwood, R. D., (eds.), Methods of Research into the Unconscious: *Applying Psychoanalytic Ideas to Social Sciences* (pp.145–168). London: Routledge.

Miller, G. (2000). *The mating mind: How sexual choice shaped the evolution of human nature*. New York: Doubleday and Co.

Miller, G. F. (2001). Aesthetic fitness: How sexual selection shaped artistic virtuosity as a fitness indicator and aesthetic preferences as mate choice criteria. *Bulletin of Psychology and the Arts, 2*, 20–25.

Miller, K. E., Brownlow, J. A., & Gehrman, P. R. (2020). Sleep in PTSD: treatment approaches and outcomes. *Current Opinion in Psychology, 34*, 12–17.

Moi, T. (1990). Representation of patriarchy: Sexuality and epistemology in Freud's Dora. In C. Bernheimer & C. Kahane (Eds.), *In Dora's Case: Freud – hysteria – feminism* (pp. 181–199). New York: Columbia University Press.

Montangero, J., Ivanyi, C. T., & de Saint-Hilaire, Z. (2003). Completeness and accuracy of morning reports after a recall cue: Comparison of dream and film reports. *Consciousness and Cognition, 12*, 49–62.

Montgomery, H. (2021). The work of dreams. In S. D'Alessandro & M. Gale (Eds.), *Surrealism beyond borders*. (pp. 228–231). New York: Metropolitan Museum of Art.

Morewedge, C. K., & Norton, M. I. (2009). When dreaming is believing: the (motivated) interpretation of dream. *Journal of Personality and Social Psychology, 96*, 249–264.

Mota, N. B., Weissheimer, J., Ribeiro, M., de Paiva, M., Avilla-Souza, J., Simabucuru, G., et al. (2020). Dreaming during the Covid-19 pandemic: Computational assessment of dream reports reveals mental suffering related to fear of contagion. *PLoS ONE, 15*, e0242903.

Mota-Rolim, S. A., Pavlou, A., Nascimento, G. C., Fontenele-Araujo, J., & Ribeiro, S. (2019). Portable devices to induce lucid dreams—Are they reliable? *Frontiers in Neuroscience, 13*, 428.

Mundy, J. (2001). Letters of desire. In J. Mundy (Ed.), *Surrealism: Desire unbound* (chapter 1). London: Tate Publishing and Princeton, NJ: Princeton University Press.

Neidhardt, E. J., Krakow, B., Kellner, R., & Pathak, D. (1992). The beneficial effects of one treatment session and recording of nightmares on chronic nightmare sufferers. *Sleep, 15*, 470–473.

Nielsen, T. A. (2000). A review of mentation in REM and NREM sleep: Covert REM sleep as a possible reconciliation of two opposing models. *Behavioral and Brain Sciences, 23*, 851–866.

Nielsen, T. (2017). The stress acceleration hypothesis of nightmares. *Frontiers in Neurology, 8*, 201.

Nielsen, T. A. (2020). The COVID-19 pandemic is changing our dreams. *Scientific American, 323* (October 1st), 31–35.

Nielsen, T. A., Kuiken, D., Alain, G., Stenstrom, P., & Powell, R. A. (2004). Immediate and delayed incorporations of events into dreams: Further replication and implications for dream function. *Journal of Sleep Research, 13*, 327–336.

Nielsen, T. A., Laberge, L., Paquet, J., Tremblay, R. E., Vitaro, F., & Montplaisir, J. (2000). Development of disturbing dreams during adolescence and their relation to anxiety symptoms. *Sleep, 23*, 727–736.

Nielsen, T. A., & Powell, R. A. (1989). The 'dream-lag' effect: A 6-day temporal delay in dream content incorporation. *Psychiatric Journal of the University of Ottawa, 14*, 561–565.

Nielsen, T. A., & Stenstrom, P. (2005). What are the memory sources of dreaming? *Nature, 437*, 1286–1289.

Nielsen, T., Stenstrom, P., Takeuchi, T., Saucier, S., Lara-Carrasco, J., Solomonova, E., & Martel, E. (2005). Partial REM-sleep deprivation increases the dream-like quality of mentation from REM sleep and sleep onset. *Sleep, 28*, 1083–1089.

Nishida, M., & Walker, M. P. (2007). Daytime naps, motor memory consolidation and regionally specific sleep spindles. *PLoS ONE, 2*, e341.

Nofzinger, E. A., Mintun, M. A., Wiseman, M. B., Kupfer, D. J., &Moore, R. Y. (1997). Forebrain activation in REM sleep: An FDG PET study. *Brain Research, 770*, 192–201.

Nolan, C. (2010). *Inception* [Film]. Warner Bros., USA.

O'Donoghue (2004). Daze of the rabblement: Early film comedy and some modernists. *Senses of cinema*, October 2004, Issue 33.

O'Pray, M. (1986). In the capital of magic: The black theatre of Jan Švankmajer. In *Jan Švankmajer: The complete short films*, pp.1–4. London: British Film Institute. Also published in *Monthly Film Bulletin*, July 1986, number 630, pp.218–219. London: British Film Institute.

Oatley, K. (1999). Why fiction may be twice as true as fact: Fiction as cognitive and emotional simulation. *Review of General Psychology, 3*, 101–117.

Oatley, K. (2011). *Such stuff as dreams: The psychology of fiction*. Chichester: Wiley.

Oatley, K. (2016). Fiction: Simulation of social worlds. *Trends in Cognitive Science, 20*, 618–628. https://doi.org/10.1016/j.tics.2016.06.002

Olsen, M. R., Schredl, M., & Carlsson, I. (2013). Sharing dreams: Frequency, motivations, and relationship intimacy. *Dreaming, 23*, 245–255. https://doi.org/10.1037/a0033392

Oneto, P. D. (2017). L'"Objet trouvé" or readymade and its implications: Virtuality and transitionality. *Wrong Wrong Magazine* (Lisbon, Portugal), 17/4/2017. https://wrongwrong.net/article/lobjet-trouve-or-readymade-and-its-implications-virtuality-and-transitionality

Pace-Schott, E. F. (2013). Dreaming as a story-telling instinct. *Frontiers in Psychology, 4*, 159.

Pagel J. F. (2003). Non-dreamers. *Sleep Medicine, 4*, 235–241.

Pagel, M. (2017). Q&A: What is human language, when did it evolve and why should we care? *BMC Biology, 15*, 64.

Pailthorpe, G. W. (1938/1939). The scientific aspect of surrealism. *London Bulletin, 7*, 10–16.

Pandya, V. (2004). Forest smells and spider webs: Ritualized dream interpretation among Andaman islanders. *Dreaming, 14*, 136–150.

Parke, A. R., & Horton, C. L. (2009). A re-examination of the interference hypothesis on dream recall and dream salience. *International Journal of Dream Research, 2*, 60–69.

Payne, J. D., Schacter, D. L., Propper, R. E., Huang, L. W., Wamsley, E. J., Tucker, M. A., Walker, M. P., & Stickgold, R. (2009). The role of sleep in false memory formation. *Neurobiology of Learning and Memory, 92*, 327–334.

Peluso, D. M. (2004). "That which I dream is true": Dream narratives in an Amazonian community. *Dreaming, 14*, 107–119.

Perogamvros, L., Dang-Vu Thien, T., Desseilles, M., & Schwartz, S. (2013). Sleep and dreaming are for important matters. *Frontiers in Psychology, 4*, 474.

Perogamvros, L., & Schwartz, S. (2012). The roles of the reward system in sleep and dreaming. *Neuroscience & Biobehavioral Reviews, 36*, 1934–1951.

Pesant, N., & Zadra, A. (2004). Working with dreams in therapy: What do we know and what should we do? *Clinical Psychology Review, 24*, 489–512.

Phillips, T. (1980). *A Humument*. London: Thames and Hudson.

Piaget, J. (1936). *Origins of intelligence in the child*. London: Routledge & Kegan Paul.

Piaget, J. (1945). *Play, dreams and imitation in childhood*. London: Heinemann.

Picard-Deland, C., & Nielsen, T. (2022). Targeted memory reactivation has a sleep stage-specific delayed effect on dream content. *Journal of Sleep Research, 31*, art. no. e13391.

Picard-Deland, C., Nielsen, T., & Carr, M. (2021). Dreaming of the sleep lab. *PLoS ONE, 16*, e0257738.

Pietrowsky, R., & Köthe, M. (2003). Personal boundaries and nightmare consequences in frequent nightmare sufferers. *Dreaming, 13*, 245–254.

Plihal, W., & Born, J. (1997). Effects of early and late nocturnal sleep on declarative and procedural memory. *Journal of Cognitive Neuroscience, 9*, 534–547.

Powell, R. A., Nielsen, T. A., Cheung, J. S., & Cervenka, T. M. (1995). Temporal delays in incorporation of events into dreams. *Perceptual and Motor Skills, 81*, 95–104.

Price, M. (2019). Early humans domesticated themselves, new genetic evidence suggests. *Science*, 4th December 2019.

Prokosch, M. D., Coss, R. G., Scheib, J. E., & Blozis, S. A. (2009). Intelligence and mate choice: Intelligent men are always appealing. *Evolution and Human Behavior, 30*, 11–20.

Propper, R. E., Stickgold, R., Keeley, R., & Christman, S. D. (2007). Is television traumatic?: Dreams, stress, and media exposure in the aftermath of September 11, 2001. *Psychological Science, 18*, 334–340.

Purcell, S., Mullington, J., Moffitt, A., Hoffmann, R., & Pigeau, R. (1986). Dream self-reflectiveness as a learned cognitive skill. *Sleep, 9*, 423–437.

Rabinovitch, C. (2020). *Duchamp's pipe: A chess romance*. Berkeley: North Atlantic Books.

Rasch, B., Büchel, C., Gais, S., & Born, J. (2007). Odor cues during slow-wave sleep prompt declarative memory consolidation. *Science, 315*(5817), 1426–1429.

Ray, M. (1928). *The starfish / L'Etoile de mer* [Film]. Produced by Man Ray. France.

Rechtschaffen A. (1978). The single-mindedness and isolation of dreams. *Sleep, 1*, 97–109.

Reid, A., Bloxham, A., Carr, M., van Rijn, E., Basoudan, N., Tulip, C., & Blagrove, M. (2022). Effects of sleep on positive, negative and neutral valenced story and image memory. *British Journal of Psychology, 113*, 777–797.

Resnais, A. (1961). *Last Year at Marienbad / L'Année Dernière À Marienbad* [Film]. Astor Pictures Corporation, Fox Lorber. France/Italy.

Resnick, J., Stickgold, R., Rittenhouse, C. D., & Hobson, J. A. (1994). Self-representation and bizarreness in children's dream reports collected in the home setting. *Consciousness and Cognition, 3*, 30–45.

Revonsuo, A. (2000). The reinterpretation of dreams: An evolutionary hypothesis of the function of dreaming. *Behavioral and Brain Sciences, 23*, 877–901.

Revonsuo, A., Tuominen, J., & Valli, K. (2016). The avatars in the machine: Dreaming as a simulation of social reality. In T. Metzinger & J. M. Windt (Eds.), *Open MIND* (pp. 1295–1322). Cambridge, MA: MIT Press.

Ribeiro, N., Gounden, Y., & Quaglino, V. (2020). A full night's sleep at home improves memory performance in an associative and relational learning task. *Dreaming*, 30, 171–188.

Richter, H. (1947). *Dreams That Money Can Buy* [Film]. Produced by Hans Richter & Kenneth Macpherson. USA.

Rimé, B. (2009). Emotion elicits the social sharing of emotion: Theory and empirical review. *Emotion Review*, 1, 60–85.

Robert, G., & Zadra, A. (2008). Measuring nightmare and bad dream frequency: impact of retrospective and prospective instruments. *Journal of Sleep Research*, 17, 132–139.

Robert, G., & Zadra, A. (2014). Thematic and content analysis of idiopathic nightmares and bad dreams. *Sleep: Journal of Sleep and Sleep Disorders Research*, 37, 409–417.

Roediger, H. L., & McDermott, K. B. (1995). Creating false memories: Remembering words not presented in lists. *Journal of Experimental Psychology: Learning, Memory and Cognition*, 21, 803–814.

Roguski, A., Rayment, D., Whone, A. L., Jones, Matt, W., & Rolinski, M. (2020). A neurologist's guide to REM sleep behavior disorder. *Frontiers in Neurology*, 11, 00610.

Rosen, M. (2021). *Many different kinds of love: A story of life, death and the NHS*. London: Ebury Press.

Ruby, P. M. (2020). The correlates of dreaming have not been identified yet. Commentary on "The neural correlates of dreaming. Nat Neurosci. 2017". *Frontiers in Neuroscience*, 14, 585470.

Rudofsky, S. F. & Wotiz, J. H. (1988). Psychologists and the dream accounts of August Kekulé. *Ambix*, 35, 31–38.

Rugoff, R. (Ed.) (2022). *Louise Bourgeois: The woven child*. Berlin: Hatje Cantz Verlag.

Ruini, C., & Mortara, C. C. (2022). Writing technique across psychotherapies—From traditional expressive writing to new positive psychology interventions: A narrative review. *Journal of Contemporary Psychotherapy*, 52, 23–34.

Rycroft, C. (1981). *The innocence of dreams*. Oxford: Oxford University Press.

Salvio, M.-A., Wood, J. M., Schwartz, J., & Eichling, P. S. (1992). Nightmare prevalence in the healthy elderly. *Psychology and Aging*, 7, 324–325.

Sanders, K. E. G., Osburn, S., Paller, K. A., & Beeman, M. (2019). Targeted memory reactivation during sleep improves next-day problem solving. *Psychological Science*, 30, 1616–1624.

Sándor, P., Szakadát, S., & Bódizs, R. (2016). The development of cognitive and emotional processing as reflected in children's dreams: Active self in an eventful dream signals better neuropsychological skills. *Dreaming*, 26, 58–78.

Sándor, P., Szakadát, S., Kertész, K., & Bódizs, R. (2015) Content analysis of 4 to 8 year-old children's dream reports. *Frontiers in Psychology*, 6, 534.

Saunders, D. T., Roe, C. A., Smith, G., & Clegg, H. (2016). Lucid dreaming incidence: A quality effects meta-analysis of 50 years of research. *Consciousness and Cognition*, 43, 197–215.

Scarpelli, S. et al. (2021). Dreams and nightmares during the first and second wave of the COVID-19 infection: A longitudinal study. *Brain Sciences*, 11, 1375.

Scarpelli, S., Bartolacci, C., D'Atri, A., Gorgoni, M., & De Gennaro, L. (2019). The functional role of dreaming in emotional processes. *Frontiers in Psychology, 10*, 459.

Scarpelli, S., D'Atri, A., Mangiaruga, A. et al. (2017). Predicting dream recall: EEG activation during NREM sleep or shared mechanisms with wakefulness? *Brain Topography, 30*, 629–638.

Schonbar R. A. (1965). Differential dream recall frequency as a component of "life style". *Journal of Consulting Psychology, 29*, 468–474.

Schnitzler, A. (1999). *Dream story.* Originally *Traumnovelle,* published 1926 in German. (Translated by J. M. Q. Davies.). London: Penguin Books.

Schrage-Früh, M. (2016). *Philosophy, dreaming and the literary imagination.* London: Palgrave Macmillan.

Schredl, M. (2003). Continuity between waking and dreaming: A proposal for a mathematical model. *Sleep and Hypnosis, 5*, 26–39.

Schredl, M. (2006). Factors affecting the continuity between waking and dreaming: Emotional intensity and emotional tone of the waking-life event. *Sleep and Hypnosis, 8*, 1–5.

Schredl, M., Berres, S., Klingauf, A., Schellhaas, S., & Göritz, A. (2014). The Mannheim Dream questionnaire (MADRE): Retest reliability, age and gender effects. *International Journal of Dream Research, 7*, 141–147.

Schredl, M., Blamo, A. E., Ehrenfeld, F., & Olivier, P. S. (2022). Dream recall frequency and sensory-processing sensitivity. *Dreaming, 32*, 15–22.

Schredl, M., & Bulkeley, K. (2019). Dream sharing frequency: Associations with sociodemographic variables and attitudes toward dreams in an American sample. *Dreaming, 29*, 211–219.

Schredl, M., & Bulkeley, K. (2020a). Lucid Nightmares: An exploratory online study. *International Journal of Dream Research, 13*, 215–219.

Schredl, M., & Bulkeley, K. (2020b). Dreaming and the COVID-19 pandemic: A survey in a U.S. sample. *Dreaming, 30*, 189–198.

Schredl, M., & Doll, E. (1998). Emotions in diary dreams. *Consciousness and Cognition, 7*, 634–646.

Schredl, M., Fröhlich, S., Schlenke, S., Stegemann, M., Voß, C., & De Gioia, S. (2015a). Emotional responses to dream sharing: A field study. *International Journal of Dream Research, 8*, 135–138.

Schredl, M., & Göritz, A. S. (2014). Umgang mit Alpträumen in der Allgemeinbevölkerung: Eine Online-Studie. [Coping with nightmares in the general population: An online study]. *Psychotherapie, Psychosomatik und Medizinische Psychologie, 64*, 192–196.

Schredl, M., & Göritz, A. S. (2018). Let's talk about dreams: An on-line survey. *International Journal of Dream Research, 11*(Suppl.1), S62–S63. Paper presented at the 35th Annual Conference of the International Association for the Study of Dreams, June 2018, Scottsdale, Arizona, US.

Schredl, M., Jochum, S., & Souguenet, S. (1997). Dream recall, visual memory, and absorption in imaginings. *Personality and Individual Differences, 22*, 291–292.

Schredl, M., Kälberer, A., Zacharowski, K., & Zimmermann, M. (2017). Pain dreams and dream emotions in patients with chronic back pain and healthy controls. *Open Pain Journal, 10*, 65–72.

Schredl, M., Kim, E., Labudek, S., Schädler, A., & Göritz, A. S. (2015b). Factors affecting the gender difference in dream sharing frequency. *Imagination, Cognition and Personality, 34*, 306–316.

Schredl, M., Schäfer, G., Hofmann, F., & Jacob, S. (1999). Dream content and personality: Thick vs. Thin boundaries. *Dreaming, 9*(4), 257–263.

Schredl, M., & Schawinski, J. A. (2010). Frequency of dream sharing: The effects of gender and personality. *American Journal of Psychology, 123,* 93–101.

Schwartz, S., Clerget, A., & Perogamvros, L. (2022). Enhancing imagery rehearsal therapy for nightmares with targeted memory reactivation. *Current Biology,* Advance online publication. doi:10.1016/j.cub.2022.09.032

Sebbag, G. (2013). The animated painting of the surrealist dreamer. In J. Jiménez (Ed.), *Surrealism and the dream* (pp. 55–74). Madrid: Museo Thyssen-Bornemisza.

Selterman, D. F., Apetroaia, A. I., Riela, S., & Aron, A. (2014). Dreaming of you: Behavior and emotion in dreams of significant others predict subsequent relational behavior. *Social Psychological and Personality Science, 5,* 111–118.

Shakespeare, W. (1600/2016). *A Midsummer Night's Dream.* (First published 1600.) B. A. Mowat & P. Werstine (eds), Folger Shakespeare Library. New York: Simon & Schuster.

Shapiro, A., Goodenough, D. R., Biederman, I., & Sleser, I. (1964). Dream recall and the physiology of sleep. *Journal of Applied Physiology, 19,* 778–783.

Sharot, S. (2015). Dreams in films and films as dreams: Surrealism and popular American cinema. *Revue Canadienne d'Études cinématographiques / Canadian Journal of Film Studies, 24*(1), 66–89.

Shen, L. (2010). On a scale of state empathy during message processing. *Western Journal of Communication, 74,* 504–524.

Sheriff, R .E. (2021). The anthropology of dreaming in historical perspective. In J. Mageo & R. E. Sheriff (eds.) *New Directions in the Anthropology of Dreaming* (chapter 2, pp.23–49). Abingdon, & New York: Routledge.

Sherman, A., & Morrissey, C. (2017). What is art good for? The socio-epistemic value of art. *Frontiers in Human Neuroscience, 11,* 411.

Shilton, D., Breski, M., Dor, D., & Jablonka, E. (2020). Human social evolution: Self-domestication or self-control? *Frontiers in Psychology, 11,* 134.

Shofty, B. *et al.* (2022). The default network is causally linked to creative thinking. *Molecular Psychiatry, 27,* 1848–1854.

Short, R. (2008a). Ocular alchemy: Surrealism's expectations of cinema. In: R. Short (ed.), *The Age of Gold, Dalí, Buñuel, Artaud: Surrealist Cinema,* Introduction, pp.5–32. Solar Books.

Short, R. (2008b). Legacy: Surrealism and cinema. In: R. Short (ed.), *The Age of Gold, Dalí, Buñuel, Artaud: Surrealist Cinema,* chapter 5, pp.175–188. Solar Books.

Siclari, F., Baird, B., Perogamvros, L., Bernardi, G., LaRocque, J. J., Riedner, B., Boly, M., Postle, B. R., & Tononi, G. (2017). The neural correlates of dreaming. *Nature Neuroscience, 20,* 872–878.

Sinclair, V. (2021). *Scansion in psychoanalysis and art: The cut in creation.* Abingdon and New York: Routledge.

Sliwinski, S. (2017). *Dreaming in dark times: Six exercises in political thought.* Minneapolis, MN: University of Minnesota Press.

Smith, B. V., & Blagrove, M. (2015). Lucid dreaming frequency and alarm clock snooze button use. *Dreaming, 25,* 291–299.

Smith, D., Schlaepfer, P., Major, K., Dyble, M., Page, A. E., Thompson, J., Chaudhary, N., Salali, G. D., Mace, R., Astete, L., Ngales, M., Vinicius, L., & Migliano, A. B. (2017). Cooperation and the evolution of hunter-gatherer storytelling. *Nature Communications, 8,* 1853.

Solms, M. (1997). *The neuropsychology of dreams: A clinico-anatomical study.* Mahwah, NJ: Lawrence Erlbaum Associates Publishers.

Solms, M. (2000). Dreaming and REM sleep are controlled by different brain mechanisms. *Behavioral and Brain Sciences, 23*, 843–850.

Spector, J. J. (1989). André Breton and the politics of dream: Surrealism in Paris, ca. 1918–1924. *American Imago, 46*, 287–317.

Sperling, G. (1960). The information available in brief visual presentations. *Psychological Monographs: General and Applied, 74*, 1–29.

Spoormaker, V. I., Schredl, M., & van den Bout, J. (2006). Nightmares: From anxiety symptom to sleep disorder. *Sleep Medicine Reviews, 10*, 19–31.

Spoormaker, V. I., & van den Bout, J. (2006). Lucid dreaming treatment for nightmares: A pilot study. *Psychotherapy and Psychosomatics, 75*, 389–394.

Spreng, R. N., McKinnon, M. C., Mar, R. A., & Levine, B. (2009). The Toronto empathy questionnaire: Scale development and initial validation of a factor-analytic solution to multiple empathy measures. *Journal of Personality Assessment, 91*, 62–71.

States, B. O. (1993). *Dreaming and storytelling.* Ithaca, NY: Cornell University Press.

Stepansky, R., Holzinger, B., Schmeiser-Rieder, A., Saletu, B., Kunze, M., & Zeitlhofer, J. (1998). Austrian dream behavior: Results of a representative population survey. *Dreaming, 8*, 23–30.

Sterpenich, V., Perogamvros, L., Tononi, G., & Schwartz, S. (2020). Fear in dreams and in wakefulness: Evidence for day/night affective homeostasis. *Human Brain Mapping, 41*, 840–850.

Stickgold, R., Hobson, J. A., Fosse, R., & Fosse, M. (2001a). Sleep, learning, and dreams: Off-line memory reprocessing. *Science, 294*(5544), 1052–1057.

Stickgold, R., Malia, A., Fosse, R., & Hobson, J. A. (2001b). Brain–mind states: I. Longitudinal field study of sleep/wake factors influencing mentation report length. *Sleep: Journal of Sleep and Sleep Disorders Research, 24*, 171–179.

Stickgold, R., & Walker, M. P. (2007). Sleep-dependent memory consolidation and reconsolidation. *Sleep Medicine, 8*, 331–343.

Stickgold, R., & Walker, M. P. (2013). Sleep-dependent memory triage: Evolving generalization through selective processing. *Nature Neuroscience, 16*, 139–145.

Stockhausen, K. (1999). *Introduction, helicopter string quartet.* (Translation by S. Stephens.) Montaigne Auvidis: Arditti Quartet Edition.

Strauch, I., & Meier, B. (1996). *In search of dreams: Results of experimental dream research.* Albany: State University of New York Press.

Strom, K. (ed.) (2023). The *Routledge Companion to Surrealism.* Abingdon & New York: Routledge.

Strunz, F. (1993). Preconscious mental activity and scientific problem-solving: A critique of the Kekulé dream controversy. *Dreaming, 3*, 281–294.

Stumbrys, T., Erlacher, D., Schädlich, M., & Schredl, M. (2012). Induction of lucid dreams: A systematic review of evidence. *Consciousness and Cognition, 21*, 1456–1475.

Stumbrys, T., Erlacher, D., & Schredl, M. (2013). Testing the involvement of the prefrontal cortex in lucid dreaming: A tDCS study. *Consciousness and Cognition, 22*(4), 1214–1222.

Stumbrys, T., Erlacher, D., & Schredl, M. (2016). Effectiveness of motor practice in lucid dreams: A comparison with physical and mental practice. *Journal of Sports Sciences, 34*, 27–34.

Sturzenacker, G. (2009). The Ullman method: Influential and often misunderstood. Paper presented at the 26th Annual Conference of the International Association for the Study of Dreams, June 2009.

Susik, A. (2016). Chance and automatism: Genealogies of the dissociative in Dada and Surrealism. In D. Hopkins (Ed.), *A companion to Dada and Surrealism*, pp.242-257. Chichester: Wiley Blackwell.

Suzuki, H., Uchiyama, M., Tagaya, H., et al. (2004). Dreaming during non-rapid eye movement sleep in the absence of prior rapid eye movement sleep. *Sleep, 27*, 1486–1490.

Švankmajer. J. (2010). *Surviving Life / Přežít svůj život* [Film]. Bontonfilm. Czech Republic/Slovakia.

Švankmajer. J. (1968). *The Flat / Byt* [Film]. Krátký film Praha. Czech Republic/Slovakia.

Taylor, F., & Bryant, R. A. (2007). The tendency to suppress, inhibiting thoughts, and dream rebound. *Behaviour Research and Therapy, 45*, 163–168.

Tedlock, B. (Ed.) (1987). *Dreaming: anthropological and psychological interpretations.* Cambridge: Cambridge University Press.

Tekriwal, A., Kern, D. S., Tsai, J., et al. (2017). REM sleep behaviour disorder: Prodromal and mechanistic insights for Parkinson's disease. *Journal of Neurology, Neurosurgery & Psychiatry, 88*, 445–451.

Timpanaro, S. (1974). *The Freudian slip: Psychoanalysis and textual criticism* (Translated by K. Soper). Atlantic Highlands: Humanities Press.

Tolton, C. D. E. (1999). Introduction: The cinema of Jean Cocteau. In C. D. E. Tolton (Ed.), *The cinema of Jean Cocteau*, pp.1–22. New York: Legas.

Tuominen, J., Stenberg, T., Revonsuo, A., & Valli, K. (2019). Social contents in dreams: An empirical test of the Social Simulation Theory. *Consciousness and Cognition, 69*, 133–145.

Tzara, T. (2013). *Seven Dada Manifestos and Lampisteries.* (Translated by B. Wright.) (First published 1924 and 1963.) London: Alma Classics.

Ullman, M. (1996/2006). *Appreciating dreams: A group approach.* Originally published by Sage, 1996. New York: Cosimo-on-Demand.

Vallat, R., Chatard, B., Blagrove, M., & Ruby, P. (2017a). Characteristics of the memory sources of dreams: A new version of the content-matching paradigm to take mundane and remote memories into account. *PLoS ONE, 12*, e0185262.

Vallat, R., Lajnef, T., Eichenlaub, J.-B., Berthomier, C., Jerbi, K., Morlet, D., & Ruby, P. M. (2017b). Increased evoked potentials to arousing auditory stimuli during sleep: Implication for the understanding of dream recall. *Frontiers in Human Neuroscience, 11*, 132.

Vallat R., & Ruby, P. M. (2019). Is it a good idea to cultivate lucid dreaming? *Frontiers in Psychology, 10*, 2585.

Vallat, R., Türker, B., Nicolas, A., & Ruby P. (2022). High dream recall frequency is associated with increased creativity and default mode network connectivity. *Nature and Science of Sleep, 14*, 265–275.

Valli, K., & Revonsuo, A. (2007). Evolutionary psychological approaches to dream content. In D. Barrett & P. McNamara (Eds.), *The new science of dreaming: Vol. 3. Cultural and theoretical perspectives* (pp. 95–116). Westport, CT: Praeger.

Valli, K., Revonsuo, A., Pälkäs, O., Ismail, K. H., Ali, K. J., & Punamäki, R. L. (2005). The threat simulation theory of the evolutionary function of dreaming: Evidence from dreams of traumatized children. *Consciousness and Cognition, 14*, 188–218.

van Eeden, F. (1913). A study of dreams. *Proceedings of the Society for Psychical Research, 26*, 431–461.

van Rijn, E., Eichenlaub, J-B., Lewis, P., Walker, M., Gaskell, M. G., Malinowski, J., & Blagrove, M. (2015). The dream-lag effect: Selective processing of personally significant events during Rapid Eye Movement sleep, but not during Slow Wave Sleep. *Neurobiology of Learning and Memory, 122,* 98–109.

van Rijn, E., Lucignoli, C., Izura, C., & Blagrove M. T. (2017). Sleep-dependent memory consolidation is related to perceived value of learned material. *Journal of Sleep Research, 26,* 302–308.

Vann, B., & Alperstein, N. (2010). Dream sharing as social interaction. *Dreaming, 10,* 111–119.

Vernon, A. (2022). *Night Terrors: Troubled Sleep and the Stories We Tell About It.* London: Icon Books.

Verweij, K. J. H., Burri, A. V., & Zietsch, B. P. (2014). Testing the prediction from sexual selection of a positive genetic correlation between human mate preferences and corresponding traits. *Evolution and Human Behavior, 35,* 497–501.

Voss, U., Holzmann, R., Tuin, I., & Hobson, J. A. (2009). Lucid dreaming: A state of consciousness with features of both waking and non-lucid dreaming. *Sleep, 32,* 1191–1200.

Wagner, U., & Born, J. (2008) Memory consolidation during sleep: Interactive effects of sleep stages and HPA regulation. *Stress, 11,* 28–41.

Wagner, U., Gais, S., & Born, J. (2001). Emotional memory formation is enhanced across sleep intervals with high amounts of rapid eye movement sleep. *Learning & Memory, 8,* 112–119.

Wagner, U., Gais, S., Haider, H., Verleger, R., & Born, J. (2004). Sleep inspires insight. *Nature, 427,* 352–355.

Walker, M. P., Brakefield, T., Seidman, J., Morgan, A., Hobson, J. A., & Stickgold, R. (2003). Sleep and the time course of motor skill learning. *Learning & Memory, 10,* 275–284.

Walker, M. P., Liston, C., Hobson, J. A., & Stickgold, R. (2002). Cognitive flexibility across the sleep-wake cycle: REM-sleep enhancement of anagram problem solving. *Cognitive Brain Research, 14,* 317–324.

Walker, M. P., & Stickgold, R. (2010). Overnight alchemy: sleep-dependent memory evolution. *Nature Reviews Neuroscience, 11,* 218.

Walker, M. P., & Van der Helm, E. (2009). Overnight therapy? The role of sleep in emotional brain processing. *Psychological Bulletin, 135,* 731–748.

Wamsley, E. J. (2014). Dreaming and offline memory consolidation. *Current Neurology and Neuroscience Reports, 14,* 433.

Wamsley, E., Donjacour, C. E. H. M., Scammell, T. E., Lammers, G. J., & Stickgold, R. (2014). Delusional confusion of dreaming and reality in narcolepsy, *Sleep, 37,* 419–422.

Wamsley, E. J., Perry, K., Djonlagic, I., Reaven, L. B., & Stickgold, R. (2010a). Cognitive replay of visuomotor learning at sleep onset: Temporal dynamics and relationship to task performance. *Sleep, 33,* 59–68.

Wamsley, E. J., & Stickgold, R. (2011). Memory, sleep and dreaming: Experiencing consolidation. *Sleep Medicine Clinics, 6,* 97–108.

Wamsley, E. J., & Stickgold, R. (2019). Dreaming of a learning task is associated with enhanced memory consolidation: Replication in an overnight sleep study. *Journal of Sleep Research, 28,* e12749.

Wamsley, E. J., Tucker, M., Payne, J. D., Benavides, J. A., & Stickgold, R. (2010b). Dreaming of a learning task is associated with enhanced sleep-dependent memory consolidation. *Current Biology, 20,* 850–855.

Watkins, C. D. (2017). Creating beauty: Creativity compensates for low physical attractiveness when individuals assess the attractiveness of social and romantic partners. *Royal Society Open Science, 4,* 160955.

Wauquier, A., Aloe, L., & Declerck, A. (1995). K-complexes: Are they signs of arousal or sleep protective? *Journal of Sleep Research, 4,* 138–143.

Wax, M. L. (2004). Dream sharing as social practice. *Dreaming, 14,* 83–93.

Wegner, D. M., Wenzlaff, R. M., & Kozak, M. (2004). Dream rebound: the return of suppressed thoughts in dreams. *Psychological Science, 15,* 232–236.

Williams, J., Carr, M., & Blagrove, M. (2021). Sensory processing sensitivity: Associations with the detection of real degraded stimuli, and reporting of illusory stimuli and paranormal experiences. *Personality and Individual Differences, 177,* 110807.

Williams, J., Merritt, J., Rittenhouse, C., & Hobson, J. A. (1992). Bizarreness in dreams and fantasies: Implications for the activation-synthesis hypothesis. *Consciousness and Cognition, 1,* 172–185.

Wilson, M. A., & McNaughton, B. L. (1994). Reactivation of hippocampal ensemble memories during sleep. *Science, 265*(5172), 676–679.

Windt, J. (2015). *Dreaming: A conceptual framework for philosophy of mind and empirical research.* Cambridge, MA: MIT Press.

Winnicott, D. W. (1953) Transitional objects and transitional phenomena—a study of the first not-me possession. *International Journal of Psychoanalysis, 34,* 89–97.

Wong, W., Noreika, V., Móró, L., Revonsuo, A., Windt, J., Valli, K., & Tsuchiya, N. (2020). The Dream Catcher experiment: Blinded analyses failed to detect markers of dreaming consciousness in EEG spectral power. *Neuroscience of Consciousness, 1,* niaa006.

Wood, J. (ed.), *Metadesigning Designing in the Anthropocene.* London: Routledge.

Wood, J. M., Bootzin, R. R., Rosenhan, D., Nolen-Hoeksema, S., & Jourden, F. (1992). Effects of the 1989 San Francisco earthquake on frequency and content of nightmares. *Journal of Abnormal Psychology, 101,* 219–224.

Wrangham, R. (2019). *The goodness paradox: The strange relationship between virtue and violence in human evolution.* New York: Vintage Books.

Wright, S. T., Kerr, C. W., Doroszczuk, N. M., Kuszczak, S. M., Hang, P. C., & Luczkiewicz, D. L. (2014). The impact of dreams of the deceased on bereavement: A survey of hospice caregivers. *The American Journal of Hospice & Palliative Care, 31,* 132–138.

Xie, L., Kang, H., Xu, Q., Chen, M. J., Liao, Y., Thiyagarajan, M., O'Donnell, J., Christensen, D. J., Nicholson, C., Iliff, J. J., Takano, T., Deane, R., & Nedergaard, M. (2013). Sleep drives metabolite clearance from the adult brain. *Science, 342*(6156), 373–377.

Yaroush, R., Sullivan, M. J., & Ekstrand, B. R. (1971). Effect of sleep on memory, II: Differential effect of the first and second half of the night. *Journal of Experimental Psychology, 88,* 361–366.

Zadra, A., & Stickgold, R. (2021). *When brains dream: Exploring the science and mystery of sleep.* New York: W.W. Norton.

Index

Note: **Bold** page numbers refer to tables and *italic* page numbers refer to figures.

Aames, D. 190
activation-synthesis hypothesis for dreaming 61
activation-synthesis theory 62, 135
Ades, D. 167
Aesthetic Sensitivity component of SPS 23
Affective Network Dysfunction model 32
After Dada (Breton) 162–163
aliquis 86
Alperstein, N. 144
'Alpine Racer' 55
American Academy of Sleep Medicine 39
Ancient Greeks 38
Andersson, R. 196
Antrobus, J. 138
Apollinaire, G. 163
apparent metaphors in dreams 138
Aristotle 38
Armitage, R. 21
Aron, E. 34
Arp, H. 162
art and socialisation of dreams 160–161
Artaud, A. 193–194
artistic creativity 137
Aserinsky, E. 42; *Regularly occurring periods of eye motility and concomitant phenomena during sleep* 60
Attitude toward Dreams questionnaire (Cernovsky) 22, 121
auditory cues 15
Aviram, L. 78

Baird, B. 5, 76
Ball, H. 162
Bardina, S. 214

Barnum/Forer effect 119
Barrett, D. 71, 175, 176, 183, 206; *Pandemic Dreams* 176
Baylor, G. W. 86
Beaulieu-Prévost, D. 22
Belicki, K. 31
Belle de Jour, film 192
Belyaev, D. 207, 208
Bergman, I. 188; *Wild Strawberries* 188–189
Bergman, M. 212
Bernal, G. G. 191
Berry, W. 160
Bertrand, O. 23
Biennale, V.: *The Milk of Dreams* 169
biopsychological trait 23
Birthday (Tanning) 167
bizarreness, in dreams 5, 62
Black, J. 9
Blagrove, M. 7, 13, 14, 34, 63, 72, 73, 94, 110, 113, 119, 120, 124, 140, 143, 145, 156, 157, *158,* 160, 176–177, 183, 206, 210
Blamo, A. E. 23
Blechner, M. J. 131
'bonding themes' 145
The Book of Dreams (Fellini) 198
Borg, I. 189
Born, J. 49, 52
Boss, M. 200, 201
boundary questionnaire 34
Bourgeois, Louise 169
Bout, J. van den 35
Boyd, B. 209, 210
brain excitation 23
brain imaging (fMRI, PET) 24, 77
brains of lucid dreamers 75–76

brain waves, in wake and sleep stage 40
Breton, A. 162–169, 193; *After Dada* 162–163; *Max Ernst* 166; *The Mediums Enter* 163; *Nadja* 165; *Object* 166; *Surrealism and Painting* 167
British Science Association 156
Bulkeley, K. 8, 71, 144, 174, 211
Bulkley, P. 8
Buñuel, L. 194, 197; *Belle de Jour* 192; *Dreams and Reveries* 197; *El Angel exterminador/The exterminating Angel* 195, 196; *My Last Breath* 194, 197; *The Phantom of Liberty* 195
Bush, G. 87

Carr, M. 23, 33–34, 74, 76, 148
Carrington, L. 169
Cartwright, R. 133
Cavallero, C. 86
Cernovsky, Z. Z. 121
Chesterton, M. 37
child development and dreaming 24–26
Chirico, G. de: *The Enigma of a Day* 165
Chytilová, V. 196
Clair, R. 193
Cocteau, J. 197–198
cognitive ability 25, 70
cognitive-experiential therapeutic method 122
Cohen, D. B. 20, 21
conceptualisation of waking life 12, 126, 135, 145, 210
conceptual metaphors 88
concrete metaphors 88
contemporary legacy of Surrealism 168–169
'contextualising' emotions 132
continuity hypothesis 12
correlational issue, in functions of dreams 132–134
Covid-19 pandemic: dreams during 174–176; sleep and dreaming during 176
Craven, W. 190
creative individuals 207
Crevel, R. 163
Cruise, T. 190
Cubism 162
cultural extensions of HSD 209
Current Biology 77
cut-up method 165–166

Dadaism 161–162, 220
Dadaist film 193

Daisies, film 196
D'Alessandro, S. 169
Dalí, S.: *Lobster Telephone* 166
Dallenbach, K. M. 48
Davidson, J. 87
'day-residue' 12
deep sleep 41
Deese-Roediger-McDermott (DRM) paradigm 54
Default Mode Network (DMN) 24
De Koninck, J. 134
Dement, W. 6
Dement, W. C. 9
Depow, G. J. 215
Desnos, R. 163
Deutsch, F. 97
Diagnostic and Statistical Manual of Mental Disorders (DSM-5) 30
Diaz, C. 190
Diekelmann, S. 52
The Discreet Charm of the Bourgeoise, film 195, 196–197
DMN *see* Default Mode Network (DMN)
Domhoff, G. W. (Bill) 5, 10–12, 124, 135, 139, 145, 199, 210; non-functional view of dreaming 151; *The scientific study of dreams: Neural networks, cognitive development, and content analysis* 10
Dora case study 91–92; first dream 93–94; life 92–93; online event 97–98; second dream 98–100; waking life circumstances 94–96
Dorus, E. 5
dream appreciation (Ullman) 94, 106, 114, 121, 122, 138, 148
dream content: dreaming and 140; dream recall and 24, 174; evolutionary pressure for 216; factors affecting 6–7; Most Recent Dream (MRD) method 10; relationship of 25; researchers 11; social and emotional characteristics of 206; task-related dream content 133; wake-life conceptualisations and 210
dream hallucination 61
dreaming 209–211; and the brain 61–62; brain injury and dream recall 62–64; child development and 24–26; during Covid-19 pandemic 176; creativity and insight 137–138; in different stages of sleep 64–65; and fiction 150–151; and higher social memory 134–135; neural basis of 66–67; NEXTUP theory

of 212; and REM sleep 60, 65–66; within-sleep and post-sleep functions of 211–213
dreaming and insight 117–119; metaphor 126–127; paintings of dreams *90, 102*; personal and group reactions 119–120; REM and NREM 123–126; waking life events 122–123
Dreaming as Story-telling (Pace-Schott) 210
Dreaming – motivated or meaningless? (Blagrove) 120
Dreaming of a learning task is associated with enhanced sleep-dependent memory consolidation (Wamsley) 55
Dreaming Souls (Flanagan) 135
dream interpretation 88
dream-lag effect 12–15, 151
DreamLight and *NovaDreamer* devices (LaBerge) 74
dream-like quality scale 65
'dream of Irma's injection' (Freud) 86
dream recall 20–22, 60, 67, 214; brain injury and 62–64; frequency 10, 21–26, 146, 175–176
Dream Reports from Different Stages of Sleep (Foulkes) 64
dreams *18, 36, 46, 172, 181, 182*; art and socialisation of 160–161; bizarreness in 5; characteristics of 4; content, factors affect 6–7; during Covid-19 pandemic 174–176; of death preparation kit *178*; Dora's first dream *90*; Dora's second dream *102*; dream-lag effect 12–15; and emotional experiences 7–10; ephemerality of 137; of family Tischler's table 83; and film 188; Freud, S. 82; function of (*see* function of dreams); individuals' reactions 148–149; in linear films 188–191; of Mai 181–184; of mother and daughter attacked on freeway *128*; *vs.* our memories 5–6; and painting *142, 154*; personal and group reactions to 119–121; phenomenology and 200–202; of pulling through from Covid *116*; of searching through keys *104*; of snowy beach *186*; socialisation of 160–161; surrealist methods and relationships to 165–167; surrealist theory and 164–165; tangential incorporation of 191–192; theories of function 130–132; threat simulation theory of 129–130; of three stages of woman *58*; unbiased sample of 10–12;

of unfair blame *204*; of walking alone and dancing with friends *80*; work techniques 84
Dreams and Hysteria (Dora case study) 92
Dreams and Reveries (Buñuel) 197
dream-sharing 216; costs and benefits of 213–214; and empathy 206–207; frequency, motivations and social effects of 144–148
dream-sharing and empathy 143–144; first experiment on 147–148; psychotherapy and relationships 151–152; second experiment on 148; testing 145–147
Dream sharing and the enhancement of empathy: Theoretical and applied implications 148
DreamsID 143, 153; collaboration 170; Covid-19 lockdown dreams project 176–177; dadaism and surrealism 161–162; science art collaboration 155–157, 159
DreamsID.com 160
DreamsID events 160–161
DreamsID YouTube channel 183
Dreams That Money Can Buy (Richter) 199
'dream-work' processes 167
Dresler, M. 62, 76
drug induction of lucid dreams 75
Duchamp, M. 163, 167, 169, 193; *Fountain* 163
Durrant, S. J. 54, 55

Earle, W. 199
Edwards, C. L. 7, 120, 122, 124, 152, 210
Eeden, F. van 70
EEG *see* electroencephalograph (EEG)
Ehrenfeld, F. 23
Eichenlaub, J. -B. 7, 15, 23, 24, 63, 67, 130
El Angel exterminador / The exterminating Angel (Buñuel) 195, 196
ELDVs *see* End-of-life dreams and visions (ELDVs)
electroencephalograph (EEG) 38
electromyograph (EMG) 38
electrooculography (EOG) 38
Ellis, L. 151
EMG *see* electromyograph (EMG)
emotional experiences 7–10
emotional memory and sleep 50
emotional regulation and processing theories of dreaming 133, 175, 211–212

empathic effect of sharing dreams 143–144, 150–151
empathy theory of dreaming 151, 206–207
The Empire of Light (Magritte) 167
end-of-life dreams and visions (ELDVs) 9, 151
Englund, R. 190
The Enigma of a Day (de Chirico) 165
Entr'acte, film 193
EOG *see* electrooculography (EOG)
ephemerality of dreams 137
epiphenomenal *vs.* functional theories of dreaming 135–136
episodic memory sources 86
Erlacher, D. 73
Ernst, M. 164, 166, 200; *Two Children are Threatened by a Nightingale* 164
evolutionary theory, aetiology of nightmares 33
experience sampling 5
The Exterminating Angel 196, 202
Eyes Wide Shut, film 189

fear memories 32, 132
Fellini, F. 198–199; *The Book of Dreams* 198
female dreams 11
fiction 209–211
Fiction: Simulation of social worlds 215
films: Cocteau 197–198; contrasting realist and oneiric films 199–200; dreams and 188; neorealist to oneiric films (Felini) 198–199; realist and non-realist dream films, history of 192; realist *versus* surrealist 192–197; Surrealist oneiric films 192–197; tangential incorporation of dreams into 191–192
Finkelstein, H.: *The Seashell and the Clergyman* 195
'first night effect' 43
Fisher, S. 63
Fitch, T. 21
Flanagan, O. 135, 139; *Dreaming Souls* 135
The flat, film 196
Flitterman-Lewis, S. 193–195
flying dream, with lucidity 68
fMRI *see* functional Magnetic Resonance Imaging (fMRI)
Fosse, M. J. 4
Foulkes, D. 24–26, 64, 199; *Dream Reports from Different Stages of Sleep* 64
Fountain (Duchamp) 163

Fouquet, N. 14
four right-left eye movements (LRLRLRLR) 70, 75
Fox, K. C. 4
Fragments of an Analysis of a Case of Hysteria ('Dora') 92
Frau, K. 94, 97–98
free association method: evaluation of 86–87; use of 82–86
French, C. 119
frequency: and characteristics, of Lucid dreams 70–72; of sharing dreams 144–145
The Freudian Slip (Timpanaro) 86
Freud, S. 12, 21, 61, 63, 81, 83, 84–86, 88, 126, 156, 157, 159, 162, 166; Dora case study 91–100; of dreams 82; *The Interpretation of Dreams* 82, 86, 92–94, 157, 219; *Introductory Lectures on Psychoanalysis* 82, 83; *The Psychopathology of Everyday Life* 83
functional Magnetic Resonance Imaging (fMRI) 77
function of dreams: correlational issue in 132–134; epiphenomenal view 135–136; insight and **138,** 138–139; possibilities for testing 136–137
functions: of consciousness 215–216; of dreaming 57, 73, 132, 206, 211–213; of dreams (*see* function of dreams); of sleep 54, 135
Funkhouser, A. 120
Futurism 162

Gackenbach, J. 72, 74
Gains from Dream Interpretation questionnaire (Hill) 121, 123
Gais, S. 49
Gale, M. 169
Gendlin, E. T. 200
General aspects of dream psychology (Jung) 110
Gestalt therapy group 35
Glass Tears (Ray) 166
Gondry, M.: *The Science of Sleep* 191
Gorgoni, M. 174
Göritz, A. S. 149
Graf, D. 213
Grant, K. 151, 167
Gray, G. 136
grief dreams 9

Hall and Van de Castle system 11
Hall, C. S. 11, 12, 33

Hall Van de Castle (HVdC) variable scores 11
Hare, B. 208
Harford, A. 189–190
Harford, B. 189–190
Hartmann, E. 4, 21, 30, 34, 55, 131, 132, 139, 199; *Making connections in a safe place: is dreaming psychotherapy?* 131
Hartnell, S. J. 72
Hearne, K. 70
Hebbian maxim 132
Helicopter Quartet, Stockhausen 138
Henley-Einion, J. 13, 110
Herr, K. 94–100, 103
high and low dream recallers: brain and sleep of 23–24; personality differences between 20–23
high-density electroencephalography 66
higher social memory, dreaming and 134–135
Highly Sensitive Person Scale (HSPS) 22, 23, 34
Hill, C. E. 120, 122, 152, 201
hippocampus 32
Hitchcock, A.: *Spellbound* 191
Hobson, J. A. 25–26, 61, 62, 65, 135, 139, 199
Hoel, E. 55, 131
Holzinger, B. 35, 94, 174
Hopkins, D. 166, 169
Horton, C. L. 126
HSD *see* human self-domestication (HSD)
HSPS *see* Highly Sensitive Person Scale (HSPS)
Hu, X. 53
human evolution 209–211
human self-domestication (HSD) 205; cultural and language extensions of 209; hypothesis of human social evolution 207–209; within-sleep and post-sleep functions of dreaming 211–213
human social evolution, HSD hypothesis of 207–209
hypnogram, stages of sleep *43*
hypotheses of dreaming 135

IASD *see* International Association for the Study of Dreams (IASD)
Ida Bauer 93, *93*
Idilio (*Idyll*) 167–168
idiopathic nightmares 30
Ijams, K. 144

imagery rehearsal therapy (IRT) 34–35
Inception, film 74, 78
individual differences of lucid dreamers 72–73
inducing lucid dreams 73–74
InfraRed Spectroscopy 77
insight: creativity and 137–138; and function of dreams **138,** 138–139; home dreams and 121–122; and metaphor 126–127; REM and NREM dreams and 123–126; waking life events and 122–123
internal Locus of Control 72
International Association for the Study of Dreams (IASD) 110, 119–120, 201
International Classification of Sleep Disorders (ICSD-3) 30
International Journal of Dream Research (Lockheart) 103
International Society for the Study of Surrealism 155, 187
The Interpretation of Dreams (Freud) 82, 86, 92–94, 157, 219
Introductory Lectures on Psychoanalysis (Freud) 82, 83
IRT *see* imagery rehearsal therapy (IRT)

Jenkins, J. G. 48
Jiménez, J. 165
Journal of Palliative Medicine (Kerr) 8
Jung, C. G. 126; *General aspects of dream psychology* 110; *On the nature of dreams* 126; *The practical use of dream analysis* 126
Jungian method 120

Kahan, T. L. 71
Kales, A. 39
K-complexes 41
Kekulé, A. 137
Kerr, C. W.: *Journal of Palliative Medicine* 8
Kezich, T. 199
King, M. 161
Kleitman, N. 42; *Regularly occurring periods of eye motility and concomitant phenomena during sleep* 60
Konkoly, K. 74, 77
Krueger, F. 190
Kubrick, S.: *Eyes Wide Shut* 189
Kuenzli, R. E. 193

LaBerge, S. 70, 71, 74, 75; *DreamLight* and *NovaDreamer* devices 74
Ladd, G. T. 42

Lakoff, G. 88
language extensions of HSD 209
La Révolution surréaliste 163, 164, 166–167
LastYear at Marienbad, film 192
Le Sang d'un Poète/The Blood of a Poet, film 197, 198
Le Testament d'Orphée/The Testament of Orpheus, film 198
Levin, R. 32
Levitan, L. 74
Lewis, P.A. 54, 55
lifestyle hypothesis 21
linear films, dreams in 188–191
Linguistic Inquiry and Word Count (LIWC) 175
Lipsky, J. 152
literary movement 167
LIWC *see* Linguistic Inquiry and Word Count (LIWC)
Lobster Telephone (Dalí) 166
Lockheart, J. 94, 103, 140, 156, *158, 159,* 160, 183; *International Journal of Dream Research* 103
Los Olvidados, film 195
Lucas, S. 169
lucid dreamers: brains of 75–76; individual differences of 72–73; personality of 72–73
lucid dream induction method 73, 78
lucid dreaming 35, 70, 72–76, 78
lucid dreams 69–70; brains of 75–76; drug induction of 75; and experimenters, communication between 77; frequency and characteristics of 70–72; induction of 73–74; personality and individual differences of 72–73; possible adverse effects of 78; technological induction of 74–75; uses of 76–77
lucidity reactivation training 74
lure, false memory 54–55
Lynch, D.: *Mulholland Drive* 191
Lynch, S. 87
Lyons, M. 215

Macêdo, T. C. F. 35, 76
Machiavellianism 215
MADRE *see* Mannheim Dream Questionnaire (MADRE)
Mageo, J. 215
Magritte, R. 165, 167, 169, 200; *The Empire of Light* 167
Making connections in a safe place: is dreaming psychotherapy? (Hartmann) 131

male dreams 11
Malinowski, J. 126
Mandela, N. 214
Manifesto of Surrealism 161, 164
Mannheim Dream Questionnaire (MADRE) 146
Marcoci, R. 168
Mar, R.A. 150
Matthews, J. H. 192, 194–196
Matthijs Bal, P. 150
Max Ernst (Breton) 166
McCarley, R.W. 61, 62, 135, 139
McNamara, P. 145, 207
McNaughton, B. L. 53–54
The Mediums Enter (Breton) 163
Meier, B. 5
Meister, S. H. 168
memory consolidation 14, 41, 48–53, 55–57, 132, 206
memory reactivation, during sleep 53
Memory, sleep and dreaming: experiencing consolidation (Wamsley and Stickgold) 56
memory triage 51
Mersky, R. R. 160
Meshes of the Afternoon, film 199
metaphor 88, 97, 118, 122, 138, 189, 220; insight and 126–127
metaphorical content in dreams 87–88
A Midsummer Night's Dream 221
MILD *see* Mnemonic Induction of Lucid Dreams (MILD)
The Milk of Dreams (Biennale) 169
Miller, L. D. 144
Mind in the Eyes test 150
Mnemonic Induction of Lucid Dreams (MILD) 73
mood disorders 50–51
Morewedge, C. K. 123
Most Recent Dream (MRD) method 10–12
Mota, N. B. 174
Mota-Rolim, S. A. 74
motivations of sharing dreams 144–145
MRD method *see* Most Recent Dream (MRD) method
Mulholland Drive, film 191
Mundy, J. 165
My Last Breath (Buñuel) 194, 197
My Nurse (Oppenheim) 166

Nadja (Breton) 165
National Health Service 173, 183
Need for Cognition 72
neural basis of dreaming 66–67

neural replay, during sleep 53–54
neurocognitive theory 62
The Neuropsychology of Dreams (Solms) 62
NEXTUP theory of dreaming (Zadra and Stickgold) 136, 139
NHS *Finding Hope* project 184
Nicolas, A. 24, 63
Nielsen, T. A. 9, 12–15, 31–32, 34, 65
A Nightmare on Elm Street, film 190
nightmares *28*, 29–31, 144, 174; definition of 30; disorder 30; distress questionnaire 31–32, 34, 176; frequency 31, 34, 35, 176; personality and susceptibility to 33–34; predisposition 32–34; stress-diathesis 33; theories of 32–33; treatments for 34–35
11/13, in dreams 7, 87
non-HSPs 23, 34
non-literal content in dreams 87–88
non-rapid eye movement (NREM) sleep 14, 30, 39–41, 52, 64–66, 136; lucid dreams 70
non-realist dream films, history of 192
Nordby, V. J. 12
Norton, M. I. 123
NREM–REM cycle 53
NREM sleep *see* non-rapid eye movement (NREM) sleep
null hypothesis 135

Oatley, K. 150, 215
Object (Breton) 166
objet trouvé/found object 157, 161, 162, 169
O'Donoghue 193
Olivier, P. S. 23
Olsen, M. R. 144
oneiric films 188, 192, 202; contrasting realist and 199–200; from neorealist to 198–199; Surrealist oneiric films 188, 192–197
On the nature of dreams (Jung) 126
Oppenheim, M.: *My Nurse* 166
O'Pray, M. 191
Orphée/Orpheus, film 198
Otto Bauer 93
Out of Body Experiences and Near-Death Experiences 61

Pace-Schott, E. F.: *Dreaming as Storytelling* 210
Pagel, J. F. 20, 63
Pagel, M. 211

Pailthorpe, G.: *The Scientific Aspect of Surrealism* 167
pain sensations 6
paintings in Surrealism 166–168
Pandemic Dreams (Barrett) 176
pandemic-period dream 175
paradoxical sleep 42
Paris Institute for Advanced Study 19
Parker, C. 169
partial correlations 31
participant's dream 13–15, 24, 49, 54, 56, 62, 64, 66, 67, 74–75, 77, 88, 119, 149, 174
Peck, G. 191
Perogamvros, L. 135
personal and group reactions, to dreams 119–121
personality: of lucid dreamers 72–73; and susceptibility, to nightmares 33–34
Pesant, N. 151
PET scan *see* positron emission tomography (PET) scan
The Phantom of Liberty, film 195
Phantoms of Surrealism 169
photography 167–168
Piaget, J. 25
Picard-Deland, C. 9, 15
positron emission tomography (PET) scan 24
possible adverse effects of lucid dreaming 78
post-traumatic nightmares 30
post-traumatic stress disorder (PTSD) nightmare 30, 214
The practical use of dream analysis (Jung) 126
predisposition to nightmares 32–34
pre-sleep mood 21
Propper, R. E. 7, 174
psychoanalysis 92, 93, 97, 98, 192
The Psychologist (Blagrove) 120
The Psychopathology of Everyday Life (Freud) 83
psychopathy 215
psychotherapy 151–152
PTSD *see* post-traumatic stress disorder (PTSD)
Purcell, S. 70, 73

Rapid Eye Movement (REM) sleep 8, 14, 24, 42–43, 50, 75, 130–131, 136, 145, 206; behaviour disorder 33; nap 66; and NREM dreams 123–126; rebound 66

Rasch, B. 53
Ray, M. 163, 166, 169, 193, 199; *Glass Tears* 166; *Ruth, Roses and Revolvers* 199–200
realist dream films, history of 192
reality-checking method 73
Rechtschaffen, A. 39; *The single-mindedness and isolation of dreams* 71
Regularly occurring periods of eye motility and concomitant phenomena during sleep (Aserinsky and Kleitman) 60
Reid, A. 50
REM-deprived participants 66
REM sleep *see* Rapid Eye Movement (REM) sleep
Resnick, J. 25–26
The Reticent Child 169
retrospective assessments of dream recall 22
Revonsuo, A. 33, 130, 139, 145; threat simulation theory 33, 139
Ribeiro, N. 56, 133
Richter, H.: *Dreams That Money Can Buy* 200
Rijn, E. van 51
Rimé, B. 211
Robert, G. 30
Rosen, M. 117–119, 177; *We're Going on a Bear Hunt* 118
Ruby, P. M. 67, 78
Ruth, Roses and Revolvers (Ray) 199–200

Sanders, B. 11–12
Sándor, P. 26, 210
Saunders, D. T. 70
Scarpelli, S. 175
scepticism 119
Schawinski, J. A. 144
schemas, abstraction of 54–55
Schneider, A. 10, 11, 145
Schnitzler, A.: *Traumnovelle* 189
Schonbar, R. 21
Schredl, M. 6–8, 12, 21, 23, 71, 144, 149, 152, 174
Schwartz, S. 135
The Science of Sleep, film 191
The Scientific Aspect of Surrealism (Pailthorpe) 167
The scientific study of dreams: Neural networks, cognitive development, and content analysis (Domhoff) 10
SCS *see* Social Content Scale (SCS)
The Seashell and the Clergyman, film 195
Sebbag, G. 163, 164

Selterman, D. F. 145
sensory memories 137
Sensory Processing Sensitivity (SPS) 22, 34
Sharot, S. 192
Sheriff, R .E. 215
Shilton, D. 209
Short, R. 193
short-term memories 137
Siclari, F. 66, 67, 136
Sievers, B. 160
signal-verified lucid dream (SVLD) 70
Sinclair, F. 165
The single-mindedness and isolation of dreams (Rechtschaffen) 71
sleep 37; and abstraction of schemas 54–55; during Covid-19 pandemic 174–176; cycle 42; emotional memory and 50; lab 70, 74; measurement of 38–39, *39*; memory reactivation during 53; and mood disorders 50–51; neural replay during 53–54; non-rapid eye movement sleep 39–41; Rapid Eye Movement sleep 42–43; spindles 41; theories of mechanism 52–53
sleep and memory 47; beneficial effect of 48; dreaming 55–57; motivation 51; sleep stages *vs.* wake for memory 48–50
sleep-dependent memory consolidation effect 56
Sleep to Remember and Sleep to Forget model 33
Sliwinski, S. 214
slow-wave sleep (SWS) 8, 41, 49
Smith, B. V. 73
Social Content Scale (SCS) 4
Social Dream Drawing 160
social effects of sharing dreams 144–145
social evolution 210, 220
social evolutionary benefits of dream-sharing 207
socialisation of dreams 160–161
Social Simulation Theory (SST) 4, 130, 134, 145, 151
Soffer-Dudek, N. 78
Solms, M. 24, 62–63, 67; *The Neuropsychology of Dreams* 62
Songs from the Second Floor, film 196–197
spandrel 135, 206
Spector, J. J. 163–164
Spellbound, film 191
Spoormaker, V. I. 35, 76
SPS *see* Sensory Processing Sensitivity (SPS)

SST *see* Social Simulation Theory (SST)
States, B. O. 150
statistical analyses 11, 146
Stenstrom, P. 13–14, 32
Stern, G. 167
Sterpenich, V. 133
Stickgold, R. 50–52, 55, 56, 64, 65, 130–132, 134–136, 139, 199, 212–213; *Memory, sleep and dreaming: experiencing consolidation* 56
Stockhausen, K. 137, 138
Strauch, I. 5
stress-diathesis 33
Strom, K. 169
Stroop task 26, 72
Strunz, F. 137
Stumbrys, T. 73
Sturzenacker, G.: *The Ullman Method: Influential and Often Misunderstood* 111
Surrealism 161–162, 170, 220; contemporary legacy of 168–169; and valuing of dreams 162–164
Surrealism and Painting (Breton) 167
Surrealism Beyond Borders 191
Surrealist movement 164
Surrealist art 167–168
Surrealist methods 165–167
Surrealist oneiric films 192–197
Surrealist theory and dreams 164–165
Surviving Life, film 191
Suzuki, H. 66
Švankmajer, J. 191, 196; *Surviving Life* 191
SVLD *see* signal-verified lucid dream (SVLD)
SWS *see* slow-wave sleep (SWS)
system consolidation process 52

tangential incorporation of dreams 191–192
Tanning, D. 167–168; *Birthday* 167
Targeted Memory Reactivation (TMR) 53
technological induction of lucid dreams 74–75
TEQ *see* Toronto Empathy Questionnaire (TEQ)
testing, for function of dreams 136–137
theories: activation-synthesis theory 62, 135; of dream function 130–132; empathy theory of dreaming 206, 207; evolutionary theory, aetiology of nightmares 33; of nightmares 32–33; of oneiric Darwinism 131; Revonsuo's threat simulation theory 33, 139;

Surrealist theory 164–165; threat simulation theory 129–130, 175
thin boundaries 21, 22, 34, 132, 146–147
threat simulation theory of dreams 129–130, 175
Timpanaro, S. 86–87, 119; *The Freudian Slip* 86
TMR *see* Targeted Memory Reactivation (TMR)
To Make a Dadaist Poem (Tzara) 166
Toronto Empathy Questionnaire (TEQ) 145
trait empathy 145–147
transcranial Direct Current Stimulation 76
Traumnovelle (Schnitzler) 189
treatments for nightmares 34–35
Tuominen, J. 4
Two Children are Threatened by a Nightingale (Ernst) 164
Tzara, T.: *To Make a Dadaist Poem* 166

Ullman dream appreciation technique 114, 138, 148
Ullman group dream discussion method 106–108, 143; characters in 110; 'If It Were My Dream' stage 110–113; initial assessment of dreamers' 110; stages of 108–109
Ullman group procedure 122
Ullman, M. 147
Ullman method 110–113, 120, 122–123, 151, 156, 157, 220
The Ullman Method: Influential and Often Misunderstood (Sturzenacker) 111
Un Chain andalou/An Andalusian dog, film 194
unequivocal REM sleep 70

Vallat, R. 6, 12, 23, 24, 78, 86
Valli, K. 130, 135, 148
Van de Castle, B. 11
Van de Castle, R. L. 33
Van der Helm, E. 33, 50
Vann, B. 144
Veltkamp, M. 150
Viridiana, film 195
virtual reality (VR) of dream 12, 74, 130, 175
visuospatial task 25
Voss, U. 75
VR of dream *see* virtual reality (VR) of dream

Wagner, U. 50
Wake Back to Bed (WBTB) method 73–74
Waking Dream Séance, Ray (1924) 163
Walker, M. P. 33, 48, 50–52, 55
Wamsley, E. J. 55, 56, 88, 130–132, 134; *Dreaming of a learning task is associated with enhanced sleep-dependent memory consolidation* 55; *Memory, sleep and dreaming: experiencing consolidation* 56
WBTB method *see* Wake Back to Bed (WBTB) method
We do not dream of the 5 Rs 4
Welsh language 51
We're Going on a Bear Hunt (Rosen) 118
Wes Craven's New Nightmare, film 190
Wessely, Z. 94
When Brains Dream: Exploring the science and mystery of sleep (Zadra) 131
Wild Strawberries (Bergman) 188–189
Williams, J. 5, 23, 34

Wilson, M. A. 53–54
Windt, J. 4
Winnicott, D. 161
wish-fulfilment 81
Wolfe, G. 20
Wolpert, E. A. 6
Wood, J. M. 31
Wood, R. 63
The Woven Child (Bourgeois) 169
Wrangham, R. 207–209
Wright, S. T. 9

YBAs *see* Young British Artists (YBAs)
YouGov 174
Young British Artists (YBAs) 169
You, the Living, film 196

Zadra, A. 22, 30, 131, 136, 139, 151, 212–213; *When Brains Dream: Exploring the science and mystery of sleep* 131
Zellenka, H. 97
Zellenka, P. 97